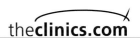

VETERINARY CLINICS

OF NORTH AMERICA

Small Animal Practice

Advances in Fluid, Electrolyte,
and Acid-Base Disorders

GUEST EDITORS
Helio Autran de Morais, DVM, PhD
Stephen P. DiBartola, DVM

May 2008 • Volume 38 • Number 3

SAUNDERS

An Imprint of Elsevier, Inc.
PHILADELPHIA   LONDON   TORONTO   MONTREAL   SYDNEY   TOKYO

W.B. SAUNDERS COMPANY
A Division of Elsevier Inc.

Elsevier, Inc., 1600 John F. Kennedy Blvd., Suite 1800, Philadelphia, PA 19103-2899

http://www.vetsmall.theclinics.com

VETERINARY CLINICS OF NORTH AMERICA:	**Volume 38, Number 3**
SMALL ANIMAL PRACTICE	**ISSN 0195-5616**
May 2008	**ISBN-13: 978-1-4160-5876-2**
Editor: John Vassallo; j.vassallo@elsevier.com	**ISBN-10: 1-4160-5876-1**

The ideas and opinions expressed in *Veterinary Clinics of North America: Small Animal Practice* do not necessarily reflect those of the Publisher. The Publisher does not assume any responsibility for any injury and/or damage to persons or property arising out of or related to any use of the material contained in this periodical. The reader is advised to check the appropriate medical literature and the product information currently provided by the manufacturer of each drug to be administered to verify the dosage, the method and duration of administration, or contraindications. It is the responsibility of the treating physician or other health care professional, relying on independent experience and knowledge of the patient, to determine drug dosages and the best treatment for the patient. Mention of any product in this issue should not be construed as endorsement by the contributors, editors, or the Publisher of the product or manufacturers' claims.

Veterinary Clinics of North America: Small Animal Practice (ISSN 0195-5616) is published bimonthly (For Post Office use only: volume 38 issue 3 of 6) by Elsevier Inc., 360 Park Avenue South, New York, NY 10010-1710. Months of issue are January, March, May, July, September, and November. Business and Editorial offices: 1600 John F. Kennedy Blvd., Suite 1800, Philadelphia, PA 19103-2899. Customer Service Office: 6277 Sea Harbor Drive, Orlando, FL 32887-4800. Periodicals postage paid at New York, NY and additional mailing offices. Subscription prices are $206.00 per year for US individuals, $327.00 per year for US institutions, $103.00 per year for US students and residents, $273.00 per year for Canadian individuals, $410.00 per year for Canadian institutions, $285.00 per year for international individuals, $410.00 per year for international institutions and $140.00 per year for Canadian and foreign students/residents. To receive student/resident rate, orders must be accompanied by name of affiliated institution, date of term, and the *signature* of program/residency coordinator on institution letterhead. Orders will be billed at individual rate until proof of status is received. Foreign air speed delivery is included in all *Clinics* subscription prices. All prices are subject to change without notice.
POSTMASTER: Send address changes to *Veterinary Clinics of North America: Small Animal Practice*, Elsevier Periodicals Customer Service, 6277 Sea Harbor Drive, Orlando, FL 32887-4800. Customer Service: 1-800-654-2452 (US). From outside the United States, call 1-407-563-6020. Fax: 1-407-363-9661. E-mail: JournalsCustomerService-usa@elsevier.com.

Veterinary Clinics of North America: Small Animal Practice is also published in Japanese by Inter Zoo Publishing Co., Ltd., Aoyama Crystal-Bldg 5F, 3-5-12 Kitaaoyama, Minato-ku, Tokyo 107-0061, Japan.

Reprints: For copies of 100 or more, of articles in this publication, please contact the Commercial Reprints Department, Elsevier Inc., 360 Park Avenue South, New York, New York 10010-1710. Tel. (212) 633-3813 Fax: (212) 462-1935, email: reprints@elsevier.com.

Veterinary Clinics of North America: Small Animal Practice is covered in *Current Contents/Agriculture, Biology and Environmental Sciences, Science Citation Index, ASCA, Index Medicus, Excerpta Medica,* and *BIOSIS*.

Printed in the United States of America.

Advances in Fluid, Electrolyte, and Acid-Base Disorders

GUEST EDITORS

HELIO AUTRAN DE MORAIS, DVM, PhD, Diplomate, American College of Veterinary Internal Medicine (Small Animal Internal Medicine); Clinical Associate Professor, Department of Medical Sciences, University of Wisconsin–Madison, Madison, Wisconsin

STEPHEN P. DIBARTOLA, DVM, Diplomate, American College of Veterinary Internal Medicine (Small Animal Internal Medicine); Professor, Department of Veterinary Clinical Sciences, The Ohio State University, Columbus, Ohio

CONTRIBUTORS

SOPHIE ADAMANTOS, BVSc, CertVA, MRCVS, Diplomate, American College of Veterinary Emergency and Critical Care; Lecturer in Emergency and Critical Care Medicine, Department of Veterinary Clinical Sciences, Royal Veterinary College, North Mymms, Hatfield, United Kingdom

HELIO AUTRAN DE MORAIS, DVM, PhD, Diplomate, American College of Veterinary Internal Medicine (Small Animal Internal Medicine); Clinical Associate Professor, Department of Medical Sciences, University of Wisconsin–Madison, Madison, Wisconsin

JONATHAN F. BACH, DVM, Diplomate, American College of Veterinary Internal Medicine (Small Animal Internal Medicine); Diplomate, American College of Veterinary Emergency and Critical Care; Clinical Assistant Professor, Department of Medical Sciences, School of Veterinary Medicine, University of Wisconsin, Madison, Wisconsin

SHANE W. BATEMAN, DVM, DVSc, Diplomate, American College of Veterinary Emergency and Critical Care; Clinical Professor, Department of Veterinary Clinical Sciences, The Ohio State University, Columbus, Ohio

JULIA A. BATES, DVM, Clinical Instructor, Department of Medical Sciences, University of Wisconsin, Madison, Wisconsin

ALEXANDER W. BIONDO, DVM, PhD, Associate Professor, Departamento de Medicina Veterinária, Universidade Federal do Paraná, Paraná, Brazil

SØREN R. BOYSEN, DVM, Diplomate, American College of Veterinary Emergency and Critical Care; Assistant Professor and Head of Emergency and Critical Care, Faculty of Veterinary Medicine, Department of Clinical Sciences, University of Montreal, Sainte Hyacinthe, Quebec, Canada

ANDREW J. BROWN, MA, VetMB, MRCVS, Diplomate, American College of Veterinary Emergency and Critical Care; Assistant Professor, Emergency and Critical Care Medicine, Department of Small Animal Clinical Sciences, College of Veterinary Medicine, Michigan State University, East Lansing, Michigan

DANIEL L. CHAN, DVM, MRCVS, Diplomate, American College of Veterinary Emergency and Critical Care; Diplomate, American College of Veterinary Nutrition; Lecturer in Veterinary Emergency and Critical Care; and Clinical Nutritionist, Department of Veterinary Clinical Sciences, The Royal Veterinary College, University of London, North Mymms, Hertfordshire, United Kingdom

DENNIS J. CHEW, DVM, Diplomate, American College of Veterinary Internal Medicine (Small Animal Internal Medicine); Professor, Department of Veterinary Clinical Sciences, College of Veterinary Medicine, The Ohio State University, Columbus, Ohio

TERESA C. DEFRANCESCO, DVM, Diplomate, American College of Veterinary Internal Medicine (Cardiology); Diplomate, American College of Veterinary Emergency and Critical Care; Associate Professor in Cardiology and Critical Care, Department of Clinical Sciences, North Carolina State University College of Veterinary Medicine, Raleigh, North Carolina

STEPHEN P. DIBARTOLA, DVM, Diplomate, American College of Veterinary Internal Medicine (Small Animal Internal Medicine); Professor, Department of Veterinary Clinical Sciences, The Ohio State University, Columbus, Ohio

KENNETH DROBATZ, DVM, MSCE, Diplomate, American College of Veterinary Internal Medicine; Diplomate, American College of Veterinary Emergency and Critical Care; Section of Critical Care, Department of Clinical Studies–Philadelphia, School of Veterinary Medicine, University of Pennsylvania, Philadelphia, Pennsylvania

DANIEL FOY, DVM, MS, Small Animal Internal Medicine Resident, Department of Medical Sciences, University of Wisconsin–Madison, Madison, Wisconsin

DEZ HUGHES, BVSc, MRCVS, Diplomate, American College of Veterinary Emergency and Critical Care; Greensborough, Victoria, Australia

REBECCA A. JOHNSON, MS, DVM, PhD, Diplomate, American College of Veterinary Anesthesiologists; Clinical Assistant Professor, Department of Surgical Sciences, University of Wisconsin–Madison, Madison, Wisconsin

CONTRIBUTORS continued

JENNIFER KAAE, VMD, Small Animal Internal Medicine Resident, Department of Medical Sciences, University of Wisconsin–Madison, Madison, Wisconsin

REBECCA KIRBY, DVM, Diplomate, American College of Veterinary Internal Medicine; Diplomate, American College of Veterinary Emergency and Critical Care; Executive Director, Animal Emergency Center and Specialty Services, Glendale, Wisconsin

MARCIA MERY KOGIKA, DVM, MS, PhD, Associate Professor, Departamento de Clínica Médica, Faculdade de Medicina Veterinária e Zootecnia, Universidade de São Paulo, Sao Paulo, Brazil

CATHY LANGSTON, DVM, Diplomate, American College of Veterinary Internal Medicine (Small Animal Internal Medicine); Head, Nephrology, Urology, and Hemodialysis Unit, Animal Medical Center, New York, New York

DOUGLASS K. MACINTIRE, DVM, MS, Diplomate, American College of Veterinary Internal Medicine; Diplomate, American College of Veterinary Emergency and Critical Care; PB Griffin Distinguished Professor in Critical Care Medicine, Department of Clinical Sciences, Auburn University Critical Care Program, College of Veterinary Medicine, Auburn University, Auburn, Alabama

KAROL A. MATHEWS, DVM, DVSc, Diplomate, American College of Veterinary Emergency and Critical Care; Professor and Service Chief, Department of Clinical Studies, Emergency and Critical Care Medicine, Ontario Veterinary College, University of Guelph, Guelph, Ontario, Canada

ELISA M. MAZZAFERRO, MS, DVM, PhD, Diplomate, American College of Veterinary Emergency and Critical Care; Director of Emergency Services, Wheat Ridge Veterinary Specialists, Wheat Ridge, Colorado

STEVEN MENSACK, VMD, Diplomate, American College of Veterinary Emergency and Critical Care; Medical Director, Pet Emergency Clinic, Inc., Ventura, California

CYNTHIA M. OTTO, DVM, PhD, Diplomate, American College of Veterinary Emergency and Critical Care; Associate Professor of Critical Care, University of Pennsylvania School of Veterinary Medicine, Philadelphia, Pennsylvania

GARRET E. PACHTINGER, VMD, Section of Critical Care, Department of Clinical Studies–Philadelphia, School of Veterinary Medicine, University of Pennsylvania, Philadelphia, Pennsylvania

ELKE RUDLOFF, DVM, Diplomate, American College of Veterinary Emergency and Critical Care; Director of Education, Animal Emergency Center and Specialty Services, Glendale, Wisconsin

MICHAEL SCHAER, DVM, Diplomate, American College of Veterinary Internal Medicine; Diplomate, American College of Veterinary Emergency and Critical Care; Professor of Medicine, Department of Small Animal Clinical Sciences, College of Veterinary Medicine, University of Florida, Gainesville, Florida

PATRICIA A. SCHENCK, DVM, PhD, Section Chief, Endocrine Diagnostic Section, Diagnostic Center for Population and Animal Health; and Assistant Professor, Department of Pathobiology and Diagnostic Investigation, Michigan State University, Lansing, Michigan

JENNIFER E. WALDROP, DVM, Diplomate, American College of Veterinary Emergency and Critical Care; Massachusetts Veterinary Referral Hospital, Woburn, Massachusetts

MICHAEL WILLARD, DVM, MS, Diplomate, American College of Veterinary Internal Medicine; Professor of Small Animal Clinical Sciences, College of Veterinary Medicine, Texas A&M University, College Station, Texas

Advances in Fluid, Electrolyte, and Acid-Base Disorders

CONTENTS — VOLUME 38 • NUMBER 3 • MAY 2008

Hypokalemia, hyperkalemia, hyponatremia, hypernatremia, hypocalcemia, and hypercalcemia are commonly seen in emergency medicine. Severe abnormalities in any of these electrolytes can cause potentially life-threatening consequences to the patient. It is essential that the clinician understand and correct (if possible) the underlying cause of each disorder and recognize the importance of the rates of correction, especially with serum sodium disorders. The recommended doses in this article might have to be adjusted to the individual patient, and these modifications must be adjusted again to the pathophysiology of the primary underlying disorder.

Chronic disorders of sodium and potassium occur and occasionally need symptomatic therapy. Hypernatremia primarily indicates loss of free water, whereas hyponatremia may be attributable to various problems. It is important not to correct major aberrations of serum sodium concentrations too quickly lest the therapy be more detrimental than the electrolyte abnormality. In distinction, hypokalemia and hyperkalemia may be corrected quickly. Hypomagnesemia is relatively common, but its clinical significance is still being determined.

Recent technologic advances have allowed the production and marketing of cage-side blood gas analyzers to private practitioners. The widespread use of cage-side portable blood gas analyzers in veterinary practices has increased the need to develop the basic skills of blood gas analysis as part of a tool kit for practicing veterinarians. Rapid expansion of emergency and critical care medicine as a specialty and increased numbers of veterinary emergency and veterinary specialty practices have occurred concurrently with the availability of blood gas analyzers that are affordable for private practitioners. As a result, evaluation of blood gas results is no longer an activity confined to academic institutions and has become a daily part of many practicing veterinarians' activities.

The recognition and management of acid-base disorders is a commonplace activity in the critical care unit, and the role of weak and strong acids in the genesis of metabolic acid-base disorders is reviewed. The clinical approach to patients with metabolic alkalosis and metabolic acidosis is discussed in this article.

Fluid Therapy

Fluid administration is a primary component of therapy in many small animal patients. Several different classes of fluid may be given, and there are multiple options within each class. The type, route, volume, and rate of fluid administered should be tailored to the patient's signalment, disease or injury state, and response to the administration of fluids. Monitoring vital parameters and bedside monitoring of laboratory variables allow assessment of fluid therapy success or failure. Successful fluid administration also requires that parenteral fluid therapy ultimately be discontinued with minimal adverse effects for the patient.

Colloids are increasingly becoming considered indispensable in the management of critically ill patients. Typical indications for colloid administration include patients with tissue edema, hypovolemia, and low oncotic pressure. Current guidelines for the use of colloids in veterinary patients balance the purported benefits of colloid fluid administration with the potential risks, such as volume overload and coagulation disturbances. This article focuses primarily on hydroxyethyl starches, because they are the most commonly used colloid in veterinary practice, and because recent advances in colloid therapy have been achieved with this colloid. Newer colloids have been modified to limit effects on the coagulation system, and they may be used to modulate the inflammatory response, which could prove to be particularly useful in the management of critically ill patients. A better understanding of how different fluids influence the host response may enable us to explore new applications of fluid replacement therapy beyond simply replenishing volume deficits.

Twenty-five percent human serum albumin (HSA) is a foreign protein and can potentially cause immune-mediated reactions. For this reason, the author only recommends 25% HSA use after risk analysis shows that the benefits outweigh the potential risks of adverse events. If it is apparent that a critically ill animal may succumb to its illness because of the problems associated with severe hypoalbuminemia, the benefit outweighs the risk. The veterinarian must inform the owner of potential delayed immune-mediated reactions, describe these lesions, and follow the case weekly to ensure that no reaction has occurred. Although there are many positive attributes to the administration of 25% HSA, there seems to be specific situations in which 25% HSA may be indicated and others in which it may not be indicated.

Complications of Fluid Therapy 607
Elisa M. Mazzaferro

The intravenous administration of fluids is one of the most important aspects of patient care in hospitalized animals. Intravenous fluids are administered to replace or prevent dehydration, treat hypovolemic shock and intravascular volume depletion, correct acid-base and electrolyte abnormalities, and maintain vascular access for administration of drugs, blood product components, and parenteral nutrition. Intravenous catheterization also can provide a means of blood sample collection, thus avoiding frequent and uncomfortable venipunctures in critically ill animals. Although the benefits of intravenous catheterization and fluid administration are numerous, inherent risks are associated with the procedures, and care must be taken to avoid potential complications.

Pediatric Fluid Therapy 621
Douglass K. Macintire

Many conditions of pediatric patients require fluid therapy. Depending on the veterinarian's assessment of hydration and perfusion status, fluids can be administered orally, subcutaneously, intraperitoneally, intravenously, or by the intraosseous route. Pediatric patients are prone to hypothermia, hypovolemia, hypoglycemia, and hypokalemia, which must be addressed during fluid therapy in pediatric patients. Typical parameters used to assess hydration status in adult animals do not always apply to pediatric patients. Veterinarians should be aware of differences between pediatric patients and adult animals in terms of physical assessment, common presentations, and fluid requirements for resuscitation and maintenance needs.

Assessment and Treatment of Hypovolemic States 629
Garret E. Pachtinger and Kenneth Drobatz

Hypovolemia and hypoperfusion are common life-threatening problems in animals presented to the emergency veterinarian. Assessment of physical findings and rapid recognition and treatment of abnormal tissue perfusion are crucial in optimizing outcome. The clinician should be familiar with the disease being treated and the types of fluids that are available. Development of a fluid therapy plan to correct life-threatening abnormalities and patient monitoring during treatment play an important role in patient outcome.

Rapid identification of these disorders and aggressive therapy to correct fluid, electrolyte, and acid-base imbalances are crucial to a successful outcome for the patient. An understanding of the pathophysiology behind the development of these endocrine disorders helps to guide therapy and improves the clinical outcome.

Fluid therapy in patients with pulmonary disease is challenging. Although a single set of rules cannot be applied to every patient, the following guidelines can be used when managing patients with pulmonary disease. Euvolemic patients with adequate tissue perfusion should be given sufficient isotonic fluid to balance insensible losses. If severe pulmonary compromise is present, cessation of all fluid therapy may be considered if the patient is able to match its losses by voluntary intake. In hypovolemic or hypotensive patients, small boluses of isotonic crystalloids or colloids should be given to restore perfusion, avoiding rates of more than 30 mL/kg an hour for isotonic crystalloids. If perfusion is not restored by adequate volume resuscitation, vasopressors or positive inotropes should be administered to prevent fluid overload and deterioration in pulmonary function.

Advanced heart failure and its treatment are often associated with a variety of hemodynamic, fluid, and electrolyte derangements. This article gives the practitioner an overview of the pathophysiology of common fluid and electrolyte alterations present in animals with heart failure, highlighting specific clinical correlates. Additionally, specific therapeutic interventions are discussed to manage these fluid and electrolyte abnormalities.

Preface

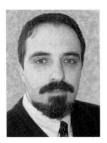 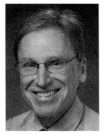

Helio Autran de Morais, DVM, PhD
Stephen P. DiBartola, DVM

Guest Editors

"Tous les liquides circulant, la liqueur du sang et les fluides intra-organiques constituent en réalité ce milieu intérieur [All circulating fluids, blood plasma and fluid within organs in reality constitutes this "milieu interieur]"

Claude Bernard

The French physiologist Claude Bernard recognized that the world inhabited by our cells is not the external world at all, but an internal world of fluids and electrolytes reminiscent of the sea from which we came. We believe that a good foundation in physiology and pathophysiology will enhance any clinician's approach to his or her patient. A conscientious, thoughtful evaluation of the laboratory results provides valuable insight into the fluid, electrolyte, and acid-base status of the patient and should improve veterinary care. With the advent of point-of-care instruments and sophisticated in-house laboratory analyzers, today's veterinarians have access to laboratory data we could only dream about 30 years ago. Puzzling over electrolyte and acid-base data is no longer just the province of those of us in academia. Now that such information is widely available, it is incumbent upon all clinicians to understand it and apply it properly. We hope that the articles collected in this edition of *Veterinary Clinics of North America: Small Animal Practice* will be helpful in that regard, and we thank all of the contributors who sacrificed their time to share their experience in managing small animal patients with fluid, electrolyte, and acid-base disturbances.

This issue is divided into three sections. First, a quick reference section provides short articles that cover the crucial information needed to quickly assess

0195-5616/08/$ – see front matter
doi:10.1016/j.cvsm.2008.03.001

the patient's acid-base and electrolyte (sodium, potassium, chloride, calcium, magnesium, and phosphorus) status. In the second section, selected diagnostic and therapeutic topics are reviewed in more depth. Finally, the last section of the issue covers general principles of fluid therapy for crystalloids, colloids, and human serum albumin and complications of fluid therapy. Finally, the use of fluid therapy in special situations, such as pediatric patients, trauma patients, renal failure, diabetic ketoacidosis, hypoadrenocorticism, gastrointestinal disease, pulmonary disease, and cardiac disease is covered. We hope you find the information in these articles useful in your daily practice of veterinary medicine, and we encourage you to contact us to make suggestions, correct errors, or provide input on controversial issues. As always, readers are encouraged to continue reading the current biomedical literature to increase understanding and move the practice of veterinary medicine forward. Finally, we thank John Vassallo at Elsevier/Saunders for suggesting this project and nurturing it to fruition.

Helio Autran de Morais, DVM, PhD
Department of Medical Sciences
University of Wisconsin–Madison
2015 Linden Drive
Madison, WI 53706, USA

E-mail address: demorais@svm.vetmed.wisc.edu

Stephen P. DiBartola, DVM
Department of Veterinary Clinical Sciences
The Ohio State University
601 Vernon L. Tharp Street
Columbus, OH 43210, USA

E-mail address: dibartola1@osu.edu

Hypoxemia: A Quick Reference

Jonathan F. Bach, DVM

Department of Medical Sciences, School of Veterinary Medicine,
University of Wisconsin, Madison, WI 53706, USA

- The partial pressure of oxygen dissolved in arterial blood (Pa_{O_2}) reflects the amount of oxygen dissolved in blood. At sea level and when breathing ambient air, hypoxemia is defined as a Pa_{O_2} of less than 80 mm Hg.
- Normally, Pa_{O_2} is approximately four- to fivefold the fraction of inspired oxygen (F_{IO_2}).
  - At sea level, the F_{IO_2} is 21% and a normal Pa_{O_2} is 80 to 100 mm Hg.

ALVEOLAR GAS EQUATION

- The alveolar gas equation uses the partial pressure of arterial carbon dioxide (Pa_{CO_2}) to estimate the partial pressure of oxygen within the alveolus (PA_{O_2}):
  - The Pa_{CO_2} is inversely proportional to ventilation, and measuring it lends direct information about the sufficiency of ventilation. An elevated Pa_{CO_2} indicates hypoventilation, whereas Pa_{CO_2} is decreased from hyperventilation.
- PA_{O_2} is estimated taking into account Pa_{CO_2}, F_{IO_2}, barometric pressure (BP), and vapor pressure of water (P_{H_2O}).

$$PA_{O_2} = F_{IO_2}(BP - P_{H_2O}) - Pa_{CO_2}/RQ$$

- Respiratory quotient (RQ) compensates for an individual's diet composition. The RQ most frequently used is 0.8. The expression F_{IO_2} (BP $-$ P_{H_2O}) is the pressure of inspired oxygen (P_{IO_2}). When a blood gas is obtained on ambient air ($F_{IO_2} = 0.21$) at sea level, the BP is often near 760 mm Hg, P_{H_2O} is approximately 47 mm Hg, and P_{IO_2} is approximately 150 mm Hg. Thus:

$$PA_{O_2} = 150 - Pa_{CO_2}/RQ$$

E-mail address: bachj@svm.vetmed.wisc.edu

0195-5616/08/$ – see front matter
doi:10.1016/j.cvsm.2008.02.001

ALVEOLAR-ARTERIAL OXYGEN DIFFERENCE

- The alveolar – arterial gas gradient (A – a) is the difference between the calculated PA_{O_2} (A) and measured Pa_{O_2} (a) obtained from the arterial blood gas. When combined, the equation reads:

$$A - a = (150 - Pa_{CO_2}/RQ) - Pa_{O_2}$$

- Ideal lungs would have an A – a gradient of 0 mm Hg. This is not the case, however, because there are normal physiologic variations throughout the lung in which ventilation and perfusion are not ideal.
  - Pressure gradients are different between dorsal and ventral lung lobes, resulting in unequal ventilation between regions.
  - The ventral regions have greater blood flow (perfusion) than the dorsal regions.
- Because of these inequalities, the normal A – a gradient in the dog is generally less than 15 to 25 mm Hg. Values greater than this indicate that a parenchymal pulmonary lesion is present, causing hypoxemia.

ANALYSIS

- Indications: Arterial blood gases should be evaluated in patients suspected of having respiratory disease to diagnose and estimate the severity of hypoxemia.
- Typical reference range: Pa_{O_2} should be greater than 80 mm Hg in patients breathing room air at sea level, whereas the A – a gradient should be less than 25 mm Hg.
- Danger values: Hypoxemia is considered severe when the Pa_{O_2} is less than 60 mm Hg.
- Artifacts: Correct sample handling is imperative for accurate Pa_{O_2} readings. Delay in measurement allows continued metabolism by the erythrocytes and reduces Pa_{O_2}. Keeping the specimen on ice allows accurate measurement to be delayed for up to 1 hour. Air bubbles introduce error and cause an increase in Pa_{O_2}.

CLINICAL APPROACH

- The causes of hypoxia include hypoventilation, low FI_{O_2}, diffusion impairment, ventilation-perfusion (V/Q) mismatch, and right-to-left shunt. Fig. 1 illustrates how the arterial blood gas results and calculation of the A – a gradient can direct the clinician to the underlying cause of a patient's hypoxemia. Supplying 28% FI_{O_2} can be achieved using a single nasal cannula and an oxygen flow rate of 50 mL/kg/min.
- Hypoventilation: When a patient has hypoventilation, the Pa_{O_2} and PA_{O_2} decrease to a similar degree that the Pa_{CO_2} and alveolar carbon dioxide (CO_2) increase. Because of these opposite and nearly equal changes, the A – a gradient does not increase. If a deviation is present in a patient with hypoventilation, concurrent diffusion impairment, V/Q mismatch, or right-to-left shunting is present. Causes of hypoventilation include centrally acting

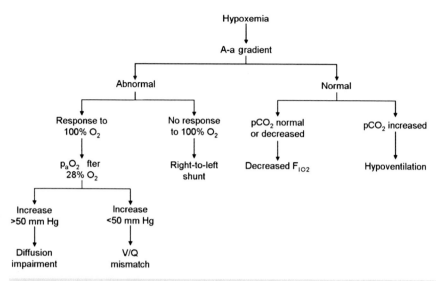

Fig. 1. Algorithm depicts the clinical approach to a patient with hypoxemia. (*Adapted from* DiBartola SP, de Morais HSA. Respiratory acid-base disorders. In: DiBartola SP, editor. Fluid therapy in small animal practice. Philadelphia: WB Saunders; 1992. p. 242; with permission.)

respiratory depressants, neuromuscular diseases inhibiting the muscles of respiration, chest wall injuries, pleural space lesions, and upper airway obstruction.

- Decreased F_{IO_2}: The most common cause of decreased F_{IO_2} is decreased BP associated with high altitude or anesthetic error, such as a low oxygen (O_2) supply source or administration of nitrogen oxide (N_2O) without O_2. As a result of the low alveolar O_2, the PaO_2 decreases, which stimulates ventilation. The hyperventilation decreases $PaCO_2$. The A − a gradient remains normal; however, the $PaCO_2$ and PaO_2 are low.
- Diffusion impairment: When there is inadequate equilibration of O_2 tension across the alveoli and capillaries, diffusion impairment is present. In normal individuals, O_2 rapidly diffuses from alveoli into the capillaries. Diffusion impairment may occur earlier in the course of pulmonary disease than V/Q mismatch. The clinical signs are mild, and by the time an owner detects clinical signs and seeks veterinary attention, his or her pet may have diffusion impairment and V/Q mismatch. Diffusion impairment is caused by thickening of the alveolar interstitial space or the capillary wall. Disease processes include interstitial edema, fibrosis, vasculitis, or emphysema.
- V/Q mismatch: V/Q mismatch is common in patients that have pulmonary disease. It occurs when regions of the lung lack ventilation or perfusion, impairing efficient gas exchange. The A − a gradient increases by abnormally low or abnormally high V/Q ratios. V/Q mismatch may occur from diseases affecting air flow (eg, asthma, bronchitis), decreased compliance (eg, pulmonary fibrosis), increased compliance (eg, emphysema), or vascular obstruction (eg, pulmonary embolism). Patients with V/Q mismatch often have

hypoxemia (low Pa_{O_2}) and hypocapnia (low Pa_{CO_2}). When they are placed on 100% O_2, their hypoxemia improves, and the Pa_{O_2} should improve by at least 50 mm Hg.

- Right-to-left shunt: In patients with right-to-left shunt, deoxygenated venous blood passes from the right heart back to the systemic circulation without exposure to ventilated lung. Normal animals have a small amount of physiologic right-to-left shunting. Causes of pathologic right-to-left shunt include alveolar collapse (eg, atelectasis), flooding of alveoli with fluid (eg, cardiogenic and noncardiogenic pulmonary edema, acute respiratory distress syndrome), alveolar consolidation (eg, pneumonia), and congenital cardiac or vascular anomalies. Patient with right-to-left shunt have low Pa_{O_2} and usually low Pa_{CO_2}, although the Pa_{CO_2} can be elevated. Because mixed venous blood is being added to the systemic circulation, the Pa_{O_2} fails to increase following administration of 100% O_2.

Further Readings

Dunphy ED, Mann FA, Dodam JR, et al. Comparison of unilateral versus bilateral nasal catheters for oxygen administration in dogs. J Vet Emerg Crit Care 2002;12(4):245–51.

Johnson RA, de Morais HA. Respiratory acid-base disorders. In: DiBartola SP, editor. Fluid, electrolyte, and acid-base disorders. 3rd edition. St. Louis (MO): Elsevier; 2006. p. 283–96.

Respiratory Alkalosis: A Quick Reference

Rebecca A. Johnson, MS, DVM, PhD

Department of Surgical Sciences, University of Wisconsin–Madison,
2015 Linden Drive, Madison, WI 53706, USA

- Respiratory alkalosis, or primary hypocapnia, occurs when alveolar ventilation exceeds that required to eliminate the carbon dioxide produced by the body.
- There is a decrease in $PaCO_2$, increase in pH, and compensatory decreases in blood HCO_3^- concentration.
- Respiratory alkalosis can be acute or chronic, with metabolic compensation initially consisting of cellular uptake of HCO_3^-, followed by longer lasting decreases in renal reabsorption of HCO_3^-.
- Chronic respiratory acidosis can be well compensated, and the arterial pH can be normal or near normal.

ANALYSIS

- Indications: Respiratory alkalosis is a common finding in critically ill patients. $PaCO_2$ should be evaluated in patients with apparent hyperventilation to diagnose respiratory alkalosis.
- Typical reference range: Normal arterial blood gas values for dogs and cats inspiring room air are presented in Table 1.
- Danger values
  - Acute respiratory alkalosis presents more danger than chronic respiratory alkalosis, because metabolic compensation is efficient in chronic disorders.
  - When arterial pH approaches approximately 7.6 or $PaCO_2$ decreases to less than 25 mm Hg, arteriolar vasoconstriction results, potentially reducing cerebral and myocardial blood flow.
- Artifacts: Correct sample handling is imperative for accurate $PaCO_2$ readings.
  - PCO_2 of room air is low, and the presence of air bubbles within the sample reduces the PCO_2 and increases pH of the blood.

E-mail address: pipob@svm.vetmed.wisc.edu

0195-5616/08/$ – see front matter
doi:10.1016/j.cvsm.2008.01.017

Table 1
Typical reference ranges for normal arterial blood gas values for dogs and cats inspiring room air

	Dog	Cat
pH	7.41 (7.35–7.46)	7.39 (7.31–7.46)
$PaCO_2$ (mm Hg)	37 (31–43)	31 (25–37)
$[HCO_3^-]$ (mEq/L)	22 (19–26)	18 (14–22)
PO_2 (mm Hg)	92 (81–103)	107 (95–118)

Data from Haskins SC. Blood gases and acid-base balance: clinical interpretation and therapeutic implications. In: Kirk RW, editor. Current veterinary therapy VIII. Philadelphia: WB Saunders; 1983. p. 201.

- Dilution of the sample by large amounts of heparin erroneously decreases PCO_2.
- Drug effects: Pharmacologic agents, such as salicylates, corticosteroids, and xanthines (eg, aminophylline), may produce respiratory alkalosis through activation of the respiratory centers.

RESPIRATORY ALKALOSIS
- Causes: Respiratory alkalosis and hypocapnia occur with alveolar hyperventilation resulting from the following (Box 1):
  - Stimulation of peripheral chemoreceptors (eg, hypoxia), pulmonary stretch receptors, or nociceptors
  - Direct activation of central respiratory centers
  - Overzealous mechanical ventilation
  - Fear, excitement, or pain
  - After treatment of metabolic acidosis, because hyperventilation may still be present for 24 to 48 hours after therapy

Box 1: Causes of respiratory alkalosis

Hypoxemia and stimulation of peripheral chemoreceptors[a]

Right-to-left shunting, decreased inspired partial pressure of oxygen (PiO_2), congestive heart failure, severe anemia, severe hypotension, decreased cardiac output, ventilation-perfusion mismatch (eg, pneumonia, pulmonary thromboembolism, pulmonary fibrosis, pulmonary edema)

Activation of stretch or nociceptors[a]

Pneumonia, pulmonary thromboembolism, interstitial lung disease, pulmonary edema

Centrally mediated hyperventilation

Liver disease, hyperadrenocorticism, sepsis, pharmacologic agents (eg, salicylates, corticosteroids, xanthines), progesterone, recovery from metabolic acidosis, central nervous system disease, exercise, heatstroke

Overzealous mechanical ventilation

Situations causing pain, fear, or anxiety[a]

[a]Most important causes in small animal medicine.

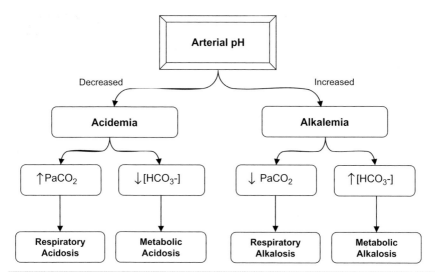

Fig. 1. Algorithm for evaluation of patients that have respiratory acid-base disorders.

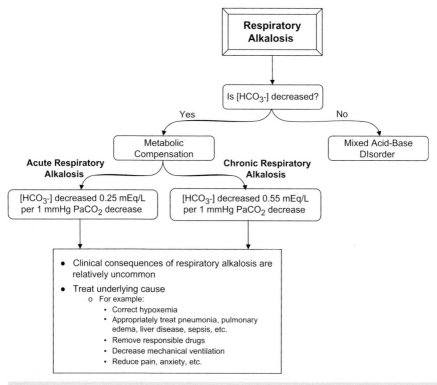

Fig. 2. Algorithm for evaluation of patients that have acute versus chronic respiratory alkalosis.

- Signs: Clinical signs in patients that have respiratory alkalosis are mainly attributable to the underlying disease process and are uncommon because of the efficient metabolic compensation that occurs.
  - Tachypnea may be the only clinical sign, especially in patients that have chronic hypocapnia.
  - In patients that have acute alkalemia, cardiac arrhythmias, confusion, and seizures from arteriolar vasoconstriction with decreased cerebral or myocardial perfusion may be seen.
- Stepwise approach: An algorithm for evaluation of general acid-base disorders, including respiratory alkalosis, is shown in Fig. 1. A more specific algorithm for the differential diagnosis of acute versus chronic respiratory alkalosis is presented in Fig. 2. Note that the decreases in HCO_3^- seen with acute metabolic compensation are similar in dogs and cats. The degree of metabolic compensation in chronic respiratory alkalosis in cats is not known, however, although the pH is frequently normal or just slightly alkalemic.

Further Readings

DiBartola SP. Introduction to acid-base disorders. In: DiBartola SP, editor. Fluid, electrolyte, and acid-base disorders. 3rd edition. St. Louis (MO): Elsevier; 2006. p. 229–51.

Haskins SC. Blood gases and acid-base balance: clinical interpretation and therapeutic implications. In: Kirk RW, editor. Current veterinary therapy VIII. Philadelphia: WB Saunders; 1983. p. 201–15.

Johnson RA, de Morais HA. Respiratory acid-base disorders. In: DiBartola SP, editor. Fluid, electrolyte, and acid-base disorders. 3rd edition. St. Louis (MO): Elsevier; 2006. p. 283–96.

Respiratory Acidosis: A Quick Reference

Rebecca A. Johnson, MS, DVM, PhD

Department of Surgical Sciences, University of Wisconsin–Madison, 2015 Linden Drive, Madison, WI 53706, USA

- Respiratory acidosis, or primary hypercapnia
  - Carbon dioxide production exceeds elimination by means of the lung, mainly attributable to alveolar hypoventilation.
    - Alveolar hypoventilation and resulting respiratory acidosis may also be associated with hypoxemia.
  - There is an increase in Pa_{CO_2}, decrease in pH, and compensatory increase in HCO_3^- concentration.
    - In acute respiratory acidosis, metabolic compensation to increase HCO_3^- concentration is attributable to cellular buffering.
    - In chronic respiratory acidosis, metabolic compensation results from renal reabsorption of HCO_3^-.

ANALYSIS
- Indications: Pa_{CO_2} should be evaluated in patients suspected of having respiratory failure or increased carbon dioxide production with concurrent alveolar hypoventilation.
- Typical reference range: Normal arterial blood gas values for dogs and cats inspiring room air are presented in Table 1.
- Danger values
  - Moderately elevated Pa_{CO_2} (60–70 mm Hg) causes sympathetic activation, increasing cardiac output and potentially causing tachyarrhythmias.
  - Cerebral blood flow and intracranial pressure increase linearly with Pa_{CO_2}.
  - Extremely high Pa_{CO_2} (>95 mm Hg) produces disorientation, narcosis, and coma.
- Artifacts: Correct sample handling is imperative for accurate Pa_{CO_2} readings.
  - P_{CO_2} increases and pH decreases as the sample waits before analysis (20–30 minutes). These changes are faster at 25°C than at 4°C.
- Drug effects: Many drugs produce respiratory acidosis by means of respiratory center depression (eg, opioids, barbiturates, inhalant anesthetics) or

E-mail address: pipob@svm.vetmed.wisc.edu

0195-5616/08/$ – see front matter
doi:10.1016/j.cvsm.2008.01.016

Table 1
Typical reference ranges for normal arterial blood gas values for dogs and cats inspiring room air

	Dog	Cat
pH	7.41 (7.35–7.46)	7.39 (7.31–7.46)
Pa_{CO_2} (mm Hg)	37 (31–43)	31 (25–37)
[HCO_3^-] (mEq/L)	22 (19–26)	18 (14–22)
P_{O_2} (mm Hg)	92 (81–103)	107 (95–118)

Data from Haskins SC. Blood gases and acid-base balance: clinical interpretation and therapeutic implications. In: Kirk RW, editor. Current veterinary therapy VIII. Philadelphia: WB Saunders; 1983. p. 201.

neuromuscular dysfunction (eg, organophosphates, aminoglycosides used in conjunction with anesthetics).

RESPIRATORY ACIDOSIS
- Causes: Most cases result from disturbances in removal of carbon dioxide by means of the lungs.
  - Respiratory acidosis and hypercapnia occur with alveolar hypoventilation resulting from any disruption in the following (Box 1):

Box 1: Causes of respiratory acidosis

Large airway obstruction[a]

 Physical or mechanical obstruction (eg, aspiration, mass lesion, plug or kink in endotracheal tube), tracheal collapse, brachycephalic syndrome, asthma, or chronic obstructive pulmonary disease

Intrinsic pulmonary and small airway disease[a]

 Severe pulmonary edema, pulmonary thromboembolism, pneumonia, asthma, or chronic obstructive pulmonary disease

Respiratory center depression[a]

 Drug induced (eg, opioids, barbiturates, inhalant anesthetics) or neurologic disease (eg, brain stem or cervical spinal cord lesion)

Restrictive extrapulmonary disorders[a]

 Diaphragmatic hernia, pleural space disease (eg, pneumothorax, pleural effusion)

Neuromuscular disease

 Myasthenia gravis, tetanus, botulism, tick paralysis, electrolyte abnormalities (eg, hypokalemia), or drug induced (eg, organophosphates, aminoglycosides used in conjunction with anesthetics)

Increased carbon dioxide production with impaired alveolar ventilation

 Heatstroke or malignant hyperthermia

Ineffective mechanical ventilation

Marked obesity (Pickwickian syndrome)

[a]Most important causes in small animal practice.

- Neural control of ventilation
- Breathing mechanics
- Alveolar gas exchange
- Acute hypercapnia and respiratory acidosis mainly result from sudden severe respiratory system (eg, pneumothorax), neurologic system (eg, spinal cord injury), or neuromuscular (eg, botulism) disease.
- Chronic respiratory acidosis has many potential causes that can lead to sustained hypercapnia (see Box 1).
- Signs: Many clinical signs in patients that have respiratory acidosis are attributable to the underlying disease process itself and not necessarily to the hypercapnia.
    - Chronic compensated patients may exhibit mild signs; thus, subjective clinical assessment of the patient is not reliable in making a diagnosis of respiratory acidosis.
    - In some patients, hypercapnia results in tachyarrhythmias (including ventricular tachycardia), increased blood pressure, and "brick-red" mucous membranes associated with vasodilation.
    - Patients may develop a fast shallow breathing pattern with inadequate tidal volumes. Their central nervous system function may deteriorate, and they may appear anxious, restless, disoriented, or somnolent.
    - In extremely acute alveolar hypoventilation (eg, cardiopulmonary arrest, airway obstruction), the patient dies from hypoxemia before hypercapnia can become severe.
- Stepwise approach: An algorithm for evaluation of general acid-base disorders, including respiratory acidosis, is shown in Fig. 1. A more specific algorithm for the differential diagnosis of acute versus chronic respiratory acidosis is presented in Fig. 2. Note that the increases in HCO_3^- seen with

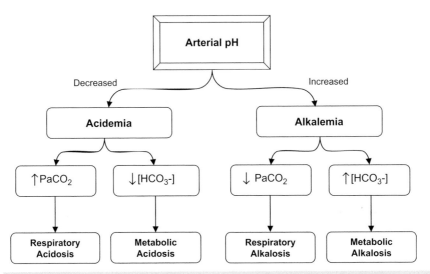

Fig. 1. Algorithm for evaluation of patients that have respiratory acid-base disorders.

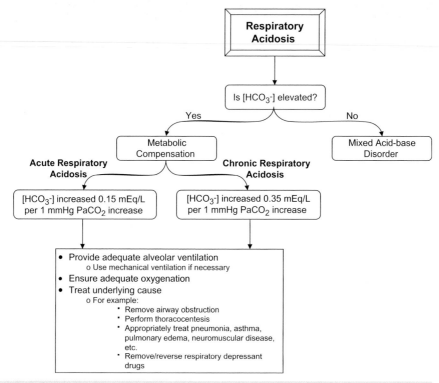

Fig. 2. Algorithm for evaluation of patients that have acute versus chronic respiratory acidosis.

acute metabolic compensation are similar in dogs and cats. The degree of metabolic compensation in chronic respiratory acidosis in cats is not known, however.

Further Readings

DiBartola SP. Introduction to acid-base disorders. In: DiBartola SP, editor. Fluid, electrolyte, and acid-base disorders. 3rd edition. St. Louis (MO): Elsevier; 2006. p. 229–51.

Haskins SC. Blood gases and acid-base balance: clinical interpretation and therapeutic implications. In: Kirk RW, editor. Current veterinary therapy VIII. Philadelphia: WB Saunders; 1983. p. 201–15.

Johnson RA, de Morais HA. Respiratory acid-base disorders. In: DiBartola SP, editor. Fluid, electrolyte, and acid-base disorders. 3rd editor. St. Louis (MO): Elsevier; 2006. p. 283–96.

Metabolic Alkalosis: A Quick Reference

Daniel Foy, DVM, MS*, Helio Autran de Morais, DVM, PhD

Department of Medical Sciences, University of Wisconsin–Madison,
2015 Linden Drive, Madison, WI 53706, USA

- Metabolic alkaloses are characterized by an increase in HCO_3^- and base excess, an increase in pH, and a compensatory increase in PCO_2.
  - Metabolic alkalosis can be identified by an increase in HCO_3^- or base excess.
  - Base excess is the amount of acid needed to return blood pH to normal. A positive base excess is associated with metabolic alkalosis.
  - There is a compensatory hypoventilation that increases PCO_2 and minimizes the change in pH.
    - In dogs, for each 1-mEq/L increase in HCO_3^-, PCO_2 increases by 0.7 mm Hg.
    - Respiratory compensation for metabolic alkalosis is similar in cats.
- Metabolic alkalosis can result from an increase in the strong ion difference (SID, or the difference between all strong cations and strong anions in blood) or a decrease in nonvolatile weak acids.

ANALYSIS

- Indications: Measurement of base excess and HCO_3^- is useful in severely ill pets at risk for developing alkalosis (eg, vomiting) or in animals that have a condition known to be associated with metabolic alkalosis or an increase in total carbon dioxide (total CO_2) concentration. Blood gas analysis is necessary to determine if the high total CO_2 is attributable to metabolic alkalosis or to compensation for respiratory acidosis.
- Typical reference range: The normal HCO_3^- concentration is approximately 19 to 23 mEq/L in dogs and 17 to 21 mEq/L in cats. The normal base excess is approximately 0 to −5 in dogs and cats. These values may vary among laboratories and analyzers. Total CO_2 is almost synonymous with HCO_3^- in samples handled anaerobically.
- Danger values: A pH greater than 7.6 indicates severe metabolic alkalosis.
- Artifacts: HCO_3^- concentration is calculated in blood gas machines based on pH and PCO_2. Thus, artifacts that interfere with PCO_2 or pH affect the estimation of HCO_3^- (see quick references on PCO_2 for further details).
- Drug effects: Sodium bicarbonate, potassium acetate, citrate or gluconate, and loop diuretics can cause metabolic alkalosis.

*Corresponding author. *E-mail address:* dfoy@svm.vetmed.wisc.edu (D. Foy).

0195-5616/08/$ – see front matter
doi:10.1016/j.cvsm.2008.01.023

METABOLIC ALKALOSIS

- Causes: Metabolic alkalosis can result from the causes listed in Box 1.
  - Increase in SID
    - Concentration alkalosis (decrease in free water, recognized by an increase in sodium concentration)
    - Hypochloremic alkalosis (decrease in chloride concentration)
      - Most common cause of metabolic alkalosis
      - Usually attributable to vomiting of stomach contents or diuretic administration
    - Chloride-resistant alkalosis is a particular kind of SID alkalosis that does not respond to chloride administration.
      - Metabolic alkalosis is usually mild, and the SID is increased as the result of a mild increase in sodium associated with a mild decrease in chloride.
  - Decrease in nonvolatile weak acids
    - Hypoalbuminemic alkalosis
      - Albumin is the only weak acid in a concentration high enough to increase blood pH when it is decreased.

Box 1: Principal causes of metabolic alkalosis

SID alkalosis

    Concentration alkalosis (recognized by ⇑ [Na$^+$])

        Pure water loss

            Water deprivation

        Hypotonic fluid loss

            Vomiting

            Diarrhea

    Hypochloremic alkalosis

        Vomiting of stomach contents[a]

        Diuretic administration (loop diuretics and thiazides)[a]

        $NaHCO_3$ administration

    Chloride-resistant hypochloremic alkalosis

        Hyperadrenocorticism

        Hyperaldosteronism

Nonvolatile ion buffer alkalosis

    Hypoalbuminemic alkalosis

        Liver failure

        Protein-losing nephropathy

        Protein-losing enteropathy

[a]Most important causes in small animal practice.

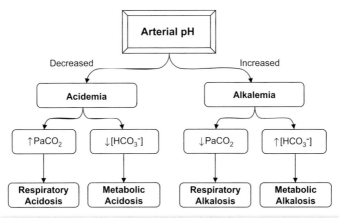

Fig. 1. Algorithm for evaluation of patients that have acid-base disorders.

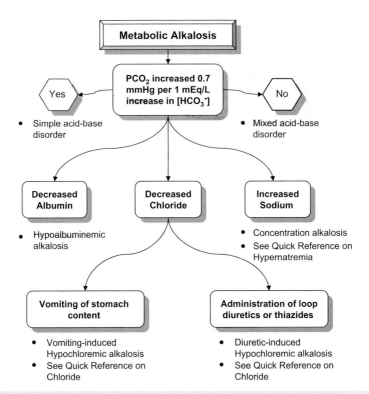

Fig. 2. Algorithm for evaluation of patients that have metabolic alkalosis.

- In vitro, a 1-g/dL decrease in albumin concentration is associated with an increase in pH of 0.093 in cats and 0.047 in dogs.
  - Hypoalbuminemia is an often overlooked cause of metabolic alkalosis.
- Signs: Clinical signs in dogs and cats with metabolic alkalosis are more likely to be caused by the underlying disease, such as muscle twitching and seizures in patients with neurologic involvement.
- Stepwise approach: An algorithm for the differential diagnosis of corrected hyperchloremia is presented in Figs. 1 and 2.

Further Readings

de Morais HA, Constable PD. Strong ion approach to acid-base disorders. In: DiBartola SP, editor. Fluid, electrolyte, and acid-base disorders. 3rd edition. St. Louis (MO): Elsevier; 2006. p. 311–21.

DiBartola SP. Metabolic acid-base disorders. In: DiBartola SP, editor. Fluid, electrolyte, and acid-base disorders. 3rd edition. St. Louis (MO): Elsevier; 2006. p. 251–83.

Metabolic Acidosis: A Quick Reference

Helio Autran de Morais, DVM, PhD

Department of Medical Sciences, University of Wisconsin–Madison,
2015 Linden Drive, Madison, WI 53706, USA

- Metabolic acidoses are characterized by a decrease in HCO_3^- and base excess, a decrease in pH, and a compensatory decrease in P_{CO_2}.
  - Metabolic acidosis can be identified by a decrease in HCO_3^- or base excess.
  - Base excess is the amount of acid needed to return blood pH to normal. The more negative the base excess, the more severe is the metabolic acidosis.
  - There is a compensatory hyperventilation that decreases P_{CO_2} and minimizes the change in pH.
    - In dogs, for each 1-mEq/L decrease in HCO_3^-, P_{CO_2} decreases by 0.7 mm Hg.
    - Cats do not seem to decrease ventilation in the face of metabolic acidosis; thus, their P_{CO_2} does not change.
- Metabolic acidosis can result from decreases in the strong ion difference (SID, or the difference between all strong cations and strong anions in blood) or an increase in nonvolatile weak acids.

ANALYSIS

- Indications: Measurement of base excess and HCO_3^- is useful in severely ill pets (eg, severe dehydration, vomiting, diarrhea, oliguria, anuria) or in animals that have a condition known to be associated with metabolic acidosis or a low total carbon dioxide (total CO_2) concentration. Total CO_2 is almost synonymous with HCO_3^- in samples handled anaerobically. A blood gas analysis is necessary to determine if the low total CO_2 is attributable to a metabolic acidosis or a compensation for respiratory alkalosis.
- Typical reference range: Normal HCO_3^- concentration is approximately 19 to 23 mEq/L in dogs and 17 to 21 mEq/L in cats. Normal base excess is approximately 0 to −5 in dogs and cats. These values may vary among laboratories and analyzers.

E-mail address: demorais@vetmed.wisc.edu

0195-5616/08/$ – see front matter
doi:10.1016/j.cvsm.2008.01.019

Box 1: Principal causes of metabolic acidosis

Strong ion difference acidosis

Dilution acidosis (recognized by ⇑ $[Na^+]$)

    With hypervolemia (gain of hypotonic fluid)

        Severe liver disease

        Congestive heart failure

    With normovolemia (gain of water)

        Psychogenic polydipsia

        Hypotonic fluid infusion

    With hypovolemia (loss of hypertonic fluid)

        Hypoadrenocorticism

        Diuretic administration

Hyperchloremic acidosis

    Diarrhea[a]

    Fluid therapy[a] (eg, 0.9% sodium chloride [NaCl], 7.2% NaCl, potassium chloride [KCl]–supplemented fluids)

    Total parenteral nutrition

    Renal failure

    Hypoadrenocorticism

Organic acidosis

    Uremic acidosis[a]

    Diabetic ketoacidosis[a]

    Lactic acidosis[a]

    Toxicities

        Ethylene glycol

        Salicylate

Nonvolatile ion buffer acidosis

Hyperphosphatemic acidosis

    Phosphate-containing enemas

    Intravenous phosphate

    Renal failure[a]

    Urethral obstruction

    Uroabdomen

[a]Most important causes in small animal practice.

- Danger values: pH less than 7.1 indicates life-threatening acidosis, which may impair myocardial contractility. HCO_3^- concentrations less than 8 mEq/L are usually associated with severe acidosis.
- Artifacts: HCO_3^- concentration is calculated in blood gas machines based on pH and P_{CO_2}. Thus, artifacts that interfere with P_{CO_2} or pH affect the estimation of HCO_3^- (see Quick References on respiratory alkalosis and respiratory acidosis elsewhere in this issue for further details).
- Drug effects: Acetazolamide and NH_4Cl may cause metabolic acidosis.

METABOLIC ACIDOSIS

- Causes: Metabolic acidosis can result from the following (Box 1):
  - Decrease in the SID (or the difference between all strong cations and strong anions in blood)
    - Dilutional acidosis (increase in free water)
    - Hyperchloremic acidosis (increase in chloride concentration)
    - Organic acidosis (increase in strong anions other than chloride)
  - Increase in nonvolatile weak acids
    - Hyperphosphatemic acidosis
  - Metabolic acidoses also can be divided based on changes in the anion gap in hyperchloremic acidosis and high anion gap acidosis.
    - The most common causes of hyperchloremic acidosis are fluid therapy and diarrhea.
    - The most common causes of high anion gap acidosis are renal failure, diabetic ketoacidosis, and lactic acidosis.
    - Hyperphosphatemia is an often overlooked cause of high anion gap acidosis.

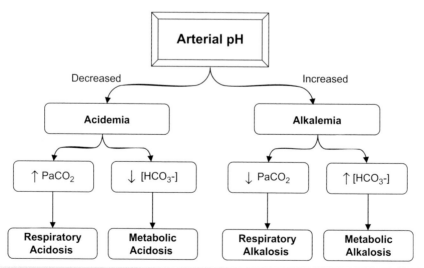

Fig. 1. Algorithm for evaluation of patients that have acid-base disorders.

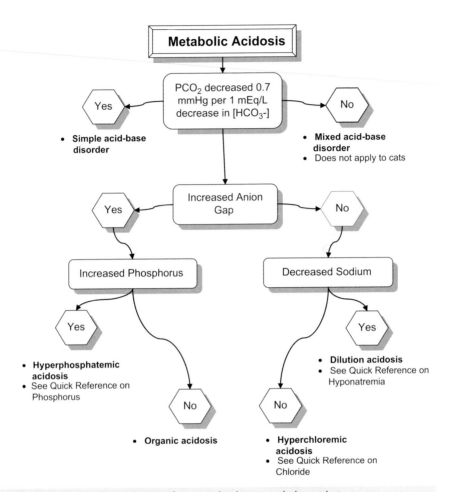

Fig. 2. Algorithm for evaluation of patients that have metabolic acidosis.

- Signs: Clinical signs in dogs and cats with metabolic acidosis are more likely to be caused by the underlying disease. Compensatory tachypnea can be observed in some patients. Severe metabolic acidosis can lead to depression.
- Stepwise approach: Algorithms for the differential diagnosis of metabolic acidosis are presented in Figs. 1 and 2.

Further Readings

de Morais HA, Constable PD. Strong ion approach to acid-base disorders. In: DiBartola SP, editor. Fluid, electrolyte, and acid-base disorders. 3rd edition. St. Louis: Elsevier; 2006. p. 311–21.

DiBartola SP. Metabolic acid-base disorders. In: DiBartola SP, editor. Fluid, electrolyte, and acid-base disorders. 3rd edition. St. Louis: Elsevier; 2006. p. 251–83.

Anion Gap and Strong Ion Gap: A Quick Reference

Jennifer Kaae, VMD*, Helio Autran de Morais, DVM, PhD

Department of Medical Sciences, University of Wisconsin–Madison,
2015 Linden Drive, Madison, WI 53706, USA

ANION GAP

- The total number of cations in the extracellular fluid always equals the total number of anions; however, not all anions and cations can be measured. This means that on a typical chemistry panel, there is an apparent gap, or difference, between the number of cations and the number of anions, and this gap is referred to as the anion gap (AG) (Fig. 1).
- Therefore, the AG represents the difference between unmeasured cations and unmeasured anions, and it can be calculated on any patient using commonly measured chemistry values as follows:
  - $AG = (Na^+ + K^+) - (Cl^- + HCO_3^-)$
  - Whenever there is an increase in unmeasured anions (eg, lactate, ketoanions) or chloride, HCO_3^- concentration decreases to maintain electroneutrality.
    - If the decrease in HCO_3^- is matched by an increase in chloride, the AG does not change and the acidosis is classified as hyperchloremic or normal AG acidosis.
    - If the acidosis is secondary to the addition of unmeasured anions, the decrease in HCO_3^- is not accompanied by an increase in chloride concentration. Thus, the AG increases, resulting in so-called "high AG acidosis."
- The AG in normal dogs and cats is mostly a result of the net negative charge of proteins, and thus is heavily influenced by protein concentration.
  - Hypoalbuminemia is the only clinically important cause of a low AG.
  - In dogs, the AG can be "corrected" for changes in protein concentration by using the following formula: AG adjusted for albumin = $AG + 4.2 \times (3.77 - [albumin])$, where [albumin] is the patient's albumin concentration.

STRONG ION GAP

- The strong ion gap (SIG) is similar to the AG in that it detects the difference between unmeasured cations and unmeasured anions, but the SIG is measured slightly differently because it takes into account the strong ion approach

*Corresponding author. E-mail address: jkaae@svm.vetmed.wisc.edu (J. Kaae).

0195-5616/08/$ – see front matter
doi:10.1016/j.cvsm.2008.01.022

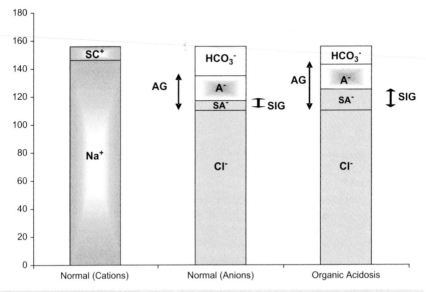

Fig. 1. Distribution of cations and anions in normal plasma and during organic acidosis, demonstrating the respective components of the AG and SIG. Notice the increase in the SIG and AG in plasma with organic acidosis because of the increase in unmeasured strong anions (SA^-). Other strong anions in normal plasma include lactate, β-hydroxybutyrate, acetoacetate, and SO_4^{2-}. Other strong cations (SC^+) in normal plasma include K^+, Ca^{2+}, and Mg^{2+}. A^- represents net negative charge of nonvolatile plasma buffers (albumin and phosphates).

to acid-base status. Using this approach, a distinction is made between strong ions, which are fully dissociated at physiologic pH, and buffer ions. The strong ions found in plasma include: Na^+, K^+, Ca^+, Mg^+, Cl^-, lactate, β-hydroxybutyrate, acetoacetate, and SO_4^{2-}. Important buffer ions are: HCO_3^-, albumin, globulins, and phosphate.

- The SIG only accounts for the differences between strong cations and strong anions (see Fig. 1). A simplified SIG can be estimated using albumin concentration and the AG as follows:
  - In dogs, SIG = [albumin] × 4.9 − AG
  - In cats, SIG = [albumin] × 7.4 − AG
  - Further information on the derivation of the simplified SIG can be found in the chapter by de Morais and Constable (2006) in the further readings section.
- The SIG increases whenever there is metabolic acidosis caused by addition of unmeasured strong ions (eg, lactic acidosis, ketoacidosis).

ANALYSIS

- Indications: An increased AG or SIG can be used to identify and differentiate disorders of metabolic acidosis.
  - For example, identifying a markedly increased AG or SIG in a critical patient should prompt the clinician to evaluate the patient's acid-base status

with a blood gas analysis and should instigate a workup to rule out causes of increased AG metabolic acidosis.
- The AG can also be used to help differentiate causes of metabolic acidosis. Finding a normal AG in a patient that has metabolic acidosis suggests that the acidosis is secondary to hyperchloremia. All other conditions causing metabolic acidosis cause the AG to be increased.
- The SIG estimates unmeasured strong anions using the strong ion approach to evaluate acid-base status. The SIG is not affected by changes in albumin or other buffer ions and may be a more accurate method of detecting unmeasured anions than the AG.
  - The simplified SIG is affected by phosphate concentration, however, and also may be increased in patients that have hyperphosphatemia.
- Typical reference range: The normal AG concentration is approximately 12 to 24 mEq/L in dogs and 13 to 27 mEq/L in cats. The normal SIG concentration is approximately 0 to −5 mEq/L in dogs and cats. These values may vary among laboratories and analyzers.
- Danger values: Danger to the patient is dictated by the underlying acid-base status and the underlying disease process. Additional diagnostic evaluation is warranted in any critical patient with an elevated AG or SIG.
- Artifacts: The AG is affected by albumin concentration, whereas the AG and SIG are both affected by hyperphosphatemia.

Box 1: Principal causes of changes in the anion gap and strong ion gap

Increased

  Organic acidosis

   Uremic acidosis[a]

   Diabetic ketoacidosis[a]

   Lactic acidosis[a]

   Renal failure[a]

  Toxicities

   Ethylene glycol

   Salicylate

  Hyperphosphatemia (hyperphosphatemic acidosis)

   Renal failure[a]

Normal

  Hyperchloremic acidosis

Decreased

  Hypoalbuminemia[a] (AG only)

  Bromide toxicity

[a]Most important causes in small animal practice.

- Albumin is the primary unmeasured ion in the AG; therefore, hypoalbuminemia causes the AG to decrease. Thus, in a hypoalbuminemic patient, the AG underestimates the severity of the patient's acidosis and the increase in unmeasured anions.
  - In dogs with a normal plasma pH, each 1-g/dL decrease in albumin results in a 4.1-mEq/L decrease in the AG.
- Severely hyperphosphatemic patients typically have metabolic acidosis and an increased AG. To calculate the SIG in a hyperphosphatemic patient accurately, the AG should first be adjusted according to the following formula:
  - AG phosphate adjusted $= AG + (2.52 - 0.58 \times$ [phosphate])
- Drug effects: Drugs that affect sodium, potassium, chloride, or bicarbonate may interfere with the AG and the SIG (see specific quick references for further details).

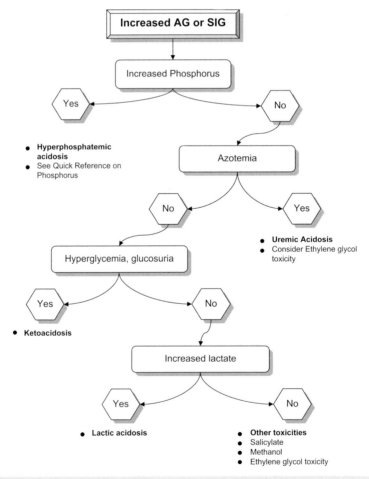

Fig. 2. Algorithm for evaluation of patients with increased AG and SIG.

CHANGES IN ANION GAP OR STRONG ION GAP

- Causes
    - Increased: High AG or SIG metabolic acidosis indicates that there are unmeasured anions in the extracellular fluid, as with ethylene glycol toxicity, uremia (sulfates and phosphates), tissue hypoxia (lactate), diabetic ketoacidosis (ketones), or salicylate intoxication (Box 1).
    - Normal: If the AG or SIG is normal in the face of metabolic acidosis, the acidosis is caused by increased chloride (a measured anion).
    - Decreased: A low AG is infrequently identified but can be seen with hypoalbuminemia. The SIG is not affected by albumin concentration. Bromide toxicity may decrease the AG and SIG because bromide is measured as chloride by most analyzers.
    - Signs: Clinical signs are attributable to the underlying disease leading to the metabolic acidosis and increase the SIG and AG.
    - Stepwise approach: Algorithms for the differential diagnosis of metabolic acidosis are presented in Fig. 1 and Fig. 2.

Further Readings

de Morais HA, Constable PD. Strong ion approach to acid-base disorders. In: DiBartola SP, editor. Fluid, electrolyte, and acid-base disorders. 3rd edition. St. Louis (MO): Elsevier; 2006. p. 311–21.

DiBartola SP. Introduction to acid-base disorders. In: DiBartola SP, editor. Fluid, electrolyte, and acid-base disorders. 3rd edition. St. Louis (MO): Elsevier; 2006. p. 229–50.

Hypercalcemia: A Quick Reference

Patricia A. Schenck, DVM, PhD[a],*, Dennis J. Chew, DVM[b]

[a]Endocrine Diagnostic Section, Diagnostic Center for Population and Animal Health,
Department of Pathobiology and Diagnostic Investigation, Michigan State University,
4125 Beaumont Road, Lansing, MI 48910, USA
[b]Department of Veterinary Clinical Sciences, College of Veterinary Medicine,
The Ohio State University, 601 Vernon L. Tharp Street, Columbus, OH 43210, USA

- Total calcium (tCa) is composed of ionized calcium (iCa), protein-bound calcium (pCa), and complexed calcium (cCa).
- iCa is the biologically active fraction.
- Major hormones involved in calcium metabolism are parathyroid hormone (PTH), calcitriol (1,25-dihydroxyvitamin D), and calcitonin.
- Major organs involved in calcium metabolism are bone, kidney, and small intestine.

ANALYSIS

- Indications: Serum tCa is measured routinely in systemic diseases. Serum iCa should be measured if tCa is elevated and in any patient that has renal disease. The simultaneous measurement of PTH along with iCa is often helpful diagnostically. The typical reference range for serum tCa and iCa in presented in Table 1.
  - To convert mmol/L to mg/dL, multiply mmol/L by 4.
  - Caution
    - Do not use adjustment formulas to "correct" the tCa to serum total protein or albumin concentration. These formulas do not accurately predict iCa concentration.
    - Do not directly compare serum iCa results with heparinized plasma or whole blood iCa results (obtained by means of a blood gas analyzer or point-of-care analyzer). The iCa concentration in heparinized plasma or whole blood is typically lower than the serum iCa concentration.
    - Do not use ethylenediaminetetraacetic acid (EDTA) plasma for iCa measurement. EDTA chelates calcium, resulting in an extremely low iCa concentration.
- Danger values
  - Interaction with phosphorus is important. If tCa (mg/dL) times the phosphorus concentration is greater than 70, tissue mineralization is likely.

*Corresponding author. E-mail address: schenck5@msu.edu (P.A. Schenck).

0195-5616/08/$ – see front matter
doi:10.1016/j.cvsm.2008.01.020

Table 1
Typical reference range (serum)

	Canine	Feline
tCa	9.0–11.5 mg/dL (2.2–3.8 mmol/L)	8.0–10.5 mg/dL (2.0–2.6 mmol/L)
iCa	5.0–6.0 mg/dL (1.2–1.5 mmol/L)	4.5–5.5 mg/dL (1.1–1.4 mmol/L)

Box 1: Causes of hypercalcemia

Nonpathologic
Nonfasting (minimal increase)
Physiologic growth of young
Laboratory error
Spurious
    Lipemia
    Detergent contamination of sample or tube

Transient or inconsequential
Hemoconcentration
Hyperproteinemia
Hypoadrenocorticism
Severe environmental hypothermia (rare)

Pathologic or consequential: persistent
Parathyroid dependent
    Primary hyperparathyroidism
        Adenoma (common)
        Adenocarcinoma (rare)
        Hyperplasia (uncommon)
Parathyroid independent
    Malignancy-associated (most common cause in dogs)
        Humoral hypercalcemia of malignancy
            Lymphoma (common)
            Anal sac apocrine gland adenocarcinoma (common)
            Carcinoma (sporadic): lung, pancreas, skin, nasal cavity, thyroid, mammary gland, adrenal medulla
            Thymoma (rare)
            Hematologic malignancies (bone marrow osteolysis, local osteolytic hypercalcemia)
            Lymphoma
            Multiple myeloma

(continued on next page)

Myeloproliferative disease (rare)

Leukemia (rare)

Metastatic or primary bone neoplasia (uncommon)

Idiopathic hypercalcemia (most common association in cats)

Chronic renal failure (with and without ionized hypercalcemia)

Hypervitaminosis D

Iatrogenic

Plants (calcitriol glycosides)

Rodenticide (cholecalciferol)

Antipsoriasis creams (calcipotriol or calcipotriene)

Granulomatous disease

Blastomycosis

Dermatitis

Panniculitis

Injection reaction

Acute renal failure (diuretic phase)

Skeletal lesions (nonmalignant) (uncommon)

Osteomyelitis (bacterial or mycotic)

Hypertrophic osteodystrophy

Disuse osteoporosis (immobilization)

Excessive calcium-containing intestinal phosphate binders

Excessive calcium supplementation (calcium carbonate)

Hypervitaminosis A

Raisin/grape toxicity

Hypercalcemic conditions in human medicine

Milk-alkali syndrome (rare in dogs)

Thiazide diuretics

Acromegaly

Thyrotoxicosis (rare in cats)

Postrenal transplantation

Aluminum exposure (intestinal phosphate binders in dogs and cats?)

- Clinical signs are usually present when serum tCa is greater than 15 mg/dL or iCa is greater than 1.8 mmol/L.
- The patient is usually critically ill whenever serum tCa is greater than 18 mg/dL or iCa is greater than 2.2 mmol/L.
- Artifacts
  - Serum iCa may be falsely elevated when stored in serum separator tubes.
  - Severe lipemia of the serum may cause a false elevation in serum tCa concentration.

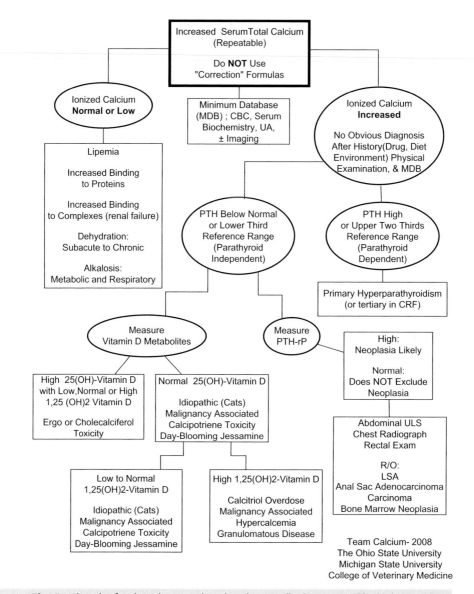

Fig. 1. Algorithm for clinical approach to disorders initially characterized by high serum tCA. CBC, complete blood cell count; CRF, corticotropin-releasing factor; LSA, lymphosarcoma; PTH-rP, parathyroid hormone related protein; R/O, rule out; UA, urinalysis; ULS, ultrasound.

CAUSES OF HYPERCALCEMIA

- In dogs, neoplasia is the most common cause of hypercalcemia, followed by hypoadrenocorticism, primary hyperparathyroidism, and renal failure (elevation of tCa but not iCa) (Box 1).
- In cats, idiopathic hypercalcemia and neoplasia are the most common causes, followed by renal failure (elevation of tCa but not iCa).

CLINICAL SIGNS

- Polyuria, polydipsia, and anorexia are most common in dogs.
- Vomiting, depression, weakness, and constipation can occur.
- Uncommon signs include cardiac arrhythmias, seizures, muscle twitching, and death.
- Cats do not exhibit polyuria, polydipsia, or vomiting as often as dogs.
- Cats with idiopathic hypercalcemia may have no clinical signs.

STEPWISE APPROACH

- An algorithm describing the clinical approach to disorders initially characterized by high total serum calcium is presented in Fig. 1.

Further Readings

Schenck PA, Chew DJ. Diseases of the parathyroid gland and calcium metabolism. In: Birchard SJ, Sherding RG, editors. Manual of small animal practice. 3rd edition. St. Louis (MO): Elsevier; 2006. p. 343–56.
Schenck PA, Chew DJ, Behrend EN. Updates on hypercalcemic disorders. In: August J, editor. Consultations in feline internal medicine. St. Louis (MO): Elsevier; 2005. p. 157–68.
Schenck PA, Chew DJ, Nagode LA, et al. Disorders of calcium: hypercalcemia and hypocalcemia. In: Dibartola S, editor. Fluid therapy in small animal practice. 3rd edition. St. Louis (MO): Elsevier; 2006. p. 122–94.

Hypocalcemia: A Quick Reference

Patricia A. Schenck, DVM, PhD[a],*, Dennis J. Chew, DVM[b]

[a]Endocrine Diagnostic Section, Diagnostic Center for Population and Animal Health,
Department of Pathobiology and Diagnostic Investigation, Michigan State University,
4125 Beaumont Road, Lansing, MI 48910, USA
[b]Department of Veterinary Clinical Sciences, College of Veterinary Medicine,
The Ohio State University, 601 Vernon L. Tharp Street, Columbus, Ohio, USA

- Total calcium (tCa) is composed of ionized calcium (iCa), protein-bound calcium (pCa), and complexed calcium (cCa).
- iCa is the biologically active fraction.
- Major hormones involved in calcium metabolism are parathyroid hormone (PTH), calcitriol (1,25-dihydroxyvitamin D), and calcitonin.
- Major organs involved in calcium metabolism are bone, kidney, and small intestine.

ANALYSIS

- Indications: Serum tCa is measured routinely in systemic diseases. Serum iCa should be measured if tCa is low and in any patient that has renal disease. The simultaneous measurement of PTH along with iCa is often helpful diagnostically. The typical reference range for serum tCa and iCa is presented in Table 1.
- To convert mmol/L to mg/dL, multiply mmol/L by 4.
- Caution
  - Do not use adjustment formulas to "correct" the tCa to serum total protein or albumin concentration. These formulas do not accurately predict iCa concentration.
  - Do not directly compare serum iCa results with heparinized plasma or whole blood iCa results (obtained by means of a blood gas analyzer or point-of-care analyzer). The iCa concentration in heparinized plasma or whole blood is typically lower than the serum iCa concentration.
  - Do not use ethylenediaminetetraacetic acid (EDTA) plasma for iCa measurement. EDTA chelates calcium, resulting in an extremely low iCa concentration.
- Danger values
  - Clinical signs are usually present when serum tCa is less than 6.0 mg/dL or iCa is less than 0.8 mmol/L.

*Corresponding author. E-mail address: schenck5@msu.edu (P.A. Schenck).

0195-5616/08/$ – see front matter
doi:10.1016/j.cvsm.2008.01.021

Table 1
Typical reference range (serum)

	Canine	Feline
tCa	9.0–11.5 mg/dL (2.2–3.8 mmol/L)	8.0–10.5 mg/dL (2.0–2.6 mmol/L)
iCa	5.0–6.0 mg/dL (1.2–1.5 mmol/L)	4.5–5.5 mg/dL (1.1–1.4 mmol/L)

Box 1: Causes of hypocalcemia

Common

Hypoalbuminemia

Chronic renal failure

Puerperal tetany (eclampsia)

Acute renal failure

Acute pancreatitis

Undefined cause (mild hypocalcemia)

Occasional

Soft tissue trauma or rhabdomyolysis

Hypoparathyroidism

    Primary

        Idiopathic or spontaneous

        Postoperative bilateral thyroidectomy

      After sudden reversal of chronic hypercalcemia

      Secondary to magnesium depletion or excess

Ethylene glycol intoxication

Phosphate enema

After $NaHCO_3$ administration

Uncommon

Laboratory error

Improper sample anticoagulant (EDTA)

Infarction of parathyroid gland adenoma

Rapid intravenous infusion of phosphates

Acute calcium—free intravenous infusion (dilutional)

Intestinal malabsorption or severe starvation

Hypovitaminosis D

Blood transfusion (citrated anticoagulant)

Hypomagnesemia

Nutritional secondary hyperparathyroidism

Tumor lysis syndrome

Human

Pseudohypoparathyroidism

Drug induced

Hypercalcitonism

Osteoblastic bone neoplasia (prostate cancer)

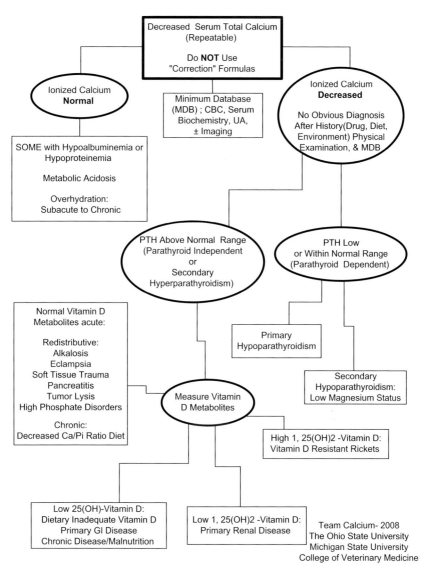

Fig. 1. Algorithm for clinical approach to disorders initially characterized by low total serum calcium. Ca, calcium; CBC, complete blood cell count; GI, gastrointestinal; Pi, phosphorous; UA, urinalysis.

- Artifacts
  - EDTA plasma yields low calcium concentrations because EDTA chelates calcium.
  - Dilution with heparin (in heparinized plasma or whole blood) gives artificially low results.

CAUSES OF HYPOCALCEMIA
Clinical Signs
- Common signs of hypocalcemia include muscle tremors and fasciculations, facial rubbing, muscle cramping, stiff gait, seizures, restlessness, aggression, hypersensitivity, and disorientation (Box 1).
- Occasional clinical signs include panting, pyrexia, lethargy, depression, anorexia, tachycardia, posterior lenticular cataracts, and prolapse of the third eyelid (cats).
- Uncommon clinical signs include polyuria, polydipsia, hypotension, respiratory arrest, or death.
- Decreased serum iCa that occurs in association with chronic renal failure rarely causes clinical signs.

STEPWISE APPROACH
- An algorithm describing the clinical approach to disorders initially characterized by low total serum calcium is presented in Fig. 1.

Further Readings

Schenck PA, Chew DJ. Diseases of the parathyroid gland and calcium metabolism. In: Birchard SJ, Sherding RG, editors. Manual of small animal practice. 3rd edition. St. Louis (MO): Elsevier; 2006. p. 343–56.

Schenck PA, Chew DJ, Behrend EN. Updates on hypercalcemic disorders. In: August J, editor. Consultations in feline internal medicine. St. Louis (MO): Elsevier; 2005. p. 157–68.

Schenck PA, Chew DJ, Nagode LA, et al. Disorders of calcium: hypercalcemia and hypocalcemia. In: Dibartola S, editor. Fluid therapy in small animal practice. 3rd edition. St. Louis (MO): Elsevier; 2006. p. 122–94.

Chloride: A Quick Reference

Alexander W. Biondo, DVM, PhD[a],[*],
Helio Autran de Morais, DVM, PhD[b]

[a]Departamento de Medicina Veterinária, Universidade Federal do Paraná,
Avenida dos Funcionários, 1540, 80.035, Curitiba, Paraná, Brazil
[b]Department of Medical Sciences, University of Wisconsin–Madison,
2015 Linden Drive, Madison, WI 53706, USA

- Chloride constitutes approximately two thirds of the anions in plasma and extracellular fluid, with a much lower intracellular concentration.
- Chloride is the major anion filtered by the glomeruli and reabsorbed in the renal tubules.
- Changes in chloride concentration are associated with metabolic acid-base disorders. Chloride is an important player in renal regulation of acid-base metabolism.

ANALYSIS

- Indications: Serum chloride concentration commonly is measured in systemic diseases characterized by vomiting, diarrhea, dehydration, polyuria, and polydipsia or in patients likely to have metabolic acid-base abnormalities.
- Typical reference range: Chloride concentration must be corrected to account for changes in plasma free water. Primary chloride disorders have abnormal corrected chloride, whereas changes in free water do not (Fig. 1). Corrected chloride can be estimated as follows:

$$[Cl^-]\text{corrected} = [Cl^-]\text{measured} \times 146/[Na^+]\text{measured(dogs)}$$

$$[Cl^-]\text{corrected} = [Cl^-]\text{measured} \times 156/[Na^+]\text{measured(cats)}$$

*Corresponding author. E-mail address: abiondo@uiuc.edu (A.W. Biondo).

0195-5616/08/$ – see front matter
doi:10.1016/j.cvsm.2008.01.015

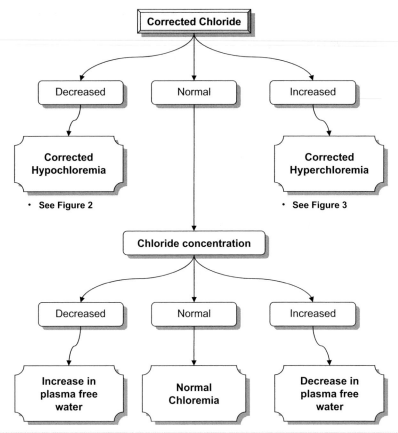

Fig. 1. Algorithm for evaluation of patients with chloride abnormalities. (*Adapted from* de Morais HSA, Biondo AW. Disorders of chloride: hyperchloremia and hypochloremia. In: DiBartola SP, editor. Fluid, electrolyte, and acid-base disorders. 3rd edition. St. Louis (MO): Elsevier; 2006. p. 84; with permission.)

- Where [Cl⁻]measured and [Na⁺]measured, respectively, are the patient's serum chloride and sodium concentrations. The values 146 and 156 reflect the mean values for serum sodium concentration in dogs and cats, respectively. Normal [Cl⁻] corrected is approximately 107 minus 113 mEq/L in dogs and 117 minus 123 mEq/L in cats. These values may vary among laboratories and analyzers.
- Danger values: Unknown. Muscle twitching or seizures in hypochloremic animals are probably attributable to metabolic alkalosis and decreased ionized calcium concentration, whereas clinical signs associated with hyperchloremia are probably attributable to hyperosmolality.
- Artifacts: Pseudohypochloremia results when chloride is measured in markedly lipemic samples by means of techniques that are not ion selective. Halides (eg, bromide, iodide, fluoride) are measured as chloride, falsely

increasing measurements even when ion-selective techniques are used. This is especially important in animals receiving potassium bromide as an anticonvulsant.

- Drug effects: Administration of chloride-containing solutions may increase chloride concentration, whereas loop diuretics and thiazides may cause excessive renal loss of chloride relative to sodium.

CORRECTED HYPOCHLOREMIA

- Causes: Corrected hypochloremia is associated with a tendency toward alkalosis (hypochloremic alkalosis) because of the increase in strong ion difference.
  - Corrected hypochloremia may result from excessive loss of chloride relative to sodium or administration of fluids containing high sodium concentration relative to chloride (Box 1).
  - The most common causes of corrected hypochloremia are chronic vomiting of gastric contents and aggressive diuretic therapy with furosemide or thiazides. Administration of sodium without chloride (eg, sodium bicarbonate) also may cause corrected hypochloremia. Hypochloremia attributable to increased renal chloride excretion is a normal adaptation that is present in chronic respiratory acidosis.
  - Persistent hypochloremia is an indication to determine serum sodium, potassium, and total carbon dioxide (TcO_2) concentrations, preferably with blood gas analysis.

Box 1: Causes of corrected hypochloremia

Excessive loss of chloride relative to sodium

Gastrointestinal loss

Vomiting of stomach contents[a]

Gastrointestinal diseases associated with hyperkalemia and hyponatremia in dogs without hypoadrenocorticism (eg, trichuriasis, salmonellosis, perforated duodenal ulcer)

Renal loss

Therapy with thiazides or loop diuretics[a]

Chronic respiratory acidosis

Hyperadrenocorticism

Excessive gain of sodium relative to chloride

Sodium bicarbonate

[a]Most important causes in small animal practice.

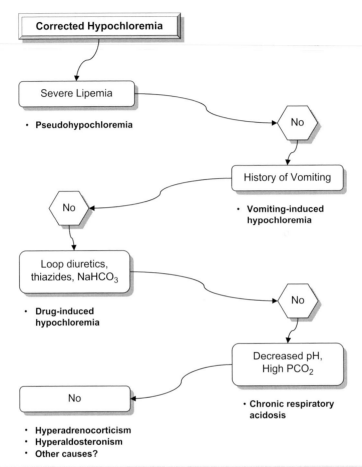

Fig. 2. Algorithm for evaluation of patients that have corrected hypochloremia. (*Adapted from* de Morais HSA, Biondo AW. Disorders of chloride: hyperchloremia and hypochloremia. In: DiBartola SP, editor. Fluid, electrolyte, and acid-base disorders. 3rd edition. St. Louis (MO): Elsevier; 2006. p. 85; with permission.)

- Signs: Clinical signs associated with pure hypochloremia in dogs and cats have not been described but probably are related to the accompanying metabolic alkalosis.
- Stepwise approach: An algorithm for the differential diagnosis of corrected hypochloremia is presented in Fig. 2.

CORRECTED HYPERCHLOREMIA

- Causes: Corrected hyperchloremia is associated with a tendency toward acidosis (hyperchloremic acidosis) because of the decrease in strong ion difference.

- Corrected hyperchloremia may result from excessive sodium loss relative to chloride, excessive chloride gain relative to sodium, or renal chloride retention (Box 2). Small bowel diarrhea causes hyperchloremic metabolic acidosis because of loss of bicarbonate-rich chloride-poor fluid. Administration of NH_4Cl, potassium chloride (KCl), cationic amino acids (eg, total parenteral nutrition), hypertonic saline, or 0.9% sodium chloride (NaCl) leads to chloride gain.
- The most common causes of corrected hyperchloremia are fluid therapy and diarrhea.
- Hyperchloremia attributable to decreased renal chloride excretion is a normal adaptation that is present in chronic respiratory alkalosis.
- Persistent hyperchloremia is an indication for determining serum sodium, potassium, and TcO_2 concentrations, preferably with blood gas analysis.
- Signs: Specific clinical signs associated with pure hyperchloremia in dogs and cats have not been reported but probably are related to the metabolic acidosis that accompanies hyperchloremia.
- Stepwise approach: An algorithm for the differential diagnosis of corrected hyperchloremia is presented in Fig. 3.

Box 2: Causes of corrected hyperchloremia

Pseudohyperchloremia

    Potassium bromide therapy

Excessive loss of sodium relative to chloride

    Diarrhea[a]

Excessive gain of chloride relative to sodium

    Exogenous intake

        Fluid therapy (eg, 0.9% NaCl, hypertonic saline, KCl-supplemented fluids)[a]

        Therapy with chloride salts (NH_4Cl, KCl)

        Total parenteral nutrition

        Salt poisoning

    Renal chloride retention

        Renal failure

        Renal tubular acidosis

        Hypoadrenocorticism

        Diabetes mellitus

        Chronic respiratory alkalosis

        Spironolactone

[a]Most important causes in small animal practice.

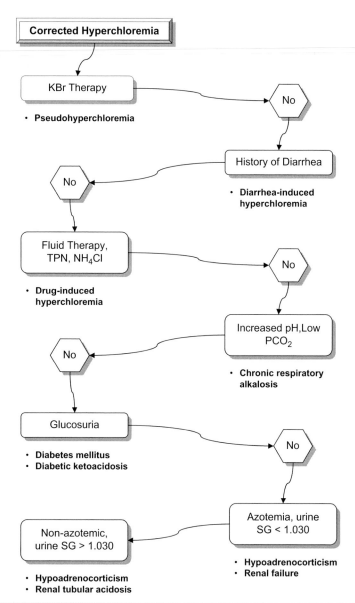

Fig. 3. Algorithm for evaluation of patients that have corrected hyperchloremia. KBr, potassium bromide; SP, specific gravity; TPN, total parenteral nutrition. (*Adapted from* de Morais HSA, Biondo AW. Disorders of chloride: hyperchloremia and hypochloremia. In: DiBartola SP, editor. Fluid, electrolyte, and acid-base disorders. 3rd edition. St. Louis (MO): Elsevier; 2006. p. 85; with permission.)

Further Readings

de Morais HA. Chloride ion in small animal practice: the forgotten ion. Journal of Veterinary Emergency and Critical Care 1992;2:11–24.

de Morais HA, Biondo AW. Disorders of chloride: hyperchloremia and hypochloremia. In: DiBartola SP, editor. Fluid, electrolyte, and acid-base disorders. 3rd edition. St. Louis (MO): Elsevier; 2006. p. 80–91.

Magnesium: A Quick Reference

Shane W. Bateman, DVM, DVSc

Department of Veterinary Clinical Sciences, The Ohio State University, 601 Vernon L. Tharp Street, Columbus, OH 43210-1089, USA

DISTRIBUTION OF MAGNESIUM
- In human beings, 1% of the total body magnesium is in the extracellular fluid (ECF), whereas the remaining 99% is intracellular.
- Approximately two thirds of body magnesium is stored with calcium and phosphorus in bones, 20% in muscles, and 11% in soft tissues other than muscles.
- Like calcium, extracellular magnesium is present in three forms:
  - Ionized or free form (55%) thought to constitute the biologically active fraction
  - Protein-bound form (20%–30%)
  - Complexed form (15%–25%)
- Magnesium is only 20% to 30% bound to protein, being less affected by changes in albumin concentration than calcium.

MAGNESIUM HANDLING
- The primary site of magnesium absorption seems to be the ileum, but the jejunum and colon also contribute substantially to net absorption.
- The kidneys control and regulate magnesium balance.
- Various segments of the nephron play an important role in magnesium homeostasis. Of the filtered magnesium:
  - 10% to 15% of magnesium is reabsorbed within the proximal tubule.
  - 60% to 70% is reabsorbed in the cortical thick ascending limb of the loop of Henle.
  - 10% to 15% is reabsorbed in the distal convoluted tubule.
  - The final concentration of magnesium in the urine is determined at the distal convoluted tubule under hormonal and nonhormonal control.

MANIFESTATIONS AND CAUSES OF MAGNESIUM DEFICIT
- Refer to Box 1.
- Cardiovascular
  - Intracellular and extracellular magnesium concentrations play an important role in cardiac excitability, contraction, and conduction through regulatory effects on calcium movement.

E-mail address: bateman.36@osu.edu

0195-5616/08/$ – see front matter
doi:10.1016/j.cvsm.2008.01.014

Box 1: Causes of magnesium deficit

Gastrointestinal
  Reduced intake, starvation, or malnutrition
  Chronic diarrhea
  Gastric suction
  Malabsorption syndromes
  Short bowel syndrome
  Gastric bypass surgery
  Colonic neoplasia
  Familial or inherited
Renal
  Diabetes mellitus or diabetic ketoacidosis
  Diuretics (except potassium-sparing agents)
  Osmotic agents (including hyperglycemia)
  Intrinsic renal causes of diuresis
    Postobstructive
    Polyuric acute failure
    Hyperaldosteronism
    Hyperthyroidism
    Renal tubular acidosis
  Concurrent electrolyte disorders
    Hypokalemia
    Hypercalcemia or hyperparathyroidism
    Hypophosphatemia
  Drugs
    Gentamicin
    Carbenicillin
    Ticarcillin
    Cyclosporin
    Cisplatin
  Postrenal transplantation
  Familial or inherited
Miscellaneous
  Excessive loss from lactation
  Redistribution
    Acute myocardial infarction
    Acute pancreatitis
    Insulin
    Catecholamine excess
  Idiopathic

Data from Bateman SW. Disorders of magnesium: magnesium deficit and excess. In: Dibartola SP, editor. Fluid, electrolyte and acid-base disorders in small animal practice. 3rd edition. Philadelphia: Elsevier; 2006. p. 218.

Table 1
Dose ranges for magnesium salts

Rapid replacement		**mEq of Mg/g of salt**	**mEq/kg/d**	**mEq/kg/h**	**mg/kg/h**
	$MgSO_4$	8.12	0.75–1	0.03–0.04	3.7–4.9
	$MgCl_2$	9.25	0.75–1	0.03–0.04	3.2–4.3
Slow replacement		**mEq of Mg/g of salt**	**mEq/kg/d**	**mEq/kg/h**	**mg/kg/h**
	$MgSO_4$	8.12	0.3–0.5	0.013–0.02	1.6–2.5
	$MgCl_2$	9.25	0.3–0.5	0.013–0.02	1.4–2.2
Emergency/ loading		**mEq/kg**	**mg/kg**	**Duration**	
	$MgSO_4$	0.15–0.3	19–37	5 min–1 h (emergency) 24 h (loading)	
	$MgCl_2$	0.15–0.3	16–32	5 min–1 h (emergency) 24 h (loading)	
Oral		**mEq/kg/d**			
	Several	1–2			

Abbreviations: h, hour; Mg, magnesium; min, minutes.
   Data from Bateman SW. Disorders of magnesium: magnesium deficit and excess. In: Dibartola SP, editor. Fluid, electrolyte and acid-base disorders in small animal practice. 3rd edition. Philadelphia: Elsevier; 2006. p. 222.

- Magnesium may act as an antiarrhythmic agent by limiting intracellular calcium overload.
- Neuromuscular
  - Magnesium depletion enhances neuronal excitability and neuromuscular transmission.
  - Magnesium acts as an analgesic by blocking N-methyl-D-aspartate (NMDA) receptors within the central nervous system.
- Electrolyte disturbances
  - Depletion of magnesium has a permissive effect on potassium exit from the cells leading to extracellular accumulation of potassium, which is subsequently lost from the body.
  - Frequently, this potassium deficiency is refractory to supplementation until the magnesium deficit also has been corrected.
  - Hypocalcemia also occurs in human beings as a concurrent electrolyte abnormality when a magnesium deficit is present.

DIAGNOSIS OF A MAGNESIUM DEFICIT

- Currently, there is no consensus regarding the best assay for diagnosis.
  - Serum magnesium does not correlate well with magnesium deficit based on clinical signs or with serum ionized magnesium.
  - Ionized serum magnesium and total serum magnesium may be useful when results are low and are consistent with clinical suspicion of a magnesium deficit.
- The magnesium retention test may be helpful in the future.

MAGNESIUM SUPPLEMENTATION

- Clinical situations in which magnesium supplementation may be considered
    - Cardiac arrhythmias
        - Torsade de pointes, digitalis toxicity, ventricular ectopy
    - Metabolic
        - Diabetic ketoacidosis, hypokalemia refractory to supplementation, hypocalcemia refractory to supplementation
- Use with caution if renal insufficiency is present.
- Refer to Table 1.

Further Readings

Bateman SW. Disorders of magnesium: magnesium deficit and excess. In: Dibartola SP, editor. Fluid, electrolyte and acid-base disorders in small animal practice. 3rd edition. Philadelphia: Elsevier; 2006. p. 210–26.

Cortes YE, Moses L. Magnesium disturbances in critically ill patients. Compend Contin Educ Pract Vet 2007;29(7):420–7.

Phosphorus: A Quick Reference

Julia A. Bates, DVM

Department of Medical Sciences, University of Wisconsin, 2015 Linden Drive,
Madison, WI 53706, USA

MAIN FUNCTIONS OF PHOSPHORUS

The main functions of phosphorus in the body are:

> To provide along with calcium the structural integrity of bones and teeth
> To supply energy in the form of adenosine triphosphate and guanosine triphosphate
> To help in the maintenance of cell membrane structure.

Distribution of phosphorus in the body is:

> Inorganic (Pi)
>> 85% in the inorganic matrix of bone
>> 14% to 15% intracellular
>> Less than 1% in the extracellular fluid and serum
>>> 10% to 20% is bound to protein
>>> The remainder circulates as free anion or is complexed to sodium, magnesium, or calcium
> Organic
>> The majority (two-thirds) is in the form of phospholipids

In its regulation, phosphorus is:

> Under the influence of parathyroid hormone, calcitriol, and calcitonin
> Absorbed from the small intestine (primarily duodenum)
>> Intestinal phosphorus absorption is increased with calcitriol
>> Intestinal phosphorus absorption is decreased with glucocorticoids, increased dietary magnesium, and hypothyroidism
> Excreted primarily by the kidneys
>> Normally, 80% to 90% of the filtered load of phosphorus is reabsorbed by the proximal tubules of the kidneys
>> Parathyroid hormone decreases phosphorus reabsorption and is the most important regulator of renal phosphate transport.

E-mail address: jabates@svm.vetmed.wisc.edu

0195-5616/08/$ – see front matter
doi:10.1016/j.cvsm.2008.02.002

ANALYSIS
Indications
Serum phosphorus concentration is commonly measured in systemic diseases characterized by anorexia, vomiting, diarrhea, or in patients with hemolysis, diabetes mellitus, renal disease, or hypercalcemia.

Typical Reference Range
The concentration of serum phosphate is generally expressed in terms of serum phosphorus mass (mg/dL). One mg/dL of phosphorus is equal to 0.32 mmol/L of phosphate. Normal serum phosphorus concentration is 2.5 mg/dL to 5.5 mg/dL (0.8 mmol/L–1.8 mmol/L) in dogs and 2.5 mg/dL to 6.0 mg/dL (0.8 mmol/L–1.9 mmol/L) in cats. These values may vary among laboratories and analyzers. They also fluctuate with age (they are higher in young animals) and dietary intake.

Danger Values
Values below 1 mg/dL are associated with hemolysis and rabdomyolysis. Severe hyperphosphatemia leads to hypocalcemia and metabolic acidosis (for each 1-mg/dL increase in phosphorus there is approximately a 0.55-mEq/L decrease in bicarbonate concentration).

Artifacts
Phosphorus concentration may be increased postprandially. Lipemia, hyperproteinemia, and hemolysis may falsely increase phosphorus concentration, whereas mannitol may falsely lower it.

Drug Effects
Antacids decrease absorption because calcium, aluminum, and magnesium bind phosphorus into insoluble complexes. Insulin and bicarbonate shift phosphorus inside the cell and may lead to hypophosphatemia. Glucose administration may lead to hypophosphatemia by inducing insulin release. Anabolic steroids and calcitriol can increase phosphorus concentration.

HYPOPHOSPHATEMIA
Causes
Hypophosphatemia may result from decreased intestinal absorption (eg, anorexia, malabsorption, vomiting, and diarrhea), increased renal excretion (eg, diabetes mellitus and diuretic administration), or from transcellular shifts (eg, insulin or bicarbonate administration). The most important causes of hypophosphatemia in dogs and cats are presented in Box 1.

Signs
Hypophosphatemia may be clinically silent in many animals. Clinical signs associated with hypophosphatemia are vague, with mild to moderately decreased phosphorus (1 mg/dL–2 mg/dL) and include weakness, disorientation, anorexia, and joint pain. Clinical signs are typically life-threatening when

---

Box 1: Common rule-outs for hypophosphatemia

Decreased gastrointestinal absorption
  Vitamin D deficiency
  Malabsorption
  Vomiting and diarrhea
  Phosphate binders and antacids
Increased excretion
  Diabetes mellitus (with or without ketoacidosis)[a]
  Primary hyperparathyroidism[a]
  Renal tubular defects
  Diuretic administration
  Hyperadrenocorticism
  Eclampsia
  Hyperaldosteronism
  Early hypercalcemia of malignancy
Transcellular shifts
  Insulin administration[a]
  Parenteral glucose administration[a]
  Bicarbonate administration[a]
  Total parenteral nutrition administration
  Refeeding syndrome
  Hypothermia
  Respiratory alkalosis
Laboratory error

[a]Most important causes in small animal practice.

---

phosphorus is less than 1 mg/dL with hemolysis, secondary to osmotic fragility, acute respiratory failure, seizures, and coma.

HYPERPHOSPHATEMIA

Causes

Hyperphosphatemia may result from increased intestinal absorption (eg, vitamin D toxicity, increased dietary phosphorus), decreased renal excretion (eg, renal failure, urinary obstruction), or from transcellular shifts (eg, hemolysis, tumor cell lysis). The most important causes of hyperphosphatemia in dogs and cats are presented in Box 2.

Box 2: Common rule-outs for hyperphosphatemia

Increased gastrointestinal absorption
  Vitamin D toxicosis
    Cholecalciferol rodenticides
    Psoriasis creams: calcipotriene
  Phosphate containing enema
Decreased excretion
  Renal
    Prerenal
      Hypoadrenocorticism
    Renal
      Acute[a]
      Chronic[a]
    Postrenal
      Uroabdomen[a]
      Urinary obstruction[a]
  Hypoparathyroidism
  Acromegaly
  Hyperthyroidism
Transcellular Shifts
  Tumor cell lysis
  Rhabdomyolysis or tissue trauma
  Hemolysis
Physiologic
  Young growing dog[a]
  Postprandial
Laboratory error
  Lipemia
  Hyperproteinemia

[a]Most important causes in small animal practice.

Signs

Hyperphosphatemia usually does not cause clinical signs. However, hyperphosphatemia may lead to hypocalcemia and its associated neuromuscular signs. Hyperphosphatemia is also a risk for soft tissue mineralization.

Stepwise Approach

An algorithm for the differential diagnosis of hyperphosphatemia is presented in Fig. 1.

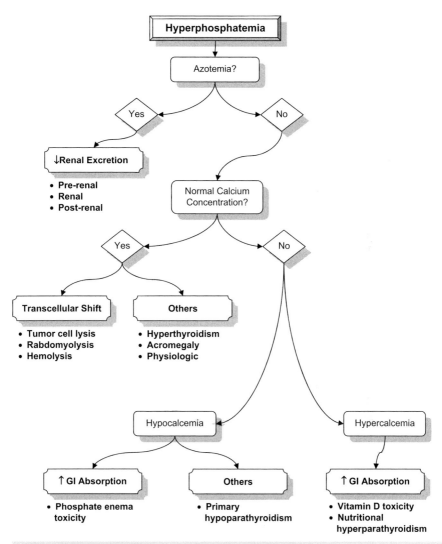

Fig. 1. Algorithm for evaluation of patients with hyperphosphatemia.

Further Readings

DiBartola W. Disorders of phosphorus: hypophosphatemia and hyperphosphatemia. In: Kersey RR, editor. Fluid therapy in small animal practice. Philadelphia: WB Saunders; 2007. p. 195–208.

Schropp DM, Kovacic J. Phosphorus and phosphate metabolism in veterinary patients. J Vet Emerg Critical Care 2007;17(2):127–34.

Hyperkalemia: A Quick Reference

Marcia Mery Kogika, DVM, MS, PhD[a],*,
Helio Autran de Morais, DVM, PhD[b]

[a]Departamento de Clínica Médica, Faculdade de Medicina Veterinária e Zootecnia,
Universidade de São Paulo, Av. Prof. Dr. Orlando Marques de Paiva, 87,
05508-270 São Paulo, SP, Brazil
[b]Department of Medical Sciences, University of Wisconsin–Madison,
2015 Linden Drive, Madison, WI 53706, USA

- Potassium is the main intracellular cation. Intracellular potassium represents approximately 95% of total body potassium. The extracellular content is much lower, but small changes in extracellular concentration can have major clinical implications.
- Total body potassium is regulated by the kidneys and colon under the influence of aldosterone.
- Intracellular potassium balance is maintained by transcellular shifts regulated mostly by insulin and catecholamines.
- Potassium maintains resting membrane potential. Changes in potassium concentration are associated with a decrease in the excitability of membranes, especially in cardiac and skeletal muscles.
- Changes in serum potassium concentration attributable to acid-base imbalance are variable and mostly clinically irrelevant.
- Hyperkalemia is uncommon if renal function and urine output are normal.

ANALYSIS

- Indications: Serum potassium should be measured in patients at high risk to have or develop hyperkalemia. This includes dogs and cats with vomiting, diarrhea, dehydration, oliguria or anuria, unexplained bradycardia, and muscular weakness. Potassium should also be measured if hypoadrenocorticism, renal failure, urethral obstruction, or uroabdomen is suspected.
- Typical reference range: Reference values for dogs and cats range from 3.5 to 5.5 mEq/L. These values may vary slightly among laboratories. Serum potassium concentrations exceed plasma concentration because potassium is released from platelets during clotting.
- Danger values: Concentrations greater than 7.5 mEq/L may be associated with substantial cardiac conduction disturbances and muscle weakness.

*Corresponding author. E-mail address: mmkogika@usp.br (M.M. Kogika).

0195-5616/08/$ – see front matter
doi:10.1016/j.cvsm.2008.01.024

Box 1: Principal causes of hyperkalemia

Pseudohyperkalemia

Thrombocytosis (usually mild but can have marked changes)

White blood cell counts greater than 100,000 cells/µL (rare but can cause significant changes)

Hemolysis in breeds or individuals with a high red blood cell potassium concentration (eg, akitas, English springer spaniels, neonates, occasional other dogs)

Decreased urinary excretion (most common)

Urethral obstruction (common and important)

Ruptured bladder or ureter (uncommon but important)

Anuric or oliguric renal failure (common and important)

Hypoadrenocorticism (uncommon but important)

Selected gastrointestinal diseases (eg, trichuriasis, salmonellosis, perforated duodenal ulcer)

Chylothorax with repeated pleural fluid drainage (rare)

Hyporeninemic hypoaldosteronism (with diabetes mellitus or renal failure) (rare)

Drugs (ACE inhibitors [eg, enalapril],[a] potassium-sparing diuretics [eg, spironolactone, amiloride, triamterene],[a] prostaglandin inhibitors,[a] or heparin[a])

Increased intake

Unlikely with normal renal or adrenal function unless administration is greatly excessive (eg, intravenous administration of fluids with high potassium chloride [KCl] concentrations, administration of large doses of potassium penicillin G)

Translocation (intracellular fluid → extracellular fluid)

Insulin deficiency (eg, diabetic ketoacidosis) (uncommon and transient)

Acute inorganic acidosis (eg, hydrogen chloride [HCl], NH_4Cl) (rare)

Massive tissue damage (eg, acute tumor lysis syndrome [rare], reperfusion of extremities after aortic thromboembolism in cats with cardiomyopathy [rare], crush injuries)

Hyperkalemic periodic paralysis (rare)

Drugs (nonspecific beta-blockers [eg, propranolol[a]])

[a]Only likely to cause hyperkalemia in conjunction with other contributing factors (eg, decreased renal function, concurrent administration of potassium supplements).

Adapted from DiBartola SP, de Morais HA. Disorders of potassium: hypokalemia and hyperkalemia. In: DiBartola SP, editor. Fluid therapy in small animal practice. 2nd edition. Philadelphia: WB Saunders; 2000. p. 100; with permission.

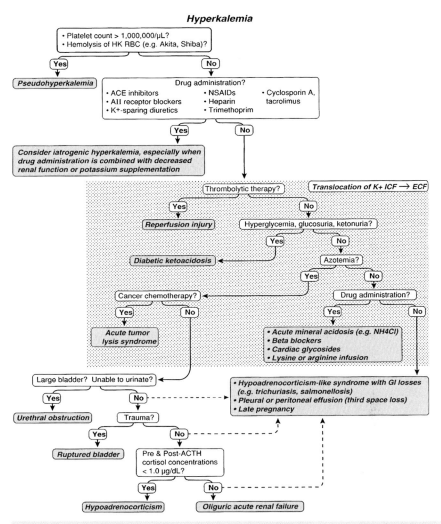

Fig. 1. Algorithm for the clinical approach for hyperkalemia. ACTH, corticotropin; ECF, extracellular fluid; GI, gastrointestinal; HK, genetic mutation associated with high intracellular potassium concentration in RBC of dogs; ICF, intracellular fluid; NSAIDs, nonsteroidal anti-inflammatory drugs; RBC, red blood cell. (*From* DiBartola SP, de Morais HA. Disorders of potassium: hypokalemia and hyperkalemia. In: DiBartola SP, editor. Fluid, electrolyte, and acid-base disorders. 3rd edition. St. Louis (MO): Elsevier; 2006. p. 112; with permission.)

- Artifacts
  - Pseudohyperkalemia, an in vitro increase in potassium concentration, may be observed in the following:
    - Hemolysis in neonates or canine breeds with high intracellular potassium (eg, akita, shiba, kindo).
    - Thrombocytosis: severe thrombocytosis may artificially increase serum potassium concentration because potassium is released from platelets

during clotting. Plasma potassium concentration should be measured in patients that have thrombocytosis.

- Leukocytosis: animals with white blood cell counts greater than 100,000 cells/μL also may have substantial hyperkalemia because of transcellular leakage of potassium.
- Use of ethylenediaminetetraacetic acid (EDTA) or potassium oxalate may markedly increase measured values.
- Drug effect: Excessive potassium administration in fluids can lead to hyperkalemia. Use of spironolactone, angiotensin-converting enzyme (ACE) inhibitors, and nonselective beta-blockers may be associated with hyperkalemia.

HYPERKALEMIA
- Causes: Hyperkalemia may result from the causes listed in Box 1.
- Stepwise approach: An algorithm for the differential diagnosis of hyperkalemia is presented in Fig. 1.
  - Increased intake of potassium if there is concomitant impairment of renal excretion or drugs that interfere with potassium renal excretion are being used.
  - Decreased urinary excretion associated with urethral obstruction, oliguric or anuric renal failure, ruptured bladder, and hypoadrenocorticism.
  - Translocation of potassium may be observed with insulin deficiency and in massive tissue breakdown (eg, acute tumor lysis syndrome, reperfusion). Translocation attributable to metabolic acidosis is only clinically important in acute mineral acidosis (eg, infusion of NH_4Cl or HCl).
  - Hyperkalemia and hyponatremia are classically found in dogs with hypoadrenocorticism. They also may occur in renal failure, secondarily in selected gastrointestinal diseases (eg, trichuriasis, salmonellosis, perforated duodenal ulcer), in ruptured bladder, and in pleural and peritoneal effusions, however.
- Signs: Muscle weakness, bradycardia, and typical electrocardiographic abnormalities.

Further Readings
DiBartola SP, de Morais HA. Disorders of potassium: hypokalemia and hyperkalemia. In: DiBartola SP, editor. Fluid, electrolyte, and acid-base disorders. 3rd edition. St. Louis (MO): Elsevier; 2006. p. 91–121.
DiBartola SP, Green RA, de Morais HA, et al. Electrolyte and acid base abnormalities. In: Willard MD, Tvedten H, editors. Small animal clinical diagnosis by laboratory methods. 4th edition. St. Louis (MO): Saunders; 2004. p. 117–34.

Hypokalemia: A Quick Reference

Marcia Mery Kogika, DVM, MS, PhD[a],*,
Helio Autran de Morais, DVM, PhD[b]

[a]Departamento de Clínica Médica, Faculdade de Medicina Veterinária e Zootecnia,
Universidade de São Paulo, Av. Prof. Dr. Orlando Marques de Paiva, 87,
05508-270 São Paulo, SP, Brazil
[b]Department of Medical Sciences, University of Wisconsin–Madison,
2015 Linden Drive, Madison, WI 53706, USA

- Potassium is the main intracellular cation. Intracellular potassium represents approximately 95% of the total body potassium.
- Despite low extracellular content, extracellular potassium concentration is maintained within narrow limits to avoid the life-threatening effects of hypokalemia or hyperkalemia.
- Potassium maintains resting membrane potential. Changes in potassium concentration are associated with a decrease in the excitability of membranes, especially in cardiac and skeletal muscles.
- Changes in serum potassium concentration attributable to acid-base imbalance are variable and mostly clinically irrelevant.

ANALYSIS

- Indications: Serum potassium should be measured in patients at high risk to have or develop hypokalemia. This includes dogs and cats with chronic or frequent vomiting, diarrhea, marked polyuria, muscle weakness, and unexplained cardiac arrhythmias and those receiving insulin, total parenteral nutrition, and diuretics.
- Typical reference range: The mean normal value expected for dogs and cats is 4.5 mEq/L (range: 3.5–5.5 mEq/L) but may vary slightly among laboratories.
  - Fractional excretion potassium (FE_K) can be used to rule out the kidneys as the source of potassium losses. FE_K is calculated as follows:

$$FE_K = \frac{U_k/S_k}{U_{Cr}/S_{Cr}} \times 100$$

where U_K is the urine concentration of potassium (mEq/L), S_K is the serum concentration of potassium (mEq/L), U_{Cr} is the urine concentration of creatinine (mg/dL), and S_{Cr} is the serum concentration of creatinine (mg/dL).

*Corresponding author. E-mail address: mmkogika@usp.br (M.M. Kogika).

0195-5616/08/$ – see front matter
doi:10.1016/j.cvsm.2008.01.026

Box 1: Principal causes of hypokalemia

Pseudohypokalemia (infrequent and rarely causing significant change)

Increased loss (most common and important category)

Gastrointestinal (FE_K <6%)

Vomiting of gastric contents (common and important)

Diarrhea (common and important)

Urinary (FE_K >20%)

Chronic renal failure in cats (common and important)

Diet-induced hypokalemic nephropathy in cats (important)

Postobstructive diuresis (common and important)

Inappropriate fluid therapy (especially with inadequate potassium supplementation) (common and important)

Diuresis caused by diabetes mellitus/ketoacidosis (common and important)

Dialysis (uncommon)

Drugs

Loop diuretics (eg, furosemide) (common and important)

Thiazide diuretics (eg, chlorothiazide, hydrochlorothiazide)

Amphotericin B

Penicillins (rare)

Albuterol overdose (rare)

Distal (type I) renal tubular acidosis (RTA) (rare)

Proximal (type II) RTA after $NaHCO_3$ treatment (rare)

Mineralocorticoid excess (rare)

Hyperadrenocorticism (mild changes)

Primary hyperaldosteronism (ie, adenoma, hyperplasia)

Translocation (extracellular fluid → intracellular fluid)

Glucose-containing fluids with or without insulin (common and important)

Total parenteral nutrition solutions (uncommon but important)

Catecholamines (rare)

Hypokalemic periodic paralysis (Burmese cats) (rare)

Decreased intake

Unlikely to cause hypokalemia by itself unless diet is severely deficient

Administration of potassium-free fluids (eg, 0.9% sodium chloride [NaCl], 5% dextrose in water)

Adapted from DiBartola SP, de Morais HA. Disorders of potassium: hypokalemia and hyperkalemia. In: DiBartola SP, editor. Fluid therapy in small animal practice. 2nd edition. Philadelphia: WB Saunders; 2000. p. 93; with permission.

Hypokalemia

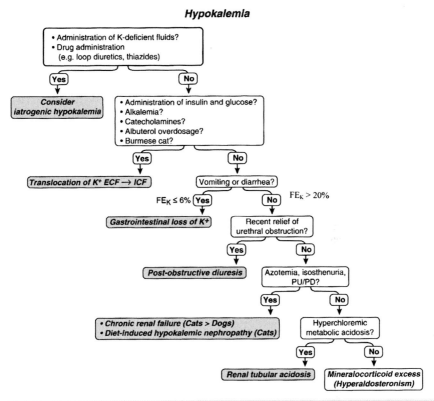

Fig. 1. Algorithm for the clinical approach to hypokalemia. (*From* DiBartola SP, de Morais HA. Disorders of potassium: hypokalemia and hyperkalemia. In: DiBartola SP, editor. Fluid, electrolyte, and acid-base disorders. 3rd edition. St. Louis (MO): Elsevier; 2006. p. 102; with permission.)

- The FE_K should be less than 6% for nonrenal sources of potassium loss. Increased values are difficult to interpret and do not necessarily mean that the kidneys are the source of potassium losses.
- Danger values: Concentrations less than 3.5 mEq/L may be associated with clinical signs. A potassium serum concentration less than 3.0 mEq/L may result in muscle weakness, cardiac arrhythmias, and polyuria, whereas rhabdomyolysis may be observed when potassium serum concentrations decrease to less than 2.0 mEq/L. Respiratory muscle paralysis may occur if potassium decreases to less than 2.0 mEq/L.
- Artifacts: Pseudohypokalemia, an in vitro decrease in potassium concentration, is uncommon and rarely leads to substantial changes in potassium concentration.
- Drug effect: Hypokalemia may occur in patients receiving diuretics, insulin, mineralocorticoids, potassium-free fluids, and sodium bicarbonate. The intracellular shift of potassium induced by sodium bicarbonate is not caused by an increase in pH.

HYPOKALEMIA

- Causes: Hypokalemia may result from the causes listed in Box 1.
  - Increased potassium loss
    - From gastrointestinal tract (FE_K <6%) in patients with vomiting or diarrhea
    - From the kidneys (FE_K >20%) in patients that have renal failure or polyuria or in those receiving diuretics or potassium-free fluids
    - Most hypokalemic patients have increased potassium losses.
  - Potassium translocation from extracellular fluid to intracellular fluid in patients receiving insulin or glucose-containing fluids
  - Decreased intake is unlikely to cause hypokalemia unless the diet is severely deficient or if potassium-free fluids are being given intravenously.
- Signs: Clinical signs vary with the severity and acuteness of K^+ depletion. Anorexia, muscular weakness, and polyuria or polydipsia are the most common signs. Generalized weakness may be observed in dogs and cats, whereas flaccid ventroflexion of the neck, forelimb hypermetria, and a broad-based hind limb stance are seen in cats with polymyopathy. Hypokalemia can lead to ventricular or supraventricular tachyarrhythmias. Hypokalemia does not cause metabolic alkalosis in dogs or cats, however.
- Stepwise approach: An algorithm for the differential diagnosis of hypokalemia is presented in Fig. 1.

Further Readings

DiBartola SP, de Morais HA. Disorders of potassium: hypokalemia and hyperkalemia. In: DiBartola SP, editor. Fluid, electrolyte, and acid-base disorders. 3rd edition. St. Louis (MO): Elsevier; 2006. p. 91–121.

DiBartola SP, Green RA, de Morais HA, et al. Electrolyte and acid base abnormalities. In: Willard MD, Tvedten H, editors. Small animal clinical diagnosis by laboratory methods. 4th edition. St. Louis (MO): Saunders; 2004. p. 117–34.

Hypernatremia: A Quick Reference

Helio Autran de Morais, DVM, PhD[a],*,
Stephen P. DiBartola, DVM[b]

[a]Department of Medical Sciences, University of Wisconsin–Madison,
2015 Linden Drive, Madison, WI 53706, USA
[b]Department of Veterinary Clinical Sciences, The Ohio State University,
601 Vernon L. Tharp Street, Columbus, OH 43210, USA

- Most sodium is located in the extracellular water. Low intracellular sodium concentration is maintained by the activity of cell membrane sodium-potassium-ATPase (N-K-ATPase).
  - Intracellular sodium for muscle is approximately 12 mEq/L, or less than 10% of its extracellular concentration.
- Serum sodium concentration is a reflection of the amount of sodium relative to the volume of water in the body and not a reflection of total body sodium content. Hypernatremic patients may have decreased, increased, or normal total body sodium content.
  - Adjustments in water balance (thirst and vasopressin [antidiuretic hormone (ADH)]) work to maintain normal serum osmolality and serum sodium concentration.
  - Adjustments in sodium balance maintain normal extracellular fluid (ECF) volume by decreasing or increasing renal sodium excretion. These adjustments include the effects of glomerulotubular balance, aldosterone, atrial natriuretic peptide, and renal hemodynamic factors.
    - ECF volume expansion increases sodium excretion, whereas ECF volume contraction decreases sodium excretion.
- Sodium and its attendant anions account for approximately 95% of the osmotically active substances in the extracellular water. Hypernatremia is associated with hyperosmolality.

ANALYSIS

- Indications: Serum sodium concentration should be measured in patients at high risk to have or develop hypernatremia. This includes dogs and cats that are dehydrated or not drinking water; those with abnormal mentation or behavior; those having seizures; and those with polyuria, polydipsia, vomiting, and diarrhea.

*Corresponding author. E-mail address: demorais@vetmed.wisc.edu (H. Autran de Morais).

0195-5616/08/$ – see front matter
doi:10.1016/j.cvsm.2008.01.025

- Typical reference range: Reference values range from 140 to 150 mEq/L for dogs and from 150 to 160 mEq/L for cats. These values may vary slightly among laboratories.
- Danger values: Clinical signs of hypernatremia are more related to rapidity of onset than to magnitude of change and associated hyperosmolality. Neurologic signs may occur with sodium concentrations greater than 170 mEq/L in dogs and greater than 175 mEq/L in cats.
- Artifacts: Samples drawn through improperly cleared intravenous catheters may yield falsely increased sodium concentrations if the fluid being administered has a high sodium content. Sodium salts of anticoagulants (eg, oxalate, fluoride, citrate) may yield increased measure values.
- Drug effect: Hypernatremia may occur with administration of fluids rich in sodium (eg, sodium bicarbonate, hypertonic saline), sodium phosphate enemas, or mineralocorticoids.

HYPERNATREMIA
- Causes: Hypernatremia may result from the causes listed in Box 1.
  - Loss of water: Pure water loss results in relative preservation of ECF volume (normovolemic hypernatremia). Normovolemic hypernatremia is relatively uncommon in small animal medicine and is usually a result of hypodipsia caused by neurologic diseases or diabetes insipidus.
  - Loss of hypotonic fluid: Hypotonic fluid loss results in decreased ECF volume (hypovolemic hypernatremia). Animals that lose hypotonic fluids and are unable to replace water are presented with hypernatremia and decreased ECF volume. The most important causes of hypovolemic hypernatremia in small animals are gastrointestinal (vomiting or diarrhea) or renal (diuretics or renal failure) losses of water and solutes.
  - Gain of sodium: Gain of salt results in increased ECF volume (hypervolemic hypernatremia). Spontaneous oral intake of sodium causing hypernatremia is uncommon in small animals. Iatrogenic overadministration of sodium-containing fluids is more common and may result in hypernatremia, particularly in cases of oliguria or marginal renal function.
- Signs: Most of the signs of hypernatremia arise from the central nervous system (CNS). The more rapid the development of hypernatremia, the more severe the neurologic signs are likely to be.
  - Acute hypernatremia results in acute hyperosmolality of ECF favoring shrinkage of brain cells. A rapid decrease in brain volume may cause rupture of cerebral vessels and focal hemorrhage.
  - If hypernatremia develops slowly, the brain has time to adapt to the hypertonic state and clinical signs are minimal or absent.
  - Anorexia, lethargy, vomiting, muscular weakness, behavioral changes, disorientation, ataxia, seizures, coma, and death have been identified in dogs and cats with hypernatremia and hypertonicity.
  - In hyponatremia secondary to hypotonic fluid losses, signs of volume depletion often are present.

Box 1: Principal causes of hypernatremia

Pure water deficit

  Primary hypodipsia

  Diabetes insipidus

  Water unavailable or patient unable to drink[a]

Hypotonic fluid loss

  Gastrointestinal[a]

    Vomiting

    Diarrhea

    Small intestinal obstruction

  Third-space loss

    Peritonitis

    Pancreatitis

  Cutaneous

    Burns

  Renal[a]

    Osmotic diuresis (mannitol infusion, hyperglycemia)

    Nonosmotic diuresis (furosemide administration)

    Chronic renal failure

    Nonoliguric renal failure

    Postobstructive diuresis

Impermeant solute gain

  Salt poisoning

  Hypertonic fluid administration (sodium bicarbonate, hypertonic saline, sodium phosphate enema)

  Hyperaldosteronism

  Hyperadrenocorticism

[a]Most important causes in small animal practice.

Modified from DiBartola SP. Disorders of sodium and water: hypernatremia and hyponatremia. In: DiBartola SP, editor. Fluid therapy in small animal practice. 3rd edition. St. Louis (MO): WB Saunders; 2006. p. 56; with permission.

- Signs of hypervolemia (eg, pulmonary edema) may be present in patients with sodium gain.
- Stepwise approach: The first step in approaching a patient that has hypernatremia is to determine the volume status (Fig. 1). Hypovolemia occurs in patients that have lost hypotonic fluids, whereas hypervolemia is associated with gain of sodium. Patients that have lost only water remain normovolemic. Signs suggestive of hypovolemia include decreased skin turgor, dry mucous membranes, delayed capillary refill time, tachycardia, and flat jugular veins.

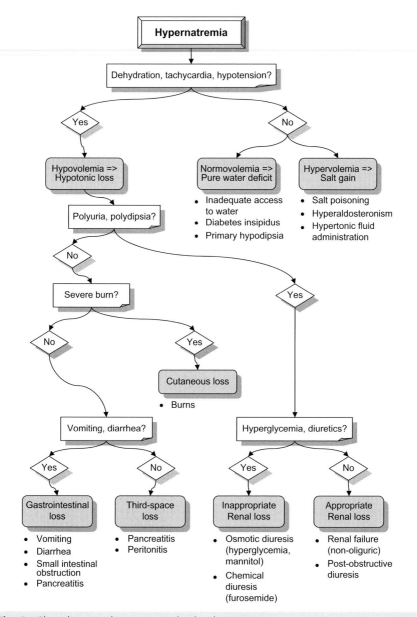

Fig. 1. Clinical approach to a patient that has hypernatremia.

Further Readings

DiBartola SP. Disorders of sodium and water: hypernatremia and hyponatremia. In: DiBartola SP, editor. Fluid, electrolyte, and acid-base disorders. 3rd edition. St. Louis (MO): Elsevier; 2006. p. 47–79.

DiBartola SP, Green RA, de Morais HA, et al. Electrolyte and acid base abnormalities. In: Willard MD, Tvedten H, editors. Small animal clinical diagnosis by laboratory methods. 4th edition. St. Louis (MO): Saunders; 2004. p. 117–34.

Hyponatremia: A Quick Reference

Helio Autran de Morais, DVM, PhD[a],*,
Stephen P. DiBartola, DVM[b]

[a]Department of Medical Sciences, University of Wisconsin–Madison,
2015 Linden Drive, Madison, WI 53706, USA
[b]Department of Veterinary Clinical Sciences, The Ohio State University,
601 Vernon L. Tharp Street, Columbus, OH 43210, USA

- Most sodium is located in the extracellular water. Low intracellular sodium concentration is maintained by the activity of cell membrane sodium-potassium-ATPase (Na-K-ATPase).
  - Intracellular sodium for muscle is approximately 12 mEq/L, or less than 10% of its extracellular concentration.
- Serum sodium concentration is a reflection of the amount of sodium relative to the volume of water in the body and not a reflection of total body sodium content. Hyponatremic patients may have decreased, increased, or normal total body sodium content.
  - Adjustments in water balance (thirst and vasopressin [antidiuretic hormone (ADH)]) work to maintain normal serum osmolality and serum sodium concentration.
  - Adjustments in sodium balance maintain normal extracellular fluid (ECF) volume by decreasing or increasing renal sodium excretion. These include the effects of glomerulotubular balance, aldosterone, atrial natriuretic peptide, and renal hemodynamic factors.
    - ECF volume expansion increases sodium excretion, whereas ECF volume contraction decreases sodium excretion.
- Sodium and its attendant anions account for approximately 95% of the osmotically active substances in the extracellular water. Hyponatremia is usually associated with hypo-osmolality.

ANALYSIS

- Indications: Serum sodium concentration should be measured in patients at high risk to have or develop hyponatremia. This includes dogs and cats with abnormal mentation or behavior; those having seizures; and those with dehydration, polyuria, polydipsia, vomiting, diarrhea, and pleural or peritoneal effusion.

*Corresponding author. E-mail address: demorais@vetmed.wisc.edu (H. Autran de Morais).

0195-5616/08/$ – see front matter
doi:10.1016/j.cvsm.2008.01.027

- Typical reference range: Reference values range from 140 to 150 mEq/L for dogs and from 150 to 160 mEq/L for cats. These values may vary slightly among laboratories.
  - Fractional excretion of sodium (FE_{Na}) can be used to determine if the kidneys are the source of excessive sodium loss. FE_{Na} is calculated as follows:

$$FE_{Na} = \frac{U_{Na}/S_{Na}}{U_{Cr}/S_{Cr}} \times 100$$

  where U_{Na} is urine concentration of sodium (mEq/L), S_{Na} is serum concentration of sodium (mEq/L), U_{Cr} is urine concentration of creatinine (mg/dL), and S_{Cr} is serum concentration of creatinine (mg/dL).
- The FE_{Na} should be less than 1% for nonrenal sources of sodium loss and 1% or greater if sodium is being lost by the kidneys.
- Danger values: Clinical signs of hyponatremia are more related to rapidity of onset than to magnitude of change and associated hypo-osmolality. Neurologic signs may occur with sodium concentrations less than 120 mEq/L in dogs and less than 130 mEq/L in cats.
- Artifacts: Historically, hyperlipidemia and hyperproteinemia could lead to underestimation of sodium concentration when flame photometry or indirect potentiometry was used. This is not a problem when ion-specific electrodes (ISE) are used. However, differences in sodium concentration are observed between machines using direct ISE (eg, point-of-care electrolyte analyzers) and those using indirect ISE (large chemistry analyzers). Samples drawn through improperly cleared intravenous catheters may yield falsely decreased sodium concentrations if the fluid being administered is low in sodium.
- Drug effect: Hyponatremia may occur with administration of fluids low in sodium (eg, 5% dextrose in water, 0.45% sodium chloride [NaCl]), loop diuretics, and thiazides. Some drugs may induce ADH secretion.

HYPONATREMIA

- Causes: Hyponatremia may result from addition of hypertonic solution without sodium (eg, mannitol, glucose), loss of salt, gain of water, or gain of hypotonic fluid (Box 1).
  - Normally, a slight reduction in sodium concentration is accompanied by excretion of dilute urine and correction of hyponatremia. Therefore, persistence of hyponatremia is associated with decreased renal water excretion (eg, renal failure), impairment of urine dilution (eg, inappropriate ADH secretion [syndrome of inappropriate secretion of antidiuretic hormone (SIADH)], slow urine flow), or excessive water intake (eg, primary polydipsia).
  - Most hyponatremic patients are hypo-osmolar, but hyperglycemia and mannitol administration may lead to hyponatremia and hyperosmolality.
  - Hyponatremia with low plasma osmolality may be accompanied by normal, decreased, or increased plasma volume. Determination of fluid volume status is therefore important to identify the cause of hyponatremia.
  - Patients that have hyponatremia and hypovolemia usually have sodium depletion caused by renal or extrarenal routes of fluid loss. The source of volume and salt loss may be identifiable on the basis of the patient history.

Box 1: Principal causes of hyponatremia

With high plasma osmolality

Hyperglycemia[a]

Mannitol infusion

With low plasma osmolality

Hypervolemia

Severe liver disease causing ascites[a]

Congestive heart failure[a]

Nephrotic syndrome causing effusion

Advanced renal failure

Normovolemia

Psychogenic polydipsia

SIADH

Antidiuretic drugs (eg, narcotics, vincristine, nonsteroidal anti-inflammatory drugs)

Myxedema

Hypotonic fluid infusion[a]

Hypovolemia

Gastrointestinal loss

Vomiting and diarrhea[a]

Diarrhea[a]

Third-space loss

Pancreatitis

Peritonitis

Uroabdomen

Cavitary effusion

Cutaneous loss

Burns

Renal loss

Hypoadrenocorticism[a]

Diuretic administration[a]

[a] Most important causes in small animal practice.
Modified from DiBartola SP. Disorders of sodium and water: hypernatremia and hyponatremia. In: DiBartola SP, editor. Fluid therapy in small animal practice. 3rd edition. St. Louis (MO): WB Saunders; 2006. p. 65; with permission.

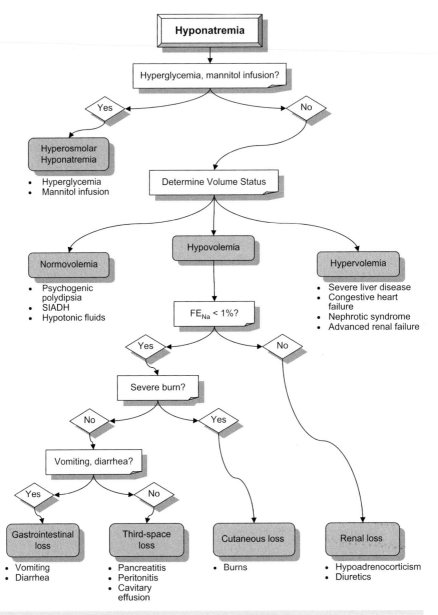

Fig. 1. Clinical approach to a patient that has hyponatremia.

- Hyponatremia with normovolemia is rare in small animal practice but may occur in patients that have psychogenic polydipsia and SIADH.
- Hyponatremia with hypervolemia occurs in animals with severe liver disease, congestive heart failure, and nephrotic syndrome. These patients have decreased effective arterial volume and a consequent reduction in glomerular filtration rate and renal plasma flow. These animals tend to have renal retention of sodium, and the FE_{NA} is usually less than 1%.
- Signs: Cerebral edema and water intoxication occur if hyponatremia develops faster than the brain's defense mechanisms can be called into play. Neurologic signs include focal and diffuse deficits, with occasional seizures. The more rapid the development of hyponatremia, the more severe the neurologic signs are likely to be.
  - Hypovolemic animals may have signs of dehydration with decreased skin turgor, tachycardia, increased packed cell volume (PCV) and total protein concentration, high urine specific gravity, and hypotension.
  - Hypervolemic patients may be presented with ascites, jugular distention, peripheral edema, or pulmonary edema.
- Stepwise approach: Determination of volume status helps to determine the cause of the hyponatremia (Fig. 1).

Further Readings

DiBartola SP. Disorders of sodium and water: hypernatremia and hyponatremia. In: DiBartola SP, editor. Fluid, electrolyte, and acid-base disorders. 3rd edition. St. Louis: Elsevier; 2006. p. 47–79.

DiBartola SP, Green RA, de Morais HA, et al. Electrolyte and acid base abnormalities. In: Willard MD, Tvedten H, editors. Small animal clinical diagnosis by laboratory methods. 4th edition. St. Louis: Saunders; 2004. p. 117–34.

Calcium: Total or Ionized?

Patricia A. Schenck, DVM, PhD[a],*, Dennis J. Chew, DVM[b]

[a]Endocrine Diagnostic Section, Diagnostic Center for Population and Animal Health, Department of Pathobiology and Diagnostic Investigation, Michigan State University, 4125 Beaumont Road, Lansing, MI 48910, USA
[b]Department of Veterinary Clinical Sciences, College of Veterinary Medicine, The Ohio State University, 601 Vernon L. Tharp Street, Columbus, OH 43210, USA

Calcium exists in three forms, or fractions, in plasma or serum: ionized (iCa; free calcium), complexed (cCa) or chelated (bound to phosphate, bicarbonate, sulfate, citrate, and lactate), and protein bound [1]. In clinically normal dogs, the protein-bound calcium, cCa, and iCa fractions account for approximately 34%, 10%, and 56% of the total serum calcium concentration, respectively [2]. In normal cats, the protein-bound calcium, cCa, and iCa fractions account for 40%, 8%, and 52% of the serum total calcium (tCa) concentration, respectively [3]. iCa is the biologically active fraction of calcium, and its homeostasis is important for many physiologic functions [4]. Calcium ions regulate homeostasis directly by binding to cell membrane receptors specific for iCa [5]. Serum iCa concentration is controlled by interacting feedback loops that involve iCa, phosphorus, parathyroid hormone (PTH), calcitriol, and calcitonin. These mechanisms help to maintain serum iCa concentration in a narrow range.

MEASUREMENT OF TOTAL CALCIUM

The calcium status of animals is usually determined on serum tCa concentration, despite the fact that only the iCa fraction is physiologically active. Fasting serum or heparinized plasma samples are suitable for analysis; oxalate, citrate, and ethylenediaminetetraacetic acid (EDTA) anticoagulants should not be used, because calcium is bound to these chemicals and becomes unavailable for analysis [6]. Hemolyzed samples yield falsely increased tCa concentrations, high concentrations of bilirubin falsely decrease tCa, and hyperlipidemia can result in spuriously high calcium concentrations [7]. Samples should not be diluted for measurement, because serum tCa concentrations may be falsely decreased. Age, diet, and fasting may have an impact on tCa measurement. Normal serum tCa concentrations in mature dogs and cats are approximately 10.0 and 9.0 mg/dL (2.5 and 2.25 mmol/L), respectively. Dogs younger than 3 months of age have slightly higher serum tCa concentrations (mean of 11.0 mg/dL or 2.75 mmol/L) than

*Corresponding author. E-mail address: schenck5@msu.edu (P.A. Schenck).

0195-5616/08/$ – see front matter
doi:10.1016/j.cvsm.2008.01.010

those of dogs older than 1 year of age (mean of 10.0 mg/dL or 2.5 mmol/L) because of bone growth. In some normal young dogs, serum tCa concentration may be as high as 12.0 to 15.0 mg/dL (3.0–5.0 mmol/L) [8].

Reliance on measurement of serum tCa is based on the assumption that it is directly proportional to iCa concentration. This assumption may lead to erroneous interpretation of laboratory data in many clinical conditions. In human beings with calcium disorders, measurement of serum tCa concentrations failed to predict serum iCa concentrations in 31% of all patients [9] and in 26% of patients that have renal disease [10]. In 1633 canine serum samples, the diagnostic disagreement between serum iCa and tCa was 27%, and in dogs with chronic renal failure, this disagreement was 36% [11]. A 40% diagnostic disagreement between serum iCa and tCa was noted in 434 cats [12]. In dogs, tCa measurement overestimated normocalcemia and underestimated hypocalcemia. In cats, hypercalcemia and normocalcemia were underestimated, and hypocalcemia was overestimated when using serum tCa to predict iCa status.

ADJUSTED TOTAL CALCIUM

Because tCa is composed of three fractions, changes in any one fraction have an impact on tCa measurement. It has been suggested that canine serum tCa concentrations should be "corrected" or "adjusted" relative to serum total protein or albumin concentration to improve diagnostic interpretation [13]. This correction seemed reasonable at the time these calculations were developed, because there is substantial binding of serum calcium to protein and 80% to 90% of the bound calcium is bound to albumin. The assumptions are that serum tCa concentrations that correct into the normal range are associated with normal iCa concentrations and results that fail to correct into the normal range represent abnormal iCa concentrations. These formulas, however, were developed without verification by iCa measurements. In 1633 canine serum samples, the use of an adjustment formula to predict iCa status showed a higher diagnostic discordance than did measurement of serum tCa alone [11]. The use of a formula to adjust tCa based on total protein had a diagnostic disagreement with iCa of 37%, and the use of a formula to adjust tCa based on albumin had a diagnostic disagreement with iCa of 38%. In 490 dogs with chronic renal failure, diagnostic disagreement between adjusted tCa and iCa measurement increased to 53%, indicating poor performance of the adjustment formulas in the prediction of iCa status. In all 1633 canine samples, the adjustment formulas overestimated hypercalcemia and normocalcemia and underestimated hypocalcemia. In dogs with chronic renal failure, the adjustment formulas overestimated hypercalcemia, with an underestimation of normocalcemia and hypocalcemia. Adjustment formulas perform poorly because they only take into account the potential protein-bound fraction of calcium and ignore the cCa. The cCa is not constant, especially in dogs with chronic renal failure, in which the cCa can range from 6% to 39% of tCa [14]. Serum tCa measurements or adjusted tCa measurements are unacceptable predictors of iCa status because of the high level of discordance, especially in patients that have chronic renal failure. Changes in serum protein concentration, individual protein-binding capacity and affinity, and alterations in cCa concentration all can change tCa independent of iCa. The use of adjustment formulas to predict iCa status is not recommended.

MEASUREMENT OF IONIZED CALCIUM

For accurate measurement of calcium status, iCa should be measured directly. iCa measurement is superior to serum tCa measurement in many conditions, including hyperparathyroidism, renal disease, hypoproteinemia, hyperproteinemia, acid-base disturbances, and critical illnesses [11,15,16]. Analyzers using an ion-selective electrode allow easy and accurate measurement of iCa [17]. Differences among analyzers exist, and reference ranges should be established for each analyzer [18].

Serum iCa concentration in normal dogs is approximately 5.0 to 5.8 mg/dL (1.25–1.45 mmol/L), and it is approximately 4.6 to 5.6 mg/dL (1.15–1.40 mmol/L) in adult cats. Young dogs and cats have serum iCa concentrations that are 0.1 to 0.4 mg/dL higher than those reported in older animals [4].

Accurate determination of iCa concentration requires that samples be collected and processed correctly. Acidic pH favors dissociation of calcium from proteins and increases the amount of iCa in the sample. Alkaline pH that occurs with loss of carbon dioxide (CO_2) favors calcium binding to protein, decreasing the amount of iCa. The mixing of serum with air (aerobic collection) results in increased pH in the sample and decreased iCa concentration. When attempting anaerobic serum collection, exposure to air in partially filled serum tubes affects iCa concentration, resulting in as much as a 0.07-mmol/L decrease in iCa concentration compared with tubes are were 100% filled [19].

Anaerobic measurement of iCa requires meticulous separation techniques. Serum should be collected directly into a serum Vacutainer tube (Becton-Dickinson, Franklin Lakes, New Jersey). Silicone separator tubes are not recommended, because serum iCa concentration may increase as a result of release of calcium from the silicone gel [20]. Blood should be allowed to clot and then be separated by centrifugation. To remove serum from the tube, a spinal needle attached to a non–air-containing syringe should be used, puncturing the red-topped stopper without exposing the sample to air. iCa in canine serum is stable for 72 hours at 23°C or 4°C and for 7 days at −10°C [21].Accurate aerobic methods for iCa measurement have been developed. The iCa concentration of an aerobically collected serum sample at any given pH can be mathematically corrected to the theoretic iCa concentration at pH 7.4 [22,23]. These correction formulas are based on the predictable linear change in iCa concentration with changes in pH. This correction to a standard pH is necessary, because samples exposed to air typically have a high pH value that affects calcium binding. iCa analyzers have a preprogrammed internal formula that makes this correction. This internal correction formula, however, should not be used, because these formulas were designed for use with human serum samples. Different species seem to have different protein-binding properties; thus, formulas should be developed and validated for each species. Excellent correlation between iCa measurement in anaerobically handled and aerobically handled samples corrected to a pH of 7.4 has been observed (P.A. Schenck, DVM, PhD, D.J. Chew, DVM, unpublished data, 2002). Although not quite as precise as anaerobic measurement, aerobic measurement under controlled conditions offers a diagnostically accurate methodology for iCa determination with simplified collection, shipping, and handling requirements.

iCa can be measured in heparinized plasma or whole blood, but there are issues that must be addressed with heparinized samples. iCa and pH are more stable in serum than in whole or heparinized blood. Serum analysis eliminates the potential interference of heparin and allows longer storage periods before analysis. In dogs, concentrations of iCa are lower by approximately 0.05 mmol/L in heparinized plasma compared with serum [19]. The amount of heparin used is critical in the measurement of iCa in blood, because heparin dilutes the sample, causing a decrease in the measured iCa concentration. Syringes containing a premeasured quantity of dry heparin are preferable to coating a syringe manually with an unknown and variable quantity of liquid heparin. Even when using syringes containing dry heparin, it is imperative to collect the same volume of blood for each sample to avoid dilutional effects. iCa concentration is underestimated when dry heparin syringes are filled with a less than recommended quantity of blood [24,25]. The type of heparin used also has an impact on iCa measurement. Zinc heparin causes an overestimation of iCa because of a decrease in pH, which displaces calcium from proteins [24,26]. Lithium heparin causes an underestimation, and electrolyte-balanced heparin may underestimate or overestimate iCa depending on whether hypocalcemia, normocalcemia, or hypercalcemia is present [24].

Portable clinical analyzers are now available for cage-side analysis of iCa concentration. These analyzers use a disposable cartridge containing an impregnated biosensor for iCa and other analytes. Heparinized whole blood is used for analysis, but iCa concentrations are typically 0.05 to 0.26 mmol/L lower in dogs and 0.05 to 0.14 mmol/L lower in cats compared with serum iCa measurement [27]. The greatest underestimation occurs when iCa concentration is greater than 1.3 mmol/L. The reported correlation for iCa concentration in heparinized whole blood comparing ion-selective electrode measurement and portable clinical analyzer methods was only 0.71 [28]. The portable clinical analyzer method results in an iCa measurement that is approximately 2.6% lower than that measured with an ion-selective electrode [29]. Because the quantity and type of heparin used and volume of blood collected have an effect on iCa measurement as discussed previously, it is best to establish a standardized protocol for blood collection when using a portable clinical analyzer. Reference ranges should be established for the analyzer using this standardized protocol, and results cannot be directly compared with ion-selective method measurements.

SUMMARY

Measurement of serum tCa has been relied on for assessment of calcium status, despite the fact that it is the iCa fraction that has biologic activity. Serum tCa does not accurately predict iCa status in many clinical conditions. Adjustment formulas developed to correct serum tCa based on total protein or albumin concentration do not improve the prediction of iCa status and, in some instances, can decrease its prediction; thus, their use should be abandoned. For accurate assessment of iCa status, iCa should be directly measured. Measurement of iCa in heparinized whole blood is problematic because of dilutional effects of heparin and the effect of the type of heparin on the measurement. Anaerobic measurement of serum iCa under controlled conditions provides the most reliable assessment of calcium status; aerobic measurement of iCa with species-specific pH correction is highly correlated with anaerobic measurements.

References

[1] Endres DB, Rude RK. Mineral and bone metabolism. In: Burtis CA, Ashwood ER, editors. Tietz textbook of clinical chemistry. 3rd edition. Philadelphia: W.B. Saunders; 1999. p. 1395–457.

[2] Schenck PA, Chew DJ, Brooks CL. Fractionation of canine serum calcium, using a micropartition system. Am J Vet Res 1996;57(3):268–71.

[3] Schenck PA, Chew DJ, Behrend EN. Updates on hypercalcemic disorders. In: August J, editor. Consultations in feline internal medicine, vol. 5. St. Louis (MO): Elsevier; 2005. p. 157–68.

[4] Schenck PA, Chew DJ, Nagode LA, et al. Disorders of calcium: hypercalcemia and hypocalcemia. In: DiBartola SP, editor. Fluid therapy in small animal practice. 3rd edition. St. Louis (MO): Elsevier; 2005. p. 122–94.

[5] Brown EM, Hebert SC. Calcium-receptor-regulated parathyroid and renal function. Bone 1997;20(4):303–9.

[6] Woo J, Cannon DC. Metabolic intermediates and inorganic ions. 17th edition. Philadelphia: W.B. Saunders Co.; 1984. p. 133–79.

[7] Meuten DJ. Hypercalcemia. Vet Clin North Am 1984;14(4):891–910.

[8] Normal blood values for cats and normal blood values for dogs. St. Louis (MO): Ralston-Purina Co.; 1975.

[9] Thode J, Juul-Jorgensen B, Bhatia HM, et al. Comparison of serum total calcium, albumin-corrected total calcium, and ionized calcium in 1213 patients with suspected calcium disorders. Scand J Clin Lab Invest 1989;49(3):217–23.

[10] Burritt MF, Pierides AM, Offord KP. Comparative studies of total and ionized serum calcium values in normal subjects and patients with renal disorders. Mayo Clin Proc 1980;55(10): 606–13.

[11] Schenck PA, Chew DJ. Prediction of serum ionized calcium concentration by serum total calcium measurement in dogs. Am J Vet Res 2005;66(8):1330–6.

[12] Schenck PA, Chew DJ. Diagnostic discordance of total calcium and adjusted total calcium in predicting ionized calcium concentration in cats with chronic renal failure and other diseases. Proceedings of the 10th Congress of the International Society of Animal Clinical Biochemistry, 2002. Gainesville, FL.

[13] Meuten DJ, Chew DJ, Capen CC, et al. Relationship of serum total calcium to albumin and total protein in dogs. J Am Vet Med Assoc 1982;180(1):63–7.

[14] Schenck PA, Chew DJ. Determination of calcium fractionation in dogs with chronic renal failure. Am J Vet Res 2003;64(9):1181–4.

[15] Gosling P. Analytical reviews in clinical biochemistry: calcium measurement. Ann Clin Biochem 1986;23:t146–56.

[16] Zaloga GP, Willey S, Tomasic P, et al. Free fatty acids alter calcium binding: a cause for misinterpretation of serum calcium values and hypocalcemia in critical illness. J Clin Endocrinol Metab 1987;64(5):1010–4.

[17] Bowers GN Jr, Brassard C, Sena SF. Measurement of ionized calcium in serum with ion-selective electrodes: a mature technology that can meet the daily service needs. Clin Chem 1986;32(8):1437–47.

[18] Hristova EN, Cecco S, Niemela JE, et al. Analyzer-dependent differences in results for ionized calcium, ionized magnesium, sodium, and pH. Clin Chem 1995;41(11):1649–53.

[19] Unterer S, Lutz H, Gerber B, et al. Evaluation of an electrolyte analyzer for measurement of ionized calcium and magnesium concentrations in blood, plasma, and serum of dogs. Am J Vet Res 2004;65(2):183–7.

[20] Larsson L, Ohman S. Effect of silicone-separator tubes and storage time on ionized calcium in serum. Clin Chem 1985;31(1):169–70.

[21] Schenck PA, Chew DJ, Brooks CL. Effects of storage on serum ionized calcium and pH values in clinically normal dogs. Am J Vet Res 1995;56(3):304–7.

[22] Lincoln SD, Lane VM. Serum ionized calcium concentration in clinically normal dairy cattle, and changes associated with calcium abnormalities. J Am Vet Med Assoc 1990;197(11): 1471–4.

[23] Nachreiner RF, Refsal KR. The use of parathormone, ionized calcium and 25-hydroxyvita-min D assays to diagnose calcium disorders in dogs. Proc Am Coll Vet Intern Med Forum, 1990.

[24] Lyon ME, Bremner D, Laha T, et al. Specific heparin preparations interfere with the simulta-neous measurement of ionized magnesium and ionized calcium. Clin Biochem 1995;28(1): 79–84.

[25] Lyon ME, Guajardo M, Laha T, et al. Electrolyte balanced heparin may produce a bias in the measurement of ionized calcium concentration in specimens with abnormally low protein concentration. Clin Chim Acta 1995;233(1–2):105–13.

[26] Lyon ME, Guajardo M, Laha T, et al. Zinc heparin introduces a preanalytical error in the measurement of ionized calcium concentration. Scand J Clin Lab Invest 1995;55(1):61–5.

[27] Grosenbaugh DA, Gadawski JE, Muir WW. Evaluation of a portable clinical analyzer in a veterinary hospital setting. J Am Vet Med Assoc 1998;213(5):691–4.

[28] Murthy JN, Hicks JM, Soldin SJ. Evaluation of i-STAT portable clinical analyzer in a neonatal and pediatric intensive care unit. Clin Biochem 1997;30(5):385–9.

[29] Lindemans J, Hoefkens P, van Kessel AL, et al. Portable blood gas and electrolyte analyzer evaluated in a multiinstitutional study. Clin Chem 1999;45(1):111–7.

Vet Clin Small Anim 38 (2008) 503–512

VETERINARY CLINICS
SMALL ANIMAL PRACTICE

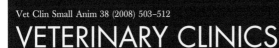

Urinary Electrolytes, Solutes, and Osmolality

Jennifer E. Waldrop, DVM

Massachusetts Veterinary Referral Hospital, 20 Cabot Road, Woburn, MA 01801, USA

U rinary tests are becoming increasingly popular because of ease of collection and some advantages to serum testing. Although plasma osmolality (POsm) and solute concentrations must exist in narrow ranges for proper cellular function, the chemical composition of urine can vary widely. The kidneys change the composition of urine to facilitate normal homeostasis and react to systemic challenges. Analysis of urine chemistry is vital in determining if the kidneys are functioning adequately for homeostasis and can appropriately respond to insult and injury.

The volume and elements that comprise urine depend on the actions of the kidneys in filtration of blood in addition to reabsorption and secretion of water and solutes. As plasma passes through the glomerulus, macromolecules (eg, proteins) and cellular elements, such as cells and proteins, are selectively retained based on charge and size. The remaining filtrate continues through the tubule and is subjected to various passive and active mechanisms that result in retention or excretion of solutes and water. The amount of solutes excreted is determined by dietary intake, renal threshold for reabsorption, hormonal influence, or a combination of these factors. Some solutes are freely filtered but neither reabsorbed nor secreted (eg, creatinine [Cr]), whereas other substances may be released by the kidney in response to damage (eg, brush border enzymes) [1,2].

Defining normal urine composition is problematic, because there can be wide intra- and interindividual variability in the amount of solutes and water in the urine of healthy animals [2–4]. Urine chemical concentrations from different breeds may even be different under normal circumstances [4,5]. This can make interpretation of urine chemistries difficult. As is the case with some other indicators in critical patients (eg, central venous pressure, lactate), trends and changes over time may be more important than individual concentrations. The use of drugs, including diuretics, parenteral nutrition, and fluid therapy, also can interfere with urine chemical analysis. This article outlines some of the clinically useful urine chemistry tests and addresses their limitations.

E-mail address: jwaldrop@intownvet.com

0195-5616/08/$ – see front matter
doi:10.1016/j.cvsm.2008.01.011

URINE SOLUTE MEASUREMENTS

The interpretation of urine chemistries can vary widely based on the urine collection method. A solute's concentration can be determined using a random sample or by 24-hour collection. Random samples can be less accurate, especially when the urine is dilute [1,6,7]. The 24-hour urine collections are laborious and usually require hospitalization, but if a urinary catheter is present, shorter timed collections may be possible [8]. Given that Cr clearance reflects glomerular filtration rate (GFR), calculation of the relative ratio of the solute to creatinine may be useful (eg, urine protein/urine creatine [UPr/Cr] ratio). By comparing the urine concentrations of the solute and Cr with the plasma concentrations, the fractional excretion (FE) can be calculated. When the FE ratio is less than 1.0, the solute has net reabsorption, and if the ratio is greater than 1.0, the solute has net secretion [1,7]. Unless used chronically, diuretics should be withheld for 6 to 8 hours before the measurement of any urine chemistry.

The equations to calculate the FE of a solute and the renal failure index (RFI) are as follows:

$$FE(solute) = U(sol) \times PCr \times 100 / P(sol) \times UCr$$

$$RFI = UNa \times PCr / UCr$$

where U(sol) is urine solute concentration, P(sol) is plasma solute concentration, PCr is plasma creatinine, UCr is urine creatinine, and UNa is urine sodium.

URINE SODIUM AND CHLORIDE

Commonly measured urine electrolytes include sodium (Na) and chloride (Cl). Evaluation of the urine concentration of these two electrolytes aids in differentiation of hypovolemia and renal tubular dysfunction in patients that have azotemia. Sodium balance is regulated by two related and interdependent systems: osmoregulation and volume regulation [1]. Serum concentration in the extracellular fluid is controlled in a narrow range by the hypothalamus. Osmoreceptors signal changes in water intake and excretion based on changes in POsm. Antidiuretic hormone (ADH) is released if water needs to be conserved and acts on the renal collecting ducts to maximize water reabsorption. ADH targets the V2 receptors on the collecting duct cells, signaling the downstream insertion of water channels, called aquaporins, into the luminal membrane. Without ADH, the aquaporins are removed and urine is maximally dilute [1,2].

By regulating the absolute amounts of Na and water, the body determines the effective circulating volume. Volume changes are sensed by stretch receptors throughout the vascular tree (eg, aortic arch, afferent arteriole, atria, carotid sinus). Changes in volume lead to secretion of various hormones to affect sodium absorption or secretion (Table 1). Cl usually follows Na, and as more solute is retained or discarded, water moves secondarily. With a substantial decrease in effective circulatory volume, volume receptors signal

Table 1
Hormonal and physiologic signals affecting renal sodium excretion

Agent	Effect
Renin	Production of angiotensin I
Angiotensin II	↑ Aldosterone release
	↑ Tubular Na reabsorption directly
Aldosterone	Distal nephron: ↑ Na/Cl reabsorption, potassium loss
Atrial natriuretic peptide	↓ Aldosterone and renin release
	Collecting duct: inhibit Na reabsorption
Dopamine	↓ Aldosterone release
Prostaglandins	↑ Increase renin release
	↑ Renal Na excretion
Sympathetic nervous system	↑ Intrarenal Na retention (α_1)
Pressure natriuresis	↑ Intrarenal Na loss
Hyperkalemia	↑ Aldosterone

the release of ADH as well, allowing further retention of water. With severe hypovolemia, the preservation of cardiac output "trumps" the moderate hypo-osmolality that may result from maximal stimulation of ADH and water retention [1,6,7].

Given maximal stimulation of the renin-angiotensin-aldosterone system (RAAS) with hypovolemia, UNa and urine chloride (UCl) concentrations should be low (<20 mEq/L) (Table 2). UNa and UCl are high (>40 mEq/L) when the kidneys are unable to respond to normal stimuli, as in acute tubular dysfunction. Acute tubular necrosis (ATN) can occur secondary to (1) renal ischemia as may occur with hypotension, hypoxia, and sepsis; (2) prolonged prerenal azotemia; or (3) endogenous or exogenous toxins, including aminoglycoside antibiotics, nonsteroidal anti-inflammatory drugs (NSAIDs), contrast media, cisplatin, and myoglobin. A high UNa can be seen in several conditions other than ATN, including postrenal causes of azotemia, hypothyroidism, hypoadrenocorticism, and diuretic use. Any defect in Na reabsorption can lead to a falsely high UNa despite hypovolemia [1,6,9].

Table 2
Summary of expected urine indices (measured and calculated) in prerenal azotemia and acute tubular necrosis

Index	Prerenal	ATN
UNa	<20 mEq/L	>40 mEq/L
UCl	<20 mEq/L	>40 mEq/L
UCr/PCr ratio	>40	<20
FENa	<1%	>2%–3%
RFI	<1	>2
UOsm/POsm ratio	>1.5	1.0–1.5

Abbreviations: ATN, acute tubular necrosis; FENa, fractional excretion of sodium; UOsm/POsm, urine osmolality–to–plasma osmolality ratio.

A gray zone exists between a UNa of 20 and 40 mEq/L, wherein overlap can occur. A low UNa can be seen in normovolemic animals when selective renal or glomerular ischemia has occurred secondary to severe decreases in renal blood flow or acute glomerulonephritis (GN). A single UNa can be measured, but 24-hour collections and comparisons with Cr clearance are most useful. Interpreting a single UNa is difficult, and comparison of a few renal indices is advised in the medical literature [1,6,8,9]. The presence of any underlying chronic renal disease negates the utility of UNa and UCl.

Alterations in urine water concentration also make interpretation of UNa difficult. A classic example is central diabetes insipidus (CDI). The lack of ADH allows maximally dilute urine and a low UNa. Most animals with CDI have achieved volume balance with severe polydipsia and are not hypovolemic unless a crisis occurs. Calculating the fractional excretion of sodium (FENa) removes water balance from the equation by adjusting for GFR. A FENa greater than 2% is consistent with a UNa greater than 30 mEq/L and indicates that the observed azotemia is not likely prerenal. Calculation of the FENa is most sensitive when polyuria is not present but may provide the most information when used in combination with other renal indices.

UCl and fractional excretion of chloride (FECl) usually add little information to that provided by UNa and FENa [1,6,7,10]. Both should be calculated and compared when trying to differentiate prerenal azotemia from ATN (see Table 2). If there is a difference of more than 15 mEq/L between UNa and UCl in a hypovolemic animal, it is likely attributable to the excretion of Na with another anion (eg, bicarbonate) or Cl with another cation (eg, ammonia). It currently is recommended in the medical literature that UCl be measured in patients that are hypovolemic but have a somewhat increased UNa. This most commonly occurs in metabolic alkalosis because of excretion of Na with bicarbonate (UCl <20 mEq/L) [6,7]. A UCl less than 20 mEq/L also can occur secondary to exogenous or endogenous corticosteroids [1].

Table 2 summarizes the expected values for urine Na and Cl indices and includes other calculations cited in the medical literature to differentiate ATN and prerenal azotemia [1,7,9]. The use of these indices in the medical field has been standardized, and there are many on-line calculators for FENa and RFI (including Refs. [11,12]). The use of these urinary indices in veterinary medicine has not been verified but may be available in some cases of acute toxic or ischemic injury to the kidneys. Urinary indices, such as UNa and FENA, should be used in conjunction with standardized testing, including PCr, blood urea nitrogen (BUN), and urine output [7,8].

There are three clinical scenarios in veterinary medicine in which measurement of UNa and UCl may be most useful: (1) NSAID toxicity, (2) monitoring aminoglycoside use, and (3) after severe hypotension. Episodes of severe hypotension may occur with shock, anesthesia, or cardiopulmonary arrest. Monitoring UNa and UCl after successful cardiopulmonary resuscitation may be helpful to monitor for signs of substantial renal damage. This has not yet been studied in veterinary medicine but could be clinically useful when multiple renal indices are measured and compared.

Common treatments for NSAID toxicity include diuresis, activated charcoal, and prostaglandin (PG) E_1 analogues. Serial measurements of BUN and PCr are monitored to determine if there is clinically relevant renal damage, because urine osmolality (UOsm) is not likely to be helpful in the face of diuresis. At presentation, many animals may have moderately concentrated urine, which can make it difficult to determine if they had limited renal function before ingesting toxic doses of NSAIDs. Measurement of UNa and UCl on entry and serially may help to indicate substantial renal toxicity before increases in BUN and PCr, which may not occur for 36 to 48 hours after ingestion. In the author's experience, urine indices have been helpful in several cases and are widely available and inexpensive.

Monitoring for aminoglycoside toxicity is also difficult, given that considerable damage may occur before the BUN and PCr are increased. Other urine markers of early renal damage include brush border enzymes, glucose, and casts. In one pediatric study, urinary losses of Na, magnesium, and calcium were significantly increased after a single dose of aminoglycosides, but renal damage was not noted in that clinical study [13]. It is not known whether urinary measurements of Na and other electrolytes can identify animals more likely to incur renal damage or may just highlight animals that are prone to urinary electrolyte wasting. Aminoglycosides are widely used in veterinary neonates (eg, septic foals, dogs with parvoviral enteritis), however, further investigation into the clinical usefulness of urine chemistries with aminoglycoside use is needed in veterinary medicine.

Sepsis is a common cause of disease in animals, and considerable renal damage can occur secondary to inflammation, thromboembolism, and decreased renal perfusion. The use of urinary indices to document ATN in sepsis is still open to debate. A recent review of the available medical literature linking urinary indices and experimental models of acute renal failure and sepsis found significant variability in the ability of urinary indices to diagnose acute renal injury [14]. Acute renal failure induced by gram-negative sepsis in ewes did not cause urinary indices to change any established pattern [15].

PCr is an established marker for GFR, as discussed previously, and is an extremely reliable marker of renal function. Small changes in PCr can indicate severe loss of function even when the PCr is in the "normal" range [8]. A comparison of UCr and PCr is another way to estimate tubular water reabsorption. Patients with prerenal causes of azotemia generally reabsorb most water and have a UCr/PCr ratio greater than 40 (see Table 2) [1].

OSMOLALITY

Osmolality is defined as the number of solute particles per kilogram of solvent. The major determinants of extracellular and intracellular fluid osmolalities are Na and potassium (K) respectively, whereas UOsm reflects a more heterogeneous mixture of solutes. Urine solutes include urea, Na, K, ammonium

(NH$_4$), Cl, and other anions [1,2,7]. UOsm can be estimated (UOsm = Urea + 2[Na+K+NH$_4$]) or measured by freezing point depression osmometry. Normal UOsm can range widely between 800 and 2500 mOsm/kg in the dog and between 600 and 3000 mOsm/kg in the cat [2,16]. In contrast, normal POsm ranges between 290 and 330 mOsm/kg for dogs and cats [2].

Urine specific gravity (Usg) is a more useful test clinically and is usually measured using a refractometer. Specific gravity is considered a valid estimation of osmolality if the urine does not have high concentrations of glucose, proteins, or molecules (eg, radiocontrast agents) [1,2,17]. UOsm can be calculated from Usg with the following equation: UOsm = (Usg − 1.000) × 40,000 (Table 3) [17].

Water can be actively reabsorbed in the presence of ADH and passively lost with large solute loads. Maximal water reabsorption can only be attained with adequate hypertonicity of the renal medulla (countercurrent multiplier effect) and appropriate responsiveness of the collecting duct cells to ADH. In the normal animal, water reabsorption or loss is determined by water intake, POsm, and effective circulating volume. The retention of some solutes, such as Na and Cl, aid in water retention [1,2].

The clinical importance of measuring UOsm is most obvious in differentiating prerenal and renal causes of azotemia and verifying that at least 33% of the kidney mass is functioning adequately. A concentrated urine sample (UOsm >1200 mOsm/kg, Usg >1.035) is found when renal concentrating function is adequate. There are conditions under which the expected UOsm may not be found, however, despite signs of azotemia or dehydration and adequate renal function. Clinically important conditions that may cause hypotonic urine include any cause of polyuria and polydipsia (eg, diabetes mellitus, hyper- or hypoadrenocorticism), medullary washout secondary to fluid administration, sepsis, and pharmacologic agents (eg, corticosteroids, diuretics).

Another common use of UOsm in combination with UNa in the medical field is for the diagnosis of the syndrome of inappropriate antidiuretic hormone secretion (SIADH), a major cause of hyponatremia in human beings. SIADH has rarely been reported in veterinary medicine and is an "umbrella" term for a variety of causes of hyponatremia [18]. When vascular volume is essentially normal but hyponatremia persists, ADH secretion is inappropriate. A diagnosis of SIADH is one of exclusion, and possible causes in people include neoplasia, central nervous system disorders (eg, stroke, masses, trauma),

Table 3
Comparison of urine osmolality and corresponding specific gravity

UOsm (mOsm/kg)	Usg
40	1.001
520	1.013
680	1.017
1600	1.040
2400	1.060

pulmonary conditions (eg, positive-pressure ventilation, infections), medications (eg, chemotherapy, tricyclic antidepressants), surgery and anesthesia, pain, and HIV infection. To diagnose SIADH, the following criteria must be met: (1) isovolemic hypotonic hyponatremia; (2) normal adrenal, renal, and thyroid function, (3) high UOsm (>100 mOsm/kg) in the presence of low POsm; (4) inappropriate natriuresis (UNa >20 mEq/L); (5) documentation of increased ADH concentration; and (6) correction of hyponatremia by water restriction [2,18].

OTHER URINE INDICES

Urine potassium (UK) and functional excretion of potassium (FEK) are affected by aldosterone and vary with dietary K intake, because serum and intracellular K concentrations are controlled in a narrow range. The most clinically useful application of UK is in the diagnosis of uroabdomen. Calculation of the abdominal fluid/peripheral blood ratio of K and Cr is highly predictive of the presence of urine in the abdomen. Schmeidt and colleagues [19] report a K ratio of greater than 1.4 (abdominal to peripheral) to be 100% sensitive and specific for dogs with uroabdomen. The measurement of plasma and urine K and Cr can be performed on an emergency basis by most in-house chemical analyzers.

Urinary calcium (UCa) and UNa may be useful to monitor the success of dietary modification in animals with urolithiasis. In the medical literature, increased UCa has been seen with many neoplastic disorders, including multiple myeloma and bone metastasis, and with corticosteroid use [6]. The clinical usefulness of UCa is limited in veterinary medicine at this time.

The loss of enzymes into the urine, or enzymuria, has been noted in a variety of renal disorders and reflects tubular cell damage [20]. Increases in urine N-acetyl-β-D-glucosaminidase (NAG) occur when more protein is presented to the renal tubular cells, and therefore increases lysosomal activity and excretion of NAG. Alkaline phosphatase and γ-glutamyl transpeptidase (GGT) are too large to be filtered through the glomerulus; therefore, their presence in urine reflects leakage from the proximal tubule brush border cells. As with other urine indices, an enzyme-to-Cr ratio may be more accurate. Establishing a baseline for enzymuria before renal injury may be a limiting factor in clinical practice.

Enzymuria has been documented as an early marker of renal disease in many species, including the dog, cat, and cow [21]. For example, renal function has been studied using urine enzymes in pyometra [22], anesthesia [23], leishmaniasis [24], and NSAID use [25]. Urine NAG is increased in some dogs with pyometra even after spaying, indicating continued renal tubular damage [22]. Urine alkaline phosphatase, GGT, and NAG have been used as early markers of aminoglycoside nephrotoxicity. In one study, a threefold increase of urine GGT over baseline preceded changes in Usg, proteinuria, and PCr concentration after administration of a toxic dose of gentamicin [26].

Novel urine indices have been used in a variety of diseases, and some may become commercially available. For example, an interesting clinical study of canine gastric dilatation and volvulus (GDV) found that urine concentrations of 11-dehydro-thromboxane B2 (11-dTXB2) were higher in affected dogs than in healthy surgical controls before and after surgery. A postoperative increase in the urine 11-dTXB2/Cr ratio was associated with an increased incidence of postoperative complications. Thromboxanes are generated after perfusion is restored to ischemic tissues, and excretion of thromboxane metabolites, such as 11-dTXB2, in the urine has been associated with myocardial infarction and atherosclerosis [27].

PROTEINURIA

UPr testing is one of the more established urine chemistries. Evidence of proteinuria can indicate loss of proteins secondary to many causes, including prerenal (eg, multiple myeloma), renal (eg, GN, tubular damage), or postrenal (eg, bladder neoplasia) disorders. Single UPr measurements are not sensitive, especially typical dipstick methods. Use of the UPr/Cr ratio is sensitive to significant protein loss, with a value of greater than 1.0 prompting immediate investigation [28,29]. Active urine sediment impairs the interpretation of the ratio, because severe infection can increase the ratio to greater than 30, but small amounts of hemorrhage, such as may occur with cystocentesis, without active pyuria may not. In an in vitro study, blood contamination of 10% total volume still only increased the UPr/Cr ratio to 1.8 [30].

Substantial proteinuria is a poor prognostic indicator in animals with chronic kidney disease (CKD) [20,28,29]. More recently, detection of microproteinuria has been advocated as an "early warning system" for CKD and other systemic diseases [28,31]. Detection of pathologic microalbuminuria (urine albumin <30 mg/dL) can be performed in-house or with more quantitative methods [20,29]. The use of the microalbumin/Cr ratio may be more accurate because it relates albumin loss to GFR.

Microalbuminuria also can be seen with many conditions that change vascular permeability. Transient microalbuminuria has been seen after exercise, surgery, burns, trauma, and pancreatitis [32]. Pathologic vascular leakage, or capillary leak syndrome, occurs systemically in response to the global release of inflammatory mediators after severe injury. Increased vascular permeability may manifest as acute respiratory distress syndrome (ARDS) or edema. Given that the kidney "is ideally placed to amplify small changes in vascular permeability" [32], microalbuminuria may occur days before other indicators of inflammation, such as C-reactive protein. A surge of microalbuminuria has been documented in posttraumatic patients that have ARDS in the first 24 hours after injury and may be an early predictor of those patients at risk for developing ARDS [33]. In another small medical study, a surge in the urine microalbumin/Cr ratio at 6 hours after admission to an intensive care unit predicted mortality [34]. Although some veterinary studies have been published examining the association of microalbuminuria and systemic disease, no study has evaluated the change in microalbuminuria that may occur with an acute systemic insult, such as septic abdomen or GDV.

SUMMARY

Urinary chemical markers are a little used clinical resource in veterinary medicine, despite their wide availability and cost-effectiveness. Interpretation of urinary chemistries should be made in light of expected renal responses and using multiple indices to avoid the limitations associated with a single urine test. Urine chemistries may be most useful in cases of acute renal damage, such as toxicities, or changes in glomerular permeability, such as capillary leak syndrome. Additional research is needed to validate the usefulness of urine chemistries to predict disease, but the veterinary clinician still can use urine chemistries in conjunction with laboratory and clinical findings.

References

[1] Rose BD, Post TW. Clinical physiology of acid-base and electrolyte disorders. 5th edition. New York: McGraw Hill; 2001.

[2] DiBartola SP. Fluid, electrolyte, and acid-base disorders in small animal practice. 3rd edition. St. Louis (MO): Elsevier; 2006 p. 26–46.

[3] van Vonderen IK, Kooistra HS, Rijnberk A. Intra- and interindividual variation in urine osmolality and urine specific gravity in healthy pet dogs of various ages. J Vet Intern Med 1997;11:30–5.

[4] Bennett SL, Abraham LA, Anderson GA, et al. Reference limits for urinary fractional excretion of electrolytes in adult non-racing Greyhound dogs. Aust Vet J 2006;84:393–7.

[5] Stevenson AE, Markwell PJ. Comparison of urine composition of healthy Labrador retrievers and Miniature Schnauzers. Am J Vet Res 2001;62:1782–6.

[6] Kamel KS, Ethier JH, Richardson RM, et al. Urine electrolytes and osmolality. Am J Nephrol 1990;10:89–102.

[7] Haskins SC. Interpretation of urine electrolyte, specific gravity and osmolality. In: Proceedings of the 12th International Veterinary Emergency and Critical Care Symposium. San Antonio; 2006. p. 631–3.

[8] Francey T. Assessment of renal function in the critical patient. In: Proceedings of the 10th International Veterinary Emergency and Critical Care Symposium. San Diego; 2004. p. 575–78.

[9] Nally JV. Acute renal failure in hospitalized patients. Clev Clin J Med 2002;69:569–74.

[10] de Morais HAS, Chew DJ. Use and interpretation of serum and urine electrolytes. Semin Vet Med Surg (Small Anim) 1992;7:262–74.

[11] Available at: http://www.intmed.mcw.edu/clincalc/fena.html. Accessed February 13, 2008.

[12] Available at: http://www.mdcalc.com/fena. Accessed February 13, 2008.

[13] Giapros VI, Cholevas VI, Andronikou AK. Acute effects of gentamicin on urinary electrolyte excretion in neonates. Pediatr Nephrol 2004;19:322–5.

[14] Bagshaw SM, Langenberg C, Wan L, et al. A systematic review of urinary findings in experimental septic acute renal failure. Crit Care Med 2007;35:1592–8.

[15] Langenberg C, Wan L, Bagshaw SM, et al. Urinary biochemistry in experimental septic acute renal failure. Nephrol Dial Transplant 2006;21:3389–97.

[16] Cottam YH, Caley P, Wamberg S, et al. Feline reference values for urine composition. J Nutr;132:1754S–6S.

[17] Chadha V, Garg U, Alon US. Measurement of urinary concentration: a critical appraisal of methodologies. Pediatr Nephrol 2001;16:374–82.

[18] Brofman PJ, Knostman KA, DiBartola SP. Granulomatous amebic meningoencephalitis causing the syndrome of inappropriate secretion of antidiuretic hormone in a dog. J Vet Intern Med 2003;17:230–4.

[19] Schmeidt C, Tobias KM, Otto CM. Evaluation of the abdominal fluid:peripheral blood creatinine and potassium ratios for diagnosis of uroperitoneum in dogs. J Vet Emerg Crit Care 2001;11:275–80.

[20] Grauer GF. Early detection of renal damage and disease in dogs and cats. Vet Clin North Am Small Anim Pract 2005;35:581–96.

[21] Sato R, Soeta S, Miyazaki M, et al. Clinical availability of urinary N-acetyl-β-D-glucosaminidase index in dogs with urinary diseases. J Vet Med Sci 2002;64:361–5.

[22] Heiene R, Moe L, Mlmen G. Calculation of urinary enzyme excretion with renal structure and function in dogs with pyometra. Res Vet Sci 2001;70:129–37.

[23] Lobetti R, Lambrechts N. Effects of general anesthesia and surgery on renal function in healthy dogs. Am J Vet Res 2000;61:121–4.

[24] Palacio J, Liste F, Gascón M. Enzymuria as an index of renal damage in canine leishmaniasis. Vet Rec 1997;140:477–80.

[25] Narita T, Tomizawa N, Sato R, et al. Effects of long-term oral administration of ketoprofen in clinically healthy beagle dogs. J Vet Med Sci 2005;67:847–53.

[26] Rivers BJ, Walter PA, O'Brien TD, et al. Evaluation of urine gamma-glutamyl transpeptidase-to-creatinine ratio as a diagnostic tool in an experimental model of aminoglycoside-induced acute renal failure in the dog. J Am Anim Hosp Assoc 1996;32:323–36.

[27] Baltzer WI, McMichael MA, Ruauz CG. Measurement of urinary 11-dehydro-thromboxane B2 excretion in dogs with gastric dilatation-volvulus. Am J Vet Res 2006;67:78–83.

[28] Lees GE, Brown SA, Elliott J, et al. Assessment and management of proteinuria in dogs and cats: 2004 ACVIM Forum Consensus Statement (Small Animal). J Vet Intern Med 2005;19: 377–85.

[29] Brunker J. Protein-losing nephropathy. Compend Contin Educ Pract Vet 2005;27:686–94.

[30] Bagley RS, Center SA, Lewis RM, et al. The effect of experimental cystitis and iatrogenic blood contamination on the urine protein/creatinine ratio in the dog. J Vet Intern Med 1991;5:66–70.

[31] Whittemore JC, Gill VL, Jensen WA, et al. Evaluation of the association between microalbuminuria and the urine albumin-creatinine ratio and systemic disease in dogs. J Am Vet Med Assoc 2006;229:958–63.

[32] Gosling P. Microalbuminuria: a marker of systemic disease. Br J Hosp Med 1995;54: 285–9.

[33] Pallister I, Gosling P, Alpar K, et al. Prediction of posttraumatic adult respiratory distress syndrome by albumin excretion rate eight hours after admission. J Trauma 1997;42:1056–61.

[34] MacKinnon KL, Molnar Z, Lowe D, et al. Use of microalbuminuria as a predictor of outcome in critically ill patients. Br J Aneasth 2000;84:239–41.

Therapeutic Approach to Electrolyte Emergencies

Michael Schaer, DVM

Department of Small Animal Clinical Sciences, College of Veterinary Medicine,
University of Florida, PO Box 100126, Gainesville, FL 32610–0126, USA

Fluid and electrolyte imbalances are encountered frequently in a variety of disorders and require the clinician's astute evaluation of the patient's fluid and electrolyte status. Disorders involving the gastrointestinal tract, kidneys, and endocrine system frequently cause abnormalities in sodium, potassium, and calcium balance and require accurate assessment of serum sodium, potassium, and calcium concentrations initially and subsequently during treatment so as to maintain electrolyte homeostasis. Failure to do so can lead to severe clinical consequences for the patient and change a diagnostic triumph into a therapeutic failure. This article discusses the therapeutic approach to serum electrolyte disorders involving sodium, potassium, and calcium.

HYPOKALEMIA

Hypokalemia occurs when the serum potassium concentration is less than 3.5 mEq/L (normal range: 3.5–5.5 mEq/L).

Etiology

The causes of hypokalemia can be classified into four major categories: (1) dilutional hypokalemia and decreased intake, (2) transcellular maldistribution, (3) loss of potassium by way of the gastrointestinal tract, and (4) loss of potassium through urine [1–7].

Clinical Findings

The clinical signs of hypokalemia occur from a disturbance in neuromuscular function attributable to impaired electrical conduction at the cell membrane level [1,5,7,8]. Neuromuscular signs are seldom present until serum potassium has decreased to 2.5 mEq/L or less. Muscle weakness and cardiac conduction abnormalities eventually occur as a result of a hyperpolarization block at the neuromuscular junction [8,9]. Other signs that can accompany severe or chronic hypokalemia include paralysis, muscle cramps, paresthesia, respiratory muscle impairment, lethargy and confusion, inability to concentrate urine, carbohydrate intolerance, anorexia, vomiting, and decreased bowel motility [7].

E-mail address: schaer@vetmed.ufl.edu

0195-5616/08/$ – see front matter
doi:10.1016/j.cvsm.2008.01.012

Hypokalemia can sustain metabolic alkalosis because of its tendency to promote renal proximal tubular HCO_3^- reabsorption. This acid-base disorder can, in turn, worsen the potassium imbalance, because the alkalosis drives potassium intracellularly [1,2,10]. The administration of intravenous 0.9% saline solution supplemented with potassium chloride while simultaneously correcting the underlying cause is essential for treating metabolic alkalosis–associated hypokalemia.

Electrocardiographic (ECG) changes first appear when the serum potassium concentration is less than 2.5 mEq/L [11,12], but their occurrence is not as reliable as the ECG changes accompanying hyperkalemia. The abnormalities include depressed ST segment; lowering, flattening, or inversion of the T wave; presence of an elevated U wave (in human beings); increased P wave amplitude; prolonged PR interval; and prolonged QRS interval. Certain cardiac arrhythmias also may occur and include sinus bradycardia, primary heart block, paroxysmal atrial tachycardia, and atrioventricular (AV) dissociation. Life-threatening arrhythmias are not commonly associated with hypokalemia.

Treatment

The treatment of chronic mild hypokalemia (3.0–3.5 mEq/L) can be accomplished with dietary measures that include the addition of potassium-rich foods, such as oranges, bananas, grapes, or nuts, to the diet. Commercial oral potassium supplement tablets and elixirs also are available [1,13]. Elixirs may induce emesis; to avoid this, they should be diluted with water. The daily dosage of these oral preparations is 0.5 to 1.0 mEq/kg mixed in food once or twice daily. A veterinary powdered supplement is commercially available (Tumil-K; Vibrac, Fort Worth, Texas) and may be given orally at a recommended dosage of 0.25 teaspoonful (2 mEq) per 4.5-kg of body weight in food twice daily. Adjust the dosage as necessary.

Parenteral Treatment of Severe Hypokalemia

The treatment of severe or acute hypokalemia with or without metabolic alkalosis requires the intravenous administration of potassium chloride solution [1,5,14]. Unfortunately, no accurate formulas exist for calculating the exact amount of potassium chloride needed to restore normal serum potassium concentrations. The excessive amounts of potassium lost through polyuria, from the gastrointestinal tract, and the commonly marked decreases accompanying the use of fluids and insulin in the treatment of diabetic ketoacidosis make the dependability of any formula unreliable. An important fact to remember is that when potassium chloride is given intravenously, the rate is more critical than the total amount administered. Under most circumstances, the rate should not exceed 0.5 mEq/kg/h. Under the most dire circumstances, however, the rate can be increased to 1.5 mEq/kg/h along with close ECG monitoring. Small animals should not receive more than 10 mEq/h for fear of fatal consequences because of the effects of a more concentrated solution on the wall of the right ventricle if the solution is given through a central intravenous line.

When administered over a 24-hour period by means of intravenous infusion in lactated Ringer's solution or isotonic saline, the milliequivalents of potassium chloride that can be safely administered are provided in Table 1. An alternate and time-tested guideline for potassium supplementation is provided in Table 2.

It is important to remember that the amounts provided in Table 1 are only ranges that must be adjusted to the specific needs of each patient. For instance, a 5-kg ketoacidotic diabetic cat with a serum potassium concentration of 2.0 mEq/L can require as much potassium chloride as 30 mEq over the first 24 hours. Potassium supplementation is a clinical exercise in titration, thereby requiring repeated monitoring of serum potassium concentrations.

Anticipated Response

The increase in serum potassium concentration occurs slowly and gradually over a few days, particularly if there are continued ongoing losses. It is important to correct any coexisting magnesium deficits, because hypomagnesemia causes additional renal potassium losses.

HYPERKALEMIA

Hyperkalemia occurs when the serum potassium concentration exceeds 5.5 mEq/L. It can become a life-threatening disorder, because myocardial toxicity can occur at serum concentrations in excess of 7.5 mEq/L. It is a serious and common enough abnormality to require prompt recognition and treatment.

Etiology

The major causes of hyperkalemia are increased potassium intake, decreased renal potassium excretion, and transcellular maldistribution. Artifactual or pseudohyperkalemia can accompany thrombocytosis or extreme leukocytosis, and it can also result from potassium escaping from red blood cells (eg, Akita breed) [1,7,15,16].

Those conditions predisposing to hyperkalemia include acute oliguric renal failure, acute obstructive uropathy, adrenal cortical insufficiency, iatrogenic overzealous administration of potassium chloride infusions, massive soft tissue trauma (in human beings), and marked metabolic acidosis, with the first three conditions being most common. Certain drugs, such as angiotensin-converting enzyme (ACE) inhibitors and trimethoprim-sulfa, and potassium-sparing diuretic agents can cause hyperkalemia [10,17–24].

In metabolic acidosis, there is a tendency for potassium to transfer from the intracellular space into the extracellular space [1,10,24]. This occurs most commonly in the presence of an inorganic acid-induced metabolic acidosis, in which the hydrogen ions tend to remain in the extracellular fluid (ECF) space as

Table 1 Recommended dose of potassium chloride according to severity and patient's weight		
	Measured serum K^+ (mEq/L)	Amount of potassium chloride per kg of body weight given over 24 hours
Mild	3.0–3.5	2–3 mEq
Moderate	2.5–3.0	3–5 mEq
Severe	<2.5	5–10 mEq

Table 2
Recommended amount of potassium chloride and rate of infusion

Serum potassium concentration (mEq/L)	Potassium chloride (mEq) to add to fluid (250 mL)	Potassium chloride (mEq) to add to fluid (1 L)	Maximal fluid infusion rate[a] (mL/kg/h)
<2.0	20	80	6
2.1–2.5	15	60	8
2.6–3.0	10	40	12
3.1–3.5	7	28	18
3.6–5.0	5	20	25

[a]So as not to exceed 0.5 mEq/kg/h.
Data from Greene RW, Scott RC. Lower urinary tract disease. In: Ettinger SJ, editor. Textbook of veterinary internal medicine. Philadelphia: WB Saunders; 1975. p. 1572.

opposed to organic acidosis, in which potassium can enter the intracellular space along with the organic anion, thus maintaining electroneutrality. Furthermore, the excretion of potassium ions by the renal tubular cells is decreased when their hydrogen ion content is increased.

Clinical Findings

The most dramatic effect of hyperkalemia occurs at the neuromuscular cell membrane [1,10]. Muscular weakness is prominent because of depolarization of the muscle cell membrane. Paralysis and paresthesias can also occur. Cardiac abnormalities can ensue when the serum potassium concentration exceeds 7.5 mEq/L. These cardiotoxic effects of hyperkalemia seem to be more severe with concomitant hyponatremia, such as seen in Addison's disease.

Various sequential ECG changes occur with progressive increases in serum potassium concentrations, thereby making electrocardiography a practical means for tentatively diagnosing and monitoring the hyperkalemic patient [12,25]. These changes include high peaked or deep T waves, prolonged PR interval, disappearance of the P wave, prolonged QRS complex, complete heart block, bradycardia, atrial standstill, ectopic beats, sine wave complexes, and ventricular fibrillation or standstill. The abnormal cardiac excitation and conduction disturbances attributable to hyperkalemia are more detrimental to the patient than are those that accompany hypokalemia.

Treatment

Any ECG abnormalities of the QRS complex require immediate treatment because of the potential for fatal arrhythmias [1,12,14,25]. Peritoneal dialysis and hemodialysis are effective approaches, but they are seldom used in most veterinary hospitals. Oral or rectal cationic exchange resins have been useful in human medicine, but these treatments are rarely used in veterinary medicine. A slow (over 3–5 minutes) intravenous push of 10% calcium gluconate at a dosage of 0.5 to 1.5 mL/kg immediately counteracts the direct cardiotoxic effects of hyperkalemia by causing decreased membrane potential and, consequently, decreased cardiac membrane excitability. This does not lower the serum potassium concentration, however. If 10% calcium chloride is used instead of calcium gluconate, only one third of the gluconate dose should be used, because the calcium chloride solution is three times as potent.

Intravenous sodium bicarbonate infusions are effective, because the resulting alkalosis attracts hydrogen ions from the cell and causes a transfer of potassium ions from the extracellular compartment into the intracellular compartment [10]. The recommended dose is 1 to 2 mEq/kg administered by intravenous push. Caution must be exercised when giving large amounts of sodium bicarbonate intravenously because of the possible induction of paradoxical cerebrospinal fluid acidosis or a hyperosmolar state ($NaHCO_3$, 40 mEq, is equivalent to 90 mOsm). Furthermore, bicarbonate administration directly after calcium treatment neutralizes the effect of calcium, because the bicarbonate alkalinizes the blood and decreases the availability of calcium ions.

An additional safe and effective treatment for hyperkalemia is the administration of dextrose and insulin infusions [14,26]. As insulin facilitates the transport of glucose into the tissues, potassium simultaneously shifts in a similar direction. Insulin also has its own independent means of moving potassium into the intracellular space because it stimulates the Na^+-H^+ antiporter and, secondarily, the Na^+-K^+-ATPase pump at the cell membranes of the insulin-dependent cells [27–31]. An antiporter is a cell membrane protein that moves two substances in opposite directions through the membrane. Because of its rapid action, regular crystalline insulin should be used at a dose of 0.5 U/kg of body weight. Dextrose at a dose of 2 g should be given simultaneously (50% dextrose solution [4 mL] = 2 g) for every calculated unit of insulin administered intravenously. A lesser amount of insulin (0.25 U/kg) and slightly more dextrose (3 g/U of insulin) should be used for the patient that has hypoadrenocorticism. Table 3 provides a summary of the treatments for hyperkalemia.

The administration of an intravenous bolus of hypertonic dextrose to a severely dehydrated patient can worsen cellular dehydration. To avoid this consequence of hyperosmolarity, the insulin and dextrose can be directly added to a bottle of lactated Ringer's or saline solution, which then is infused at a moderate rate during the initial volume repletion stages of fluid therapy. In critical situations involving a severely dehydrated patient, one quarter to one half of

Table 3
Acute management of hyperkalemia

Drug	Onset of action	Duration and comments
Calcium gluconate	Within minutes	Response lasts up to 30 minutes Does not lower the serum potassium concentration
Sodium bicarbonate	Within 15 minutes	Effect lasts approximately 30 minutes Can decrease ionized calcium availability
Insulin-dextrose	By 30 minutes	Effect lasts 30 minutes to 1 hour Lowers potassium concentration by an average of 1 mEq/L

the calculated amounts of insulin and dextrose may be given by intravenous push, with the remainder added to the infusion bottle for slower intravenous administration. This application of insulin-dextrose infusions has provided satisfactory results when used in critically ill hyperkalemic patients. Although there is some concern over the effects of potassium ions in lactated Ringer's solution when given to an oliguric or anuric patient, the effect of the potassium chloride at a rate of 1 mEq per 250 mL is diluted out for all practical purposes, especially in a patient with normal or increased urine output.

The loop diuretic furosemide enhances renal potassium excretion, and can therefore be used after the calcium and glucose-insulin treatment. This particular treatment is ineffective in renal failure because of the poor renal tubular response to furosemide.

HYPONATREMIA

Etiology

True hyponatremia results from sodium loss or water gain. Depending on the associated pathophysiology, it can occur in the overhydrated, dehydrated, or euhydrated patient and be classified according to the hydration state, plasma osmolarity, or plasma volume status (Tables 4 and 5) of the patient [32–43].

Hyponatremia does not always imply a total body sodium deficit, as illustrated in common sodium-retaining conditions, such as congestive heart failure, hepatic fibrosis, and the nephrotic syndrome, in which total body sodium

Table 4
Classification of hyponatremia according to hydration status

Type		Urine sodium concentration	Total body sodium
I	Hyponatremia in the overhydrated patient		
	1. Congestive heart failure	↓	↑
	2. Hepatic fibrosis	↓	↑
	3. Nephrotic syndrome	↓	N
	4. Compulsive water drinking	↓	N
	5. Iatrogenic water loading	↓ or ↑	N
	6. Syndrome of inappropriate ADH secretion	↑	↑
	7. Renal failure	↑ or ↓	↓ or ↑
II	Hyponatremia in the dehydrated patient		
	1. Salt-losing nephritis	↑	↓—
	2. Adrenocortical sufficiency	↑	↓
	3. Diuretic excess	↑	↓
	4. Extrarenal losses (vomiting or diarrhea)	↓	↓
	5. Osmotic diuresis	↑	↓
III	Hyponatremia in the euhydrated patient		
	1. Pseudohyponatremia, hyperlipidemia	Varies with sodium load	N
	2. Pseudohyponatremia, hyperproteinemia	Varies with sodium load	N
	3. Resetting of the osmostat	Varies with sodium load	N

Abbreviation: N , normal.

Table 5
Classification of hyponatremia according to plasma osmolarity and volume status

Plasma osmolarity		Example	Water and Na$^+$ status
1	Euosmolar	Pseudohyponatremia: hyperlipidemia, hyperproteinemia	Water normal, Na$^+$ normal
2	Hyperosmolar	Acutely extreme hyperglycemia	Water and Na$^+$ excess
3	Hypo-osmolar	Hypovolemic (overt volume contraction): gastrointestinal loss, hemorrhage, Addison's disease, third space loss	Water and Na$^+$ depleted
		Hypervolemic (overtly edematous): congestive heart failure, cirrhosis, nephrotic	Water and Na$^+$ excess
		Euvolemic (volume status clinically normal but mildly hypervolemic): SIADH, myxedema	Water excess, Na$^+$ depleted

Abbreviation: SIADH, syndrome of inappropriate antidiuretic hormone secretion.

actually is increased. In these conditions, the sodium is diluted out by water retention caused by excess antidiuretic hormone (ADH) secretion [32].

Pathophysiology

The most pronounced effects of hyponatremia occur when serum sodium concentrations decrease to lower than 120 mEq/L in less than 12 to 24 hours. The brain is most vulnerable to the adverse effects of acute hyponatremia.

Brain

As the serum sodium concentration decreases, the osmotic gradient that develops across the blood-brain barrier causes water to move into the brain, causing signs of mental depression, irritability, seizures, and coma. The severity of signs depends on the rate and magnitude of the decrease in the serum sodium concentration. A rapid decrease to 110 mEq/L over 2 hours can cause brain edema and death in experimental animals. The patient is less symptomatic if the decrease occurs over days to weeks because of certain compensatory mechanisms that are described elsewhere [44].

The adaptive changes that protect the brain against excessive swelling also render it susceptible to dehydration during the correction of hyponatremia. The rate of increase of brain intracellular potassium and organic osmolytes during correction of the hyponatremia is much slower than the rate of loss of these substances during the development of the problem. If correction of the low serum sodium concentration occurs more rapidly ($>$0.5–1.0 mEq/L/h) than the brain can recover solute, the higher plasma osmolality may dehydrate and injure the brain, producing osmotic demyelination syndrome or central pontine myelinosis [44–53].

Cardiovascular system

The cardiovascular response to hyponatremia depends primarily on the effective arterial blood volume, which may be increased, decreased, or normal depending on the underlying disorder. In volume-depleted patients, hyponatremia can cause a further decrease in the intravascular volume by allowing movement of water out of the ECF space into the intracellular fluid (ICF) space.

Hyponatremia in the hypervolemic patient takes place in the setting of heart failure accompanied by increases in plasma concentrations of ADH and aldosterone. Its presence often points to a guarded prognosis.

Clinical Findings

The clinical signs of hyponatremia depend on the underlying pathophysiologic condition and its effects on the extracellular volume. There are no ECG signs of hyponatremia. With hypovolemic hyponatremia, the patient seems weak and mentally depressed in addition to showing signs of dehydration and hypovolemia (eg, rapid and weak pulses, prolonged capillary refill time, cold extremities, hypotension).

Patients that have hypervolemic hyponatremia reflect their underlying conditions, causing sodium and water retention as seen in heart failure, cirrhosis, and nephrotic syndrome. Each of these syndromes is characterized clinically by the presence of edema, ascites, pleural effusion, or some combination of these abnormalities.

The euvolemic patient that has hyponatremia might show mild interstitial fluid accumulation as found in hypothyroid myxedema.

Patients that become acutely hyponatremic because of the rapid infusion of hypotonic solutions show signs reflecting their rapid onset of cerebral edema, such as mental dullness that progresses to stupor and coma with or without seizures [45,46].

Treatment of Hyponatremia

The medical management of hyponatremia is determined by the status of the ECF volume (low, normal, or high) and by the presence or absence of neurologic signs. Symptomatic hyponatremia requires more aggressive treatment than asymptomatic hyponatremia [47], but the potential risk for demyelinating encephalopathy (central pontine myelinosis) limits the rate of increase in serum sodium concentration [44,45]. When the decrease in serum sodium concentration occurs over a period of 48 hours or more and the serum sodium concentration is less than 120 mEq/L, the rate of increase in serum sodium concentration should not exceed 0.5 mEq/L/h, with a maximum of only 10 to 12 mEq/L of sodium increase during the 24-hour period. In light of this complication, the following guidelines can be used based on brain status [48–54].

Low Extracellular Volume

Infuse hypertonic saline (3% sodium chloride at a rate of 2 mL/kg) in symptomatic patients and isotonic saline in asymptomatic patients. The need for restoring blood pressure while avoiding too rapid an increase in serum sodium concentration is most challenging in the patient that has hypoadrenocorticism and a serum sodium concentration less than 120 mEq/L. Adding a natriuretic drug, such as furosemide, to the treatment once blood pressure is safely restored helps to prevent an excessively rapid increase in serum sodium concentration [14].

Normal Extracellular Volume
Combine furosemide diuresis with infusion of hypertonic saline (3% sodium chloride at a rate of 2 mL/kg) in symptomatic patients or isotonic saline in asymptomatic patients [14].

High Extracellular Volume
Use furosemide-induced diuresis in asymptomatic patients. In symptomatic patients, combine furosemide diuresis with judicious use of hypertonic saline [14].

Calculating the Sodium Replacement Rate
1. The estimated effect of infusate at a rate of 1 L on serum sodium concentration can be expressed using the following equation [54]:

$$\Delta \text{Serum Na}^+ = \frac{\text{Infusate Na}^+ - \text{Serum Na}}{\text{TBW} + 1} \qquad (1)$$

where infusate Na^+ is sodium concentration of the corrective fluid and TBW is total body water ($0.6 \times$ body weight [kg]).

2. Calculating the volume of fluid infusion required to meet a specific change in the early treatment period for hyponatremia can be expressed using the following equation:

$$\frac{\text{Change in serum Na}^+ \text{ targeted for given treatment period}}{\text{Output of Na}^+ \text{infusion formula in}(1)} =$$
Volume of infusion required $\qquad (2)$

The sodium content of the various available fluid products is provided in Table 6.

3. The safe infusion rate of the prescribed volume in equation 2 is given so as not to exceed a change in the serum sodium of 0.5 mEq/L/h or 10 to 12 mEq/L in 24 hours.

The formulas previously provided to treat hyponatremia can be confusing and impractical for the clinician. A simpler approach using 3% saline (513 mEq/L) is provided [55]:

- Administer the 3% saline at a rate of 1 to 2 mL/kg of body weight per hour to increase the serum sodium concentration by 1 to 2 mEq/L/h.
- Give twice this rate (2–4 mL/kg/h) for a limited period in patients with hyponatremia-induced coma or seizures.
- Give half this infusion rate (0.5 mL/kg/h) if clinical signs are minimal.

Table 6
Na$^+$ content and distribution of various parenteral fluids

Infusate	Infusate Na$^+$ (mEq/L)	ECF distribution (%)
5% NaCl	855	100
3% NaCl	513	100
0.9% NaCl	154	100
Lactated Ringer's solution	130	97
0.45% NaCl	77	73
0.2% NaCl	34	55
5% Dextrose	0	40

Abbreviation: NaCl, sodium chloride.

- Give furosemide with the saline to promote free water excretion and prevent ECF volume expansion.
- The rate of change of serum sodium concentration must be monitored every 2 to 3 hours and the infusion adjusted as needed.

HYPERNATREMIA

This electrolyte disorder occurs when the serum sodium concentration is greater than 150 mEq/L. It may result from a loss of water or a gain in sodium. When hypernatremia is attributable to a loss of water, the ICF and ECF compartments are diminished in volume. When it is attributable to a gain of salt, the ECF is increased, whereas the ICF volume is decreased [56–58].

Etiology
These are classified in Table 7 [56–70].

Pathophysiology
Because sodium ions do not freely penetrate tissue cell membranes, the ECF and plasma volume tend to be maintained in hypernatremic dehydration until the water loss is greater than 10% of the body weight. Shock is an infrequent occurrence.

Massive brain hemorrhage or multiple small hemorrhages and thromboses may occur when hypernatremia acutely causes enough cellular dehydration

Table 7
Classification of causes of hypernatremia

Volume	Total body sodium	Clinical conditions
Hypovolemic	Low	Renal losses: diuresis
		Extrarenal losses: gastrointestinal
Euvolemic	Normal	Renal water loss: diabetes insipidus
		Extrarenal water loss: hypodipsia
Hypervolemic	Increased	Acute renal failure
		Excess sodium intake

and resultant brain shrinkage to cause tearing of cerebral blood vessels [14,56,70]. This type of pathologic change occurs at serum sodium concentrations greater than 190 mEq/L. If the hypernatremia is gradual in onset and persists for more than a few days, brain dehydration may resolve and brain water content may return to normal or nearly normal levels because of the accumulation in the brain cells of amino acids known as "idiogenic osmoles." The formation of these idiogenic osmoles increases intracellular osmolality, attracts water back into the brain cells, and restores the cellular volume.

Rapid correction of chronic hypernatremia can cause seizures and severe neurologic sequelae. Unless hypernatremia is of short duration (1–2 days), idiogenic osmoles presumably are present in brain cells. Consequently, overly rapid rehydration and lowering of the serum sodium concentration causes brain cells to swell [56,70].

Rapid correction of acute (onset <24 hours) hypernatremia is better tolerated by the patient, because idiogenic osmoles are not yet present in brain cells [14,56].

Clinical Signs

The clinical signs of hypernatremia depend on the cause. Hypertonic encephalopathy causes brain hemorrhages and signs that include lethargy, confusion or coma, seizures, muscle weakness, myoclonus, and low-grade fever [56,70]. There are no ECG abnormalities associated with hypernatremia. Urine volume is decreased and specific gravity is increased, except when hypernatremia is attributable to hypotonic urine losses (eg, diabetes insipidus) and solvent drag accompanying osmotic diuresis. Intravascular volume overload can occur when concentrated saline solutions are given too rapidly intravenously.

Differential Diagnosis

The differential diagnosis includes various causes of metabolic encephalopathy (see the section on hyponatremia) and diffuse cerebral cortical disease.

Treatment

Treatment entails correcting the underlying cause and providing low-solute–containing or solute-free fluid. If the hypernatremia is mild (<160 mEq/L), water can be given orally if the clinical circumstances permit. In more severe cases in which the patient is hypovolemic, isotonic solutions should be administered initially. After hypotension is corrected, 5% dextrose in water or 2.5% dextrose in 0.45% saline should be given intravenously to correct the water deficit. The following formula can be used to estimate the water deficit: The water deficit is equal to

$$\left[TBW \times \left(\frac{Serum\ Na^+}{140} \right) - 1 \right] \tag{3}$$

where TBW is total body water ($0.6 \times$ body weight [kg]).

To avoid potentially detrimental effects to the brain from osmotic dysequilibrium, it is best to replace the patient's water deficits slowly over a 48- to 72-hour period. After first correcting any hypovolemia and dehydration, the rate of change in serum sodium concentration should not exceed 0.5 mEq/L/h and not exceed a total of 12 mEq over the first 24 hours. This recommendation applies to chronic-onset hypernatremia, in which the increase in serum sodium concentration has occurred over a period exceeding 24 hours [14,56,70].

HYPOCALCEMIA

Hypocalcemia usually is defined as a total serum calcium concentration of less than 8 mg/dL in dogs and less than 7.0 mg/dL in cats. Clinical signs usually do not occur until the total serum calcium concentration is less than 6.5 mg/dL. In terms of ionized calcium concentration, hypocalcemia occurs at concentrations less than 1.25 mmol/L in dogs and less than 1.1 mmol/L in cats [71,72].

Etiology

Hypocalcemia in dogs and cats can be attributable to hypoparathyroidism, hypoproteinemia [73], vitamin D deficiency, hyperphosphatemia [74–76], malabsorption, acute pancreatitis [77], or chronic renal disease. Postparturient hypocalcemic tetany commonly occurs in small-breed dogs, but it can also occur in cats and large-breed dogs as well [78,79]. Prepartum eclampsia can also occur [75]. Primary hypoparathyroidism can affect dogs and cats [71,72,80–84].

Pathophysiology

In dogs, normal ionized calcium concentrations are 4.5 to 6.0 mg/dL or 1.25 to 1.45 mmol/L [71,72]. Serious physiologic effects usually do not occur until ionized calcium concentrations are less than 1 to 2 mmol/L. In cats, normal ionized calcium concentrations are 4.6 to 5.4 mg/dL (1.15–1.35 mmol/L). The severity of the signs depends greatly on the rapidity of the decrease in calcium concentration, and rapid decreases lead to more substantial pathophysiologic changes. As serum calcium concentrations decrease, neuronal membranes become increasingly more permeable to sodium, enhancing excitation. Potassium and magnesium ions have an antagonistic effect on this excitation. Decreased ionized calcium concentrations decrease the strength of myocardial contraction primarily by inhibiting relaxation.

Signs

Clinical signs are primarily attributable to neuromuscular irritability [70–72]. Tetany is the major clinical sign, but there are other possible signs, including seizures, mental irritability, muscle weakness, mental depression, and anxiety. The electrocardiogram usually is normal but can demonstrate a prolonged QT interval. Hyperkalemia and hypomagnesemia potentiate the cardiac and neuromuscular irritability of hypocalcemia.

Diagnosis

In acute hypocalcemic conditions, such as eclampsia or acute hyperphosphatemia, the cause usually is obvious and seldom requires a diagnostic medical workup. Primary hypoparathyroidism can be diagnosed by radioimmunoassay to determine plasma parathyroid hormone (PTH) concentration.

Treatment

Symptomatic acute hypocalcemia is a medical emergency that requires immediate administration of 10% calcium gluconate solution [71,72]. A safe dosage for dogs and cats is 1.0 to1.5 mL/kg given slowly intravenously over a 20- to 30-minute period. Heart rate should be monitored periodically. If bradycardia occurs, the calcium infusion must be discontinued until a normal cardiac rate and rhythm ensue. Maintenance treatment for hypocalcemia is provided with 10% calcium gluconate solution at a dosage of 5 to 10 mL/kg given slowly intravenously in lactated Ringer's solution or isotonic (0.9%) sodium chloride maintenance infusions over a 24-hour period or at a dosage of 2 mL/kg given intravenously over a 6- to 8-hour period and repeated as necessary. Calcium gluconate solution should not be given subcutaneously because it can cause severe inflammatory calcinosis cutis [85]. Repeated determinations of serum calcium concentrations are essential to avoid iatrogenic hypercalcemia. Calcium solutions should not be added to bicarbonate-containing solutions so as to avoid precipitation of calcium carbonate.

For emergency treatment of eclampsia in a small animal weighing less than 10 kg when no laboratory facilities are available, 10% calcium gluconate at a dose of 1 mL can be given intravenously, immediately followed by additional 0.5-mL doses administered intravenously every 30 seconds. This treatment is discontinued when the tetanic contractions cease or the patient vomits. After treatment of eclampsia in bitches, the puppies should be weaned and begun on an orphan feeding program. Returning them to the bitch for continued nursing may cause relapsing hypocalcemia.

The use of oral vitamin D and its analogues is not covered in this section because they are more commonly used for the treatment of chronic hypocalcemia [71,72].

HYPERCALCEMIA

Definition

Hypercalcemia in dogs occurs when the total serum calcium concentration exceeds 12 mg/dL or the ionized calcium concentration exceeds 1.45 mmol/L. In cats, hypercalcemia occurs when the total serum calcium concentration exceeds 11 mg/dL (1.4 mmol/L) [71,72].

Etiologies

In dogs, the most frequent causes of hypercalcemia include primary hyperparathyroidism [72] and hypercalcemia of malignancy, with the latter being most common [72,86–98]. Osteolytic metastasis of malignant neoplasms, renal-associated hyperparathyroidism [97], and granulomatous diseases also can cause hypercalcemia [99–104]. Minor increases in serum calcium concentration can occur in patients that have Addison's disease [72], but this is of no clinical relevance and is easily rectified with fluid therapy. Other possible causes include hypervitaminosis D, day-blooming jessamine ingestion, antipsoriasis creams (eg, calcipotriol, calcipotriene) [105,106], grape ingestion [107], and the newer cholecalciferol-containing rodenticides [108–111].

In the cat, the most frequent cause is hypercalcemia of malignancy, but primary hyperparathyroidism also can occur. In addition, cats can develop an idiopathic hypercalcemia [112].

Hypercalcemia can have adverse effects on the neuromuscular, cardiovascular, gastrointestinal, renal, and skeletal systems, and these are described elsewhere [71,72].

Signs

The patient that has long-term or marked (>15 mg/dL) hypercalcemia can show anorexia, nausea, vomiting, weakness, abdominal pain, constipation, polyuria, polydipsia, dehydration, or depression.

Diagnosis

The initial medical workup should be extensive if the history does not provide an obvious cause for hypercalcemia, such as vitamin D overdose or ongoing chronic renal insufficiency causing secondary hyperparathyroidism. The medical evaluation should include serum concentrations of calcium, phosphorus, sodium, potassium, chloride, creatinine, urea nitrogen, alkaline phosphatase, and proteins. A complete urinalysis, hemogram, chest and abdominal radiographs, and abdominal or cervical ultrasonograms [113] also should be performed. Further evaluation might require renal creatinine and phosphate clearance determinations and radioimmunoassay determinations of PTH, vitamin D, and parathyroid hormone–related peptide (PTH-rp) [114–118]. A bone marrow aspirate and biopsy are indicated for suspected myelophthisic disease. Paraneoplastic syndromes can cause increased plasma concentrations of PTH-rp. The initial objectives are to stabilize the patient while determining the cause of the hypercalcemia. When all extraparathyroid causes of hypercalcemia are eliminated, the primary focus should be on the parathyroid glands. The cardinal diagnostic features of primary hyperparathyroidism are inappropriately increased PTH concentrations in the face of hypercalcemia. A normal PTH concentration in an animal with hypercalcemia is inappropriate [72]. PTH concentrations should be low and PTH-rp increased in hypercalcemia of malignancy [72].

Treatment

The four management objectives include (1) correct dehydration, (2) promote calciuresis, (3) inhibit accelerated bone resorption, and (4) treat the underlying disorder. Even when the cause of hypercalcemia turns out to be a surgical disorder, the following medical guidelines should be followed to normalize serum calcium concentration as quickly as possible.

1. Saline infusion. Because hypercalcemia is a medical emergency, treatment must not be delayed while the cause is being determined. The most important therapeutic measure is to rehydrate the patient [72,119]. Because urinary calcium excretion is enhanced by saline infusion and because 0.9% sodium

competitively inhibits renal tubular reabsorption of calcium, isotonic sodium chloride solution administered intravenously is the fluid of choice. The infusion rate should be rapid enough to produce intense diuresis, but care must be taken to avoid plasma volume overload. If possible, central venous pressure (CVP) measurements should be taken intermittently and the infusion slowed down or discontinued when the CVP is greater than 10 cm H_2O. Once the plasma space is adequately volume expanded, as evidenced by euhydration and normal capillary refill time (<2 seconds), repeated injections of furosemide can be given intravenously to enhance the diuresis. If fluid tolerance is not a major concern, furosemide should not be used. It should be held in reserve in case signs of fluid overload become apparent. Serum electrolytes must be monitored and supplemented (especially potassium) accordingly. Progressive hypernatremia (>158 mEq/L) warrants discontinuing the saline infusion.

2. Glucocorticoids are particularly beneficial when treating hypercalcemia associated with lymphoma or other malignant tumors associated with a paraneoplastic syndrome [72,120]. When lymphoma is suspected, it is best to obtain a tissue diagnosis before corticosteroid administration. The actions of glucocorticoids in inhibiting the growth of neoplastic lymphoid tissue account for their beneficial effects in treating patients that have hematologic cancers, such as lymphoma and multiple myeloma. Glucocorticoids also help to lower serum calcium concentration by decreasing bone resorption, decreasing intestinal calcium absorption, and increasing calcium excretion. In general, patients that have nonhematologic cancers do not respond well to glucocorticoids, nor do those with primary hyperparathyroidism. By counteracting the effect of vitamin D, glucocorticoids are efficacious in treating hypercalcemia caused by hypervitaminosis D. They may be particularly useful for the treatment of cholecalciferol rodenticide intoxication, granulomatous disease, and idiopathic hypercalcemia in cats.

3. Other therapeutic measures for hypercalcemia include mithramycin (plicamycin) [121], calcitonin, and bisphosphonates (eg, etidronate disodium, pamidronate) [119,122–126]. The use of these agents must be given with patient monitoring. The bisphosphonates bind to hydroxyapatite in bone and inhibit dissolution of bone crystal. They act by inhibiting osteoclast function and viability. The absorption of the earlier bisphosphonate products from the gastrointestinal tract was poor, making intravenous administration the preferred route for therapy. There are currently several products available for oral use, including alendronate, etidronate, and tiludronate. Dosages vary because of potency variations among the various products. Experience with this class of drugs is limited in veterinary patients. Gastrointestinal adverse effects, especially esophagitis, occur commonly in human patients. Pamidronate is a bisphosphonate that is currently available in the United States for parenteral use. The recommended dosage of pamidronate in dogs is 1.2 to 2.0 mg/kg administered intravenously mixed in saline and given over 2 hours. It has been used effectively to treat hypervitaminosis D intoxication. Mithramycin, an inhibitor of RNA synthesis in osteoclasts, is an effective treatment for hypercalcemia at an dosage of 25 μg/kg of body weight administered intravenously over a period of 4 to 6 hours. A single dose often is sufficient for restoring normocalcemia. Serum calcium

concentration begins to decrease as early as 12 hours after administration of the drug, and its effect can last from a few days to several weeks. Side effects (eg, hepatotoxicity, nephrotoxicity, thrombocytopenia) are unlikely when only a single dose is used, but this drug should always be used with extreme caution. Calcitonin inhibits bone resorption by inhibiting the activity and formation of osteoclasts [119]. It usually is administered subcutaneously or intramuscularly at a dosage of 4 to 8 U/kg every 8 hours. Calcitonin is the most rapidly acting hypocalcemic agent, causing the serum calcium concentration to decrease within a few hours after its administration. The nadir of the serum calcium concentration is reached within 12 to 24 hours. Its effect is rather transient, and the maximum reduction in serum calcium concentration is not as large as that seen with the bisphosphonates and mithramycin. Sodium bicarbonate has been used in the crisis management of hypercalcemia [72]. It is theoretically best used in patients that have coexisting metabolic acidosis, because acidosis increases ionized calcium concentration and bicarbonate lowers it. A dose of 1 to 4 mEq/kg has been recommended. The reduction in total serum calcium concentration is slight. Sodium bicarbonate is most likely to help when combined with other treatments.

4. Surgical excision of the parathyroid tumor or any hyperplastic parathyroid tissue is the preferred treatment for primary hyperparathyroidism [127]. Other techniques for treatment include ethanol injection and guided radio-frequency heat ablation [128–130]. Because the uninvolved parathyroid glands are atrophied as a result of the negative feedback effects from hypercalcemia, postoperative hypocalcemia should be anticipated as a potentially life-threatening complication. Hypocalcemia can occur several hours after parathyroid tumor removal and must be counteracted by slowly infusing 10% calcium gluconate at a dosage of 2 mL/kg given intravenously every 6 hours immediately after surgery (see section on hypocalcemia treatment). This infusion should be titrated according to need during the subsequent postoperative days. Dihydrotachysterol treatment might also be required for several days to weeks after surgery to maintain low normal serum calcium concentrations. The dosage is titrated to effect according to the results of periodic determinations of serum calcium concentration.

References

[1] DiBartola SP. Hypokalemia and hyperkalemia. In: DiBartola SP, editor. Fluid, electrolytes, and acid-base disorders. 3rd edition. St. Louis: Saunders-Elsevier; 2006. p. 91–121.

[2] Boag AK, Coe RJ, Martinez TA, et al. Acid-base and electrolyte abnormalities in dogs with gastrointestinal foreign bodies. J Vet Intern Med 2005;19:816–21.

[3] Nardone DA, McDonald WJ, Girard DE. Mechanisms in hypokalemia: clinical correlation. Medicine (Baltimore) 1978;57(5):435–46.

[4] Knochel JP. Diuretic-induced hypokalemia. Am J Med 1984;77(5A):18–27.

[5] Gennari FJ. Current concepts: hypokalemia. N Engl J Med 1998;339(7):451–8.

[6] Dow SW, Fettman MJ, LeCouteur RA, et al. Potassium depletion in cats: renal and dietary influences. J Am Vet Med Assoc 1987;191(12):1569–74.

[7] Brown RS. Potassium homeostasis and clinical implications. Am J Med 1984;77(5A):3–10.

[8] Dow SW, LeCouteur RA, Fettman MJ, et al. Potassium depletion in cats: hypokalemic polymyopathy. J Am Vet Med Assoc 1987;191(12):1563–8.

[9] Harrington ML, Bagley RL, Braund KG. Suspect hypokalemic myopathy in a dog. Progress in Veterinary Neurology 1996;7(4):130–2.

[10] Adrogue HJ, Madias NE. Changes in plasma potassium concentration during acute acid-base disturbances. Am J Med 1981;71:456–67.

[11] Fitzovich DE, Hamaguchi M, Tull WB, et al. Chronic hypokalemia and the left ventricular responses to epinephrine and preload. J Am Coll Cardiol 1991;18(4): 1105–11.

[12] Diercks DB, Shumaik GM, Harrigan RA, et al. Electrocardiographic manifestations: electrolyte abnormalities. J Emerg Med 2004;27(2):153–60.

[13] Theisen SK, DiBartola SP, Radin MJ, et al. Muscle potassium content and potassium gluconate supplementation in normokalemic cats with naturally occurring chronic renal failure. J Vet Intern Med 1997;11(4):212–7.

[14] Londner M, Hammer D, Kelen GD. Fluid and electrolyte problems. In: Tintinalli JE, Kalen GD, Stapezynski SS, editors. Emergency medicine—a comprehensive study guide. 6th edition. New York: McGraw-Hill; 2004. p. 167–79.

[15] Henry CJ, Lanevschi A, Marks SL, et al. Acute lymphoblastic leukemia, hypercalcemia, and pseudohyperkalemia in a dog. J Am Vet Med Assoc 1996;208(2):237–9.

[16] Degen M. Pseudohyperkalemia in Akitas. J Am Vet Med Assoc 1987;190(5):541–3.

[17] Dhein CR, Wardrop KJ. Hyperkalemia associated with potassium chloride administration in a cat. J Am Vet Med Assoc 1995;206(10):1565–6.

[18] Alappan R, Perazella MA, Buller GK. Hyperkalemia in hospitalized patients treated with trimethoprim-sulfamethoxazole. Ann Intern Med 1996;124(3):316–20.

[19] Williams ME, Gervino EV, Rosa RM, et al. Catecholamine modulation of rapid potassium shifts during exercise. N Engl J Med 1985;312(13):823–7.

[20] Greenberg S, Reiser IW, Chou S-Y, et al. Trimethoprim-sulfamethoxazole induces reversible hyperkalemia. Ann Intern Med 1993;110:291–5.

[21] Schepkens H, Vanholder R, Billiouw J-M, et al. Life-threatening hyperkalemia during combined therapy with angiotensin-converting enzyme inhibitors and spironolactone: an analysis of 25 cases. Am J Med 2001;110:438–41.

[22] Perazella MA. Drug-induced hyperkalemia: old culprits and new offenders. Am J Med 2000;109:307–14.

[23] Palmer BF. Managing hyperkalemia caused by inhibitors of the renin-angiotensin-aldosterone system. N Engl J Med 2004;351:585–92.

[24] Lee JA, Drobatz KJ. Characterization of the clinical characteristics, electrolytes, acid-base, and renal parameters in male cats with urethral obstruction. Journal of Veterinary Emergency and Critical Care 2003;13(4):227–33.

[25] Ettinger PO, Regan TJ, Oldewurtel HA. Hyperkalemia, cardiac conduction, and the electrocardiogram: a review. Am Heart J 1974;88(3):360–71.

[26] Schaer M. Hyperkalemia and hypernatremia. In: Ettinger ST, editor. Textbook of veterinary internal medicine. 4th edition. Philadelphia: WB Saunders; 1994. p. 46–9.

[27] Hiatt N, Yamakawa T, Davidson MB. Necessity for insulin in transfer of excess infused K to intracellular fluid. Metabolism 1974;23(1):43–9.

[28] Blumberg A, Weidmann P, Shaw S, et al. Effect of various therapeutic approaches on plasma potassium and major regulating factors in terminal renal failure. Am J Med 1988;85:507–12.

[29] Cox M, Sterns RH, Singer I. The defense against hyperkalemia: the roles of insulin and aldosterone. N Engl J Med 1978;299(10):525–32.

[30] Hiatt N, Morgenstern L, Davidson MB, et al. Role of insulin in the transfer of infused potassium to tissue. Horm Metab Res 1973;5:84–8.

[31] DeFronzo RA, Smith D. Clinical disorders of hyperkalemia. In: Narins RC, editor. Maxwell and Kleeman's clinical disorders of fluid and electrolyte metabolism. 5th edition. New York: McGraw-Hill; 1994. p. 697–754.

[32] Sterns RH, Ocdol H, Schrier RW, et al. Hyponatremia: pathophysiology, diagnosis, and therapy. In: Narins RG, editor. Maxwell and Kleeman's clinical disorders of fluid and electrolyte metabolism. 5th edition. New York: McGraw-Hill; 1994. p. 697–954.

[33] Anderson RJ, Chung H-M, Kluge R, et al. Hyponatremia: a prospective analysis of its epidemiology and the pathogenetic role of vasopressin. Ann Intern Med 1985;102: 164–8.

[34] Cadnapaphornchai MA, Schrier RW. Pathogenesis and management of hyponatremia. Am J Med 2000;109:688–92.

[35] Cluitmans FHM, Meinders AE. Management of severe hyponatremia—rapid or slow correction. Am J Med 1990;88:161–6.

[36] Hsu Y-J, Chiu J-S, Lu K-C, et al. Biochemical and etiological characteristic of acute hyponatremia in the emergency department. J Emerg Med 2005;29(4):369–74.

[37] Schaer M, Halling KB, Collins KE, et al. Combined hyponatremia and hyperkalemia mimicking acute hypoadrenocorticism in three pregnant dogs. J Am Vet Med Assoc 2001;218(6):897–9.

[38] Willard MD, Fossum TW, Torrance A, et al. Hyponatremia and hyperkalemia associated with idiopathic or experimentally induced chylothorax in four dogs. J Am Vet Med Assoc 1991;199(3):353–8.

[39] Beck LH, Lavizzo-Mouray R. Geriatric hyponatremia. Ann Intern Med 1987;107(5): 768–9.

[40] Steele A, Gowrishankar M, Abrahamson S, et al. Postoperative hyponatremia despite near-isotonic saline infusion: a phenomenon of desalination. Ann Intern Med 1997;126:20–5.

[41] Toll J, Barr SC, Hickford FH. Acute water intoxication in a dog. J Vet Emerg Crit Care 1999;9(1):19–24.

[42] Jacobson S, Kiechle FL. Stat lab rounds—when a low sodium is not hyponatremia. Emerg Med 1982;14:159–63.

[43] Lipschutz JH, Arieff AI. Reset osmostat in a healthy patient. Ann Intern Med 1994;120(7): 574–6.

[44] Fraser CL, Arieff AI. Epidemiology, pathophysiology, and management of hyponatremic encephalopathy. Am J Med 1997;102:67–77.

[45] Laureno R. Central pontine myelinolysis following rapid correction of hyponatremia. Ann Neurol 1983;13(5):232–42.

[46] Tien R, Kucharczyk W, Kucharczyk J. Hyponatremic encephalopathy: is central pontine myelinolysis a component? Am J Med 1992;92:513–22.

[47] Laureno R, Karp BI. Myelinolysis after correction of hyponatremia. Ann Intern Med 1997;126(1):57–62.

[48] Arieff AI. Hyponatremia, convulsions, respiratory arrest, and permanent brain damage after elective surgery in healthy women. N Engl J Med 1986;314(24):1529–35.

[49] Sterns RH, Riggs JE, Schochet SS Jr, et al. Osmotic demyelination syndrome following correction of hyponatremia. N Engl J Med 1986;314:1535–42.

[50] Lohr JW. Osmotic demyelination syndrome following correction of hyponatremia: association with hypokalemia. Am J Med 1994;96:408–13.

[51] O'Brien DP, Kroll RA, Johnson GC, et al. Myelinolysis after correction of hyponatremia in two dogs. J Vet Intern Med 1994;8(1):40–8.

[52] Churcher RK, Wason ADJ, Eaton A. Suspected myelinolysis following rapid correction of hyponatremia in a dog. J Am Anim Hosp Assoc 1999;35:492–7.

[53] Ayus JC, Wheeler JM, Arieff AI. Postoperative hyponatremic encephalopathy in menstruant women. Ann Intern Med 1992;117:891–7.

[54] Androgué HJ, Madias NE. Hyponatremia. N Engl J Med 2000;342(21):1581–9.

[55] Ellison DH, Berl T. The syndrome of inappropriate antidiuresis. N Engl J Med 2007;356(20):2064–72.

[56] Androgué HJ, Madias NE. Hypernatremia. N Engl J Med 2000;342(20):1493–9.

[57] Palevsky PM, Bhagrath R, Greenberg A. Hypernatremia in hospitalized patients. Ann Intern Med 1996;124(2):197–203.
[58] Marks SL, Taboada J. Hypernatremia and hypertonic syndromes. Vet Clin North Am Small Anim Pract 1998;28(3):533–44.
[59] Sullivan SA, Harmon BG, Purinton PT, et al. Lobar holoprosencephaly in a Miniature Schnauzer with hypodipsic hypernatremia. J Am Vet Med Assoc 2003;223(12):1783–7.
[60] Hawks D, Giger U, Miselis R, et al. Essential hypernatremia in a young dog. J Small Anim Pract 1991;32:420–4.
[61] DiBartola SP, Johnson SE, Johnson GC, et al. Hypodipsic hypernatremia in a dog with defective osmoregulation of antidiuretic hormone. JAVMA 1994;204(6):922–5.
[62] Dow SW, Fettman MJ, LeCouteur RA, et al. Hypodipsic hypernatremia and associated myopathy in a hydrocephalic cat with transient hypopituitarism. J Am Vet Med Assoc 1987;191(2):217–21.
[63] Holloway S, Schaer M. Challenging cases in internal medicine: what's your diagnosis? Vet Med 1990;85(10):1064–74.
[64] DeRubertia FR, Michelis MF, Davis BB. "Essential" hypernatremia. Report of three cases and review of the literature. Arch Intern Med 1974;134:889–95.
[65] Crawford MA, Kittleson MD, Fink GD. Hypernatremia and adipsia in a dog. J Am Vet Med Assoc 1984;184(7):818–21.
[66] Reidarson TH, Weis DJ, Hardy RM. Extreme hypernatremia in a dog with central diabetes insipidus: a case report. J Am Anim Hosp Assoc 1990;26:89–92.
[67] Khanna C, Boermans HJ, Wilcock B. Fatal hypernatremia in a dog from salt ingestion. J Am Anim Hosp Assoc 1997;33:113–7.
[68] Hammond DN, Moll GW, Robertson GL, et al. Hypodipsic hypernatremia with normal osmoregulation of vasopressin. N Engl J Med 1986;315(7):433–6.
[69] Miler PD, Krebs RA, Neal BJ, et al. Hypodipsia in geriatric patients. Am J Med 1982;73: 354–6.
[70] Morrison G, Singer I. Hyperosmolal states. In: Narins RG, editor. Maxwell and Kleeman's clinical disorders of fluid and electrolyte metabolism. 5th edition. New York: McGraw-Hill; 1994. p. 617–58.
[71] Dhupa N, Proulx J. Hypocalcemia and hypomagnesemia. Vet Clin North Am 1998;28(3): 587–608.
[72] Schenck PA, Chew DJ, Nagode LA, et al. Disorder of calcium: hypercalcemia and hypocalcemia. In: DiBartola SP, editor. Fluid, electrolyte and acid-base disorders in small animal practice. 3rd edition. St. Louis: Saunders-Elsevier; 2006. p. 122–94.
[73] Meuten DJ, Chew DJ, Capen CC, et al. Relationship of serum total calcium to albumin and total protein in dogs. J Am Vet Med Assoc 1982;180(1):63–7.
[74] Biberstein M, Parker BA. Enema-induced hyperphosphatemia. Am J Med 1985;79: 645–6.
[75] Jorgensen LS, Center SA, Randolph JF, et al. Electrolyte abnormalities induced by hypertonic phosphate enemas in two cats. J Am Vet Med Assoc 1985;187(12):1367–8.
[76] Levitt M, Gessert C, Finberg L. Inorganic phosphate (laxative) poisoning resulting in tetany in an infant. J Pediatr 1973;82(1):479–81.
[77] Wills TB, Bohn AA, Martin LG. Hypocalcemia in a critically ill patient. J Vet Emerg Crit Care 2005;15(2):136–42.
[78] Drobatz DJ, Casey KK. Eclampsia in dogs: 31 cases (1995–1998). J Am Vet Med Assoc 2000;217(2):216–9.
[79] Fascetti AJ, Hickman MA. Preparturient hypocalcemia in four cats. J Am Vet Med Assoc 1999;215(8):1127–9.
[80] Peterson ME, James KM, Wallace M, et al. Idiopathic hypoparathyroidism in five cats. J Vet Intern Med 1991;5:47–51.
[81] Peterson ME. Treatment of canine and feline hypoparathyroidism. J Am Vet Med Assoc 1982;181(11):1434–6.

[82] Bassett JR. Hypocalcemia and hyperphosphatemia due to primary hypoparathyroidism in a six-month-old kitten. J Am Anim Hosp Assoc 1998;34:503–7.

[83] Bruyette DS, Feldman EC. Primary hypoparathyroidism in the dog. Report of 15 cases and review of 13 previously reported case. J Vet Intern Med 1988;2:7–14.

[84] Sherding RG, Meuten DJ, Chew DJ, et al. Primary hypoparathyroidism in the dog. J Am Vet Med Assoc 1980;176(5):439–44.

[85] Schaer M, Ginn PE, Fox LE, et al. Severe calcicosis cutis associated with treatment of hypoparathyroidism in a dog. J Am Anim Hosp Assoc 2001;37:364–9.

[86] Ralston SH, Gallacher SJ, Patel U, et al. Cancer-associated hypercalcemia: morbidity and mortality. Clinical experience in 126 treated patients. Ann Intern Med 1990;112: 499–504.

[87] Klausner JS, Bell FW, Hayden DW, et al. Hypercalcemia in two cats with squamous cell carcinomas. J Am Vet Med Assoc 1990;196(1):103–5.

[88] Weir EC, Norrdin RW, Matus RE, et al. Humoral hypercalcemia of malignancy in canine lymphosarcoma. Endocrinology 1988;122:602–8.

[89] Ross JT, Scavelli TD, Matthiesen DT, et al. Adenocarcinoma of the apocrine glands of the anal sac in dogs: a review of 32 cases. J Am Anim Hosp Assoc 1991;27:349–55.

[90] Osborne CA, Stevens JB. Pseudohyperparathyroidism in the dog. J Am Vet Med Assoc 1973;162(2):125–34.

[91] Breslau NA, McGuire JL, Zerwekh JE, et al. Hypercalcemia associated with increased serum calcitriol levels in three patients with lymphoma. Ann Intern Med 1984;100(1):1–7.

[92] Grain E Jr, Walder EJ. Hypercalcemia associated with squamous cell carcinoma in a dog. J Am Vet Med Assoc 1982;181(2):165–6.

[93] Nafe LA, Patnaik AK, Lyman R. Hypercalcemia associated with epidermoid carcinoma in a dog. J Am Vet Med Assoc 1980;176(11):1253–4.

[94] Wilson RB, Bronstad DC. Hypercalcemia associated with nasal adenocarcinoma in a dog. J Am Vet Med Assoc 1983;182(11):1246–7.

[95] Sheafor SE, Gamblin RM, Couto CG. Hypercalcemia in two cats with multiple myeloma. J Am Anim Hosp Assoc 1996;32:503–8.

[96] Savary KCM, Price GS, Vaden SL. Hypercalcemia in cats: a retrospective study of 71 cases (1991–1997). J Vet Intern Med 2000;14:184–9.

[97] Pressler BM, Rotstein DS, Law JM, et al. Hypercalcemia and high parathyroid hormone-related protein concentration associated with malignant melanoma in a dog. J Am Vet Med Assoc 2002;221(2):263–5.

[98] Marx SJ. Hyperparathyroid and hypoparathyroid disorders. N Engl J Med 2000;343(25): 1863–75.

[99] Gkonos PJ, London R, Hendler ED. Hypercalcemia and elevated 1,25-dihydroxyvitamin D levels in a patient with end-stage renal disease and active tuberculosis. N Engl J Med 311(26):1683–5.

[100] Fradkin JM, Braniecki AM, Craig TM, et al. Elevated parathyroid hormone-related protein with hypercalcemia in two dogs with schistosomiasis. J Am Anim Hosp Assoc 2001;37:349–55.

[101] Leman J Jr, Gray RW. Calcitriol, calcium and granulomatous disease. N Engl J Med 1984;311(17):111–6.

[102] Murray JJ, Heim CR. Hypercalcemia in disseminated histoplasmosis. Aggravation by vitamin D. Am J Med 1985;78:881–4.

[103] Parker MS, Dokoh S, Woolfenden JM, et al. Hypercalcemia in coccidioidomycosis. Am J Med 1984;76:341–4.

[104] Mealey KL, Willard MD, Nagode LA, et al. Hypercalcemia associated with granuloma-tous disease in a cat. J Am Vet Med Assoc 1999;215(7):959–62.

[105] Pesillo SA, Khan SA, Rozanski EA, et al. Calcipotriene toxicosis in a dog successfully treated with pamidronate disodium. J Vet Emerg Crit Care 2002;12(3):177–81.

[106] Fan TM, Simpson KW, Trasti S, et al. Calcipotriol activity in a dog. J Small Anim Pract 1998;39:581–6.

[107] Mazzaferro EM, Eubig PA, Hackett TB, et al. Acute renal failure associated with raisin or grape ingestion in 4 dogs. J Vet Emerg Crit Care 2004;14(3):203–12.

[108] Fooshee SK, Forrester SD. Hypercalcemia secondary to cholecalciferol rodenticide toxicosis in two dogs. J Am Vet Med Assoc 1990;196(8):1265–8.

[109] Moore FM, Kudisch M, Richter K, et al. Hypercalcemia associated with rodenticide poisoning in three cats. J Am Vet Med Assoc 1988;193(9):1099–100.

[110] Gunther R, Felice LJ, Nelson RK, et al. Toxicity of a vitamin D_3 rodenticide to dogs. J Am Vet Med Assoc 1988;193(2):211–4.

[111] Dougherty SA, Center SA, Dzanis DA. Salmon calcitonin as adjunct treatment for vitamin D toxicosis in a dog. J Am Vet Med Assoc 1990;196(8):1269–72.

[112] Midkiff AM, Chew DJ, Randolph JF, et al. Idiopathic hypercalcemia in cats. J Vet Intern Med 2000;14:619–26.

[113] Wisner ER, Nyland TG, Feldman EC, et al. Ultrasonographic evaluation of the parathyroid glands in hypercalcemic dogs. Vet Radiol Ultrasound 1993;34(2):108–11.

[114] Mundy GR, Guise TA. Hypercalcemia of malignancy. Am J Med 1997;103:134–45.

[115] Kremer R, Shustik C, Tabak T, et al. Parathyroid-hormone-related peptide in hematologic malignancies. Am J Med 1996;100:406–10.

[116] Broadus AE, Mangin M, Ikeda K, et al. Humoral hypercalcemia of cancer. Identification of a novel parathyroid hormone-like peptide. N Engl J Med 1988;319(9):556–63.

[117] Budayr AA, Nissenson RA, Klein RF, et al. Increased serum levels of a parathyroid hormone-like protein in malignancy-associated hypercalcemia. Ann Intern Med 1989;111:807–12.

[118] Strewler GJ. The physiology of parathyroid hormone-related protein. N Engl J Med 2000;342(3):177–84.

[119] Bilezikian JP. Management of acute hypercalcemia. N Engl J Med 1992;326(18): 1196–203.

[120] Binstock ML, Mundy GR. Effect of calcitonin and glucocorticoids in combination on the hypercalcemia of malignancy. Ann Intern Med 1980;93:269–72.

[121] Rosol TJ, Chew DJ, Hammer AS, et al. Effect of mithramycin on hypercalcemia in dogs. J Am Anim Hosp Assoc 1994;30:244–50.

[122] Hostutler RA, Chew DJ, Jaeger JQ, et al. Uses and effectiveness of pamidronate disodium for treatment of dogs and cats with hypercalcemia. J Vet Intern Med 2005;19:29–33.

[123] Fan TM, de Lorimier L-P, Charney SC, et al. Evaluation of intravenous pamidronate administration in 33 cancer-bearing dogs with primary or secondary bone involvement. J Vet Intern Med 2005;19:74–80.

[124] Milner RJ, Farese J, Henry CJ, et al. Bisphosphonates and cancer. J Vet Intern Med 2004;18:597–604.

[125] Mundy GR, Ibbotson DJ, D'Souza SM, et al. The hypercalcemia of cancer. Clinical implications and pathogenic mechanisms. N Engl J Med 1984;310(26):1718–26.

[126] Nussbaum SR, Younger J, VandePol CJ, et al. Single-dose intravenous therapy with pamidronate for the treatment of hypercalcemia of malignancy: comparison of 30-, 60-, and 90-mg dosages. Am J Med 1993;95:297–304.

[127] Berger B, Feldman EC. Primary hyperparathyroidism in dogs: 21 cases (1976–1986). J Am Vet Med Assoc 1987;191(3):350–6.

[128] Pollard RE, Long CD, Nelson RW, et al. Percutaneous ultrasonographically guided radiofrequency heat ablation for treatment of primary hyperparathyroidism in dogs. J Am Vet Med Assoc 2001;218:1106–10.

[129] Long CD, Goldstein RE, Hornof WJ, et al. Percutaneous ultrasound-guided chemical parathyroid ablation for treatment of primary hyperparathyroidism in dogs. J Am Vet Med Assoc 1999;215(2):217–21.

[130] Rasor L, Pollard R, Feldman EC. Retrospective evaluation of three treatment methods for primary hyperparathyroidism in dogs. J Am Anim Hosp Assoc 2007;43:70–7.

Therapeutic Approach to Chronic Electrolyte Disorders

Michael Willard, DVM, MS

College of Veterinary Medicine, Texas A&M University, College Station, TX 77843-4474, USA

The first and foremost consideration in treating chronic electrolyte disorders is to find the underlying cause and resolve it. This article focuses on the therapeutic approach to patients with chronic electrolyte aberrations that have not yet been diagnosed, that need therapy while being diagnosed, or that remain undiagnosed after an appropriate diagnostic effort. The frequency of the disorder and the need for treatment are considered for each electrolyte disorder.

SODIUM

Hypernatremia tends to be seen in patients receiving inappropriate fluid therapy or those that have excessive free water loss. Comatose patients that are receiving inadequate water and those with gastrointestinal or renal losses that are not receiving enough fluids or improper fluids are typical examples of such patients [1]. The occasional dog with severe diuresis (eg, diabetes insipidus) is hypernatremic, as is the pet with primary hyperaldosteronism (a rare disorder in dogs and cats). A major cause of chronic hypernatremia of sufficient magnitude to require protracted symptomatic treatment is hypodipsia [2,3]. Rarely, miniature schnauzers have a central nervous system (CNS) lesion that causes them to drink insufficient amounts of water [4]. Conceivably, patients with other neurologic diseases that have chronically had inadequate intake of water also have chronic hypernatremia [5–7].

Clinical signs of CNS dysfunction are a clinical concern when the serum sodium concentration approaches and exceeds 170 mEq/L [8,9]. Chronic hypernatremia of sufficient magnitude (ie, >165 mEq/L) to warrant therapy specifically directed at the electrolyte abnormality itself is relatively rare. When it is severe enough to treat (eg, hypodipsic schnauzers), therapy consists of administering free water. Free water can be supplied parenterally or enterally. If free water is supplied parenterally, 5% dextrose in water (by itself or combined in some proportion with lactated Ringer's or physiologic saline solution) is administered slowly. Calculating maintenance (44–66 mL/kg/d

E-mail address: mwillard@cvm.tamu.edu

0195-5616/08/$ – see front matter
doi:10.1016/j.cvsm.2008.01.013

depending on size) and deficit water requirements is relatively straightforward. Alternatively, one may calculate the free water deficit more precisely by using the formula: Water Deficit = Weight (kg) × {(current [Na]/previous [Na]) − 1}, where Na is sodium [1]. Estimating the need, administering fluids with free water, and then periodically rechecking the serum sodium concentration usually are adequate to achieve remission. One may administer 5% dextrose in water or 0.45% saline in 2.5% dextrose. If necessary, customized fluids may be designed by mixing lactated Ringer's solution and 5% dextrose in varying proportions.

It is crucial that the serum sodium concentration not be lowered too fast if the hypernatremia is chronic and severe. One should repeatedly measure serum sodium concentration while administering fluids to correct hypernatremia. "Chronic" in the context of hypernatremia can mean a sodium level greater than 165 mEq/L that persists for more than 2 to 3 days (as opposed to weeks, which is the definition of chronic for most other disorders). Patients with hypernatremia greater than 165 mEq/L for this long have had the brain adapt by increasing its osmolality [1]. If severe hypernatremia is corrected too fast, the brain does not have a chance to adjust its osmolality. The result can be severe cerebral edema that can be fatal. No work has been done in dogs and cats to determine exactly how fast one can safely lower serum sodium concentration in patients with severe hypernatremia into the normal range, but extrapolation from human medicine suggests that 48 hours is probably an appropriate length of time when correcting hypernatremia in such patients [1].

If the patient's condition is such that return of hypernatremia is expected as the result of a CNS disease that continues to cause hypodipsia, one should also plan on increasing daily water intake after the initial correction of the hypodipsia. One may place maintenance amounts of water into the food (ie, prepare a slurry). Alternatively, one also may give water by means of an esophagostomy tube.

In the rare case in which hypernatremia is attributable to retention of sodium in the body (eg, hyperaldosteronism) as opposed to loss of free water, one can administer drugs to increase loss of salt from the body. Diuretics (eg, furosemide, thiazides) should cause loss of sodium from the body and help to lessen concurrent hypertension, which typically is present.

Hyponatremia is probably more common than hypernatremia. There are more causes of hyponatremia, the causes are more common, and the causes tend to be chronic in nature (eg, hypervolemia associated with cirrhosis, congestive heart failure, nephrotic syndrome) [1]. Ascites attributable to any cause can be associated with hyponatremia, and this seems to be more of a problem in severe or rapidly developing ascites. It is important not to supplement sodium in these patients because they often are already hypervolemic and adding sodium worsens hypervolemia. Typically, hyponatremia in patients that are hypervolemic is ignored while the underlying problem is being treated.

Hyponatremia in hypoadrenal patients is caused by loss of salt from the body, and these patients need therapy (often on an emergent basis) consisting of parenteral administration of electrolyte solutions and hormone replacement.

Despite the fact that hypoadrenal patients often are severely dehydrated, incorrect fluid therapy can be detrimental [10]. As mentioned for hypernatremia, the speed with which the hyponatremia occurs and is corrected is more predictive of problems than is the magnitude of the hyponatremia. Also, as with hypernatremia, the term *chronic* does not mean that the serum sodium concentration has been low for 2 to 3 weeks. Rather, having a sodium concentration less than 125 mEq/L for 3 to 4 days qualifies as chronic. If the sodium concentration in a dog is 130 mEq/L or greater, there is minimal concern with how fast the serum sodium concentration is corrected. Patients with sodium concentrations less than 120 mEq/L, and especially those in which the serum sodium concentration is less than 115 mEq/L, are at risk for iatrogenic CNS disease, however. Correcting the sodium concentration too quickly can cause CNS myelinolysis, which often causes clinical signs of CNS dysfunction that occur 3 to 5 days after the event [11,12]. No definitive work has been done in dogs and cats, but it has been suggested that chronic hyponatremia should not be corrected at a rate any faster than 10 mEq/L/d [1].

Hyponatremia attributable to the syndrome of inappropriate antidiuretic hormone (ADH) secretion is a rare disorder in veterinary medicine [13]. It is one of the causes of hyponatremia in a normovolemic patient. Such patients are best treated with water restriction.

POTASSIUM

Hyperkalemia is primarily attributable to decreased renal excretion, adrenal failure, or drug administration [14]. Because hyperkalemia can be life threatening, symptomatically correcting the potassium concentration often is important. Although care must be taken not to change serum sodium concentrations too fast, there is no such concern when correcting abnormal serum potassium concentrations. It is usually prudent to treat patients with serum potassium concentrations greater than 6.5 mEq/L symptomatically. If the serum potassium concentration is greater than 7.5 mEq/L, it is important to act quickly to correct it to a more normal concentration. Serum potassium concentrations greater than 8.5 mEq/L are immediately life threatening and constitute an emergency. Aggressive administration of potassium-free parenteral fluids (eg, physiologic saline solution) is usually sufficient to bring the patient out of immediate danger, assuming that the kidneys are functioning properly. Aggressive fluid therapy dilutes the potassium and enhances renal excretion. If the serum potassium concentration is 8.5 mEq/L or greater or if there is clinical evidence of marked cardiotoxicity (eg, bradycardia), intravenous administration of insulin (regular insulin at a rate of 0.5–1 U/kg of body weight) plus glucose (dextrose at a rate of 2 g/U of insulin administered) lowers the serum potassium concentration while waiting for therapy directed at the underlying cause (eg, intravenous fluids, desoxycorticosterone pivalate) to take effect [15]. In patients that are moribund, one may administer 10% calcium gluconate intravenously to effect (while monitoring by electrocardiography) to antagonize cardiotoxicity until other therapy can lower the serum potassium concentration [16].

Occasionally, patients that have renal disease present with hyperkalemia. Most of these patients are in severe renal failure (eg, preterminal chronic failure, oliguric acute renal failure) [14], and treatment of hyperkalemia consists of fluid therapy (with or without the drugs mentioned previously) and, occasionally, peritoneal dialysis. Less commonly, patients with renal disease that are not in severe failure have persistent mild hyperkalemia. These patients seldom have serum potassium concentrations of sufficient magnitude to cause morbidity or mortality, and hence may just need to be periodically monitored. If the hyperkalemia is worrisome, administration of furosemide or thiazides would be a reasonable consideration.

Chronic idiopathic hyperkalemia is exceedingly rare but has been reported (ie, idiopathic hyperkalemic periodic paralysis [17]). Too few cases have been reported in veterinary medicine to make any definitive recommendations. One should treat the patient as described previously if there is danger of cardiotoxicity. Otherwise, extrapolating from human medicine, one may anticipate that chronic administration of diuretics (eg, furosemide, thiazide) should help to control the serum potassium concentration to a reasonable degree. If idiopathic hyperkalemia does not respond to this approach, fludrocortisone acetate can be administered to determine if the hyperkalemia is mineralocorticoid responsive. Exchange resins (eg, polystyrene sulfonate) have seldom been used in veterinary medicine. In human medicine, these resins are administered orally or rectally [18]. They can cause constipation in addition to adding substantial amounts of sodium to the body.

Hypokalemia is primarily attributable to loss of potassium from the body by way of the gastrointestinal tract or the kidneys or as a result of drug administration. Like hyperkalemia, marked hypokalemia can cause substantial clinical signs and needs to be corrected quickly if it is so low (ie, <2.5 mEq/L) as to make severe weakness (including respiratory paralysis) likely.

Although not as common now as it was several years ago, severe life-threatening chronic hypokalemia can occur in cats with renal loss of potassium caused by renal tubular dysfunction [19]. This renal dysfunction was associated with being fed diets low in potassium. Many cats were so weak as to have difficulty in standing or holding up their heads. There is also a rare syndrome of periodic hypokalemic paralysis in cats, specifically the Burmese breed [20,21].

In patients that have muscular weakness because of hypokalemia, it is critical to increase the serum potassium concentration quickly. Parenteral administration classically is used when one wants to increase the serum potassium concentration quickly. The serum potassium concentration in cats, however, may actually decrease somewhat before it increases, even when administering fluids with potassium chloride at doses of 30 and 40 mEq/L. If the patient is already critically ill from hypokalemia, even a little additional decrease in the serum potassium concentration can be lethal (eg, respiratory paralysis). If parenteral administration is chosen, supplementing fluids with potassium chloride at a dose of 60 to 80 mEq/L may be necessary. Oral administration of potassium chloride solution (diluted 1:1 in water) sometimes may be more effective and safer than parenteral administration of potassium [22]. Oral administration of potassium may be as effective or more effective than parenteral administration in people [23]. Numerous oral potassium supplements can be used [14]. In general, the potassium chloride solutions marketed for people have a bitter taste and must be diluted before the patient accepts them. Avoid pills that may adhere to the mucosa of the gastrointestinal tract and cause ulceration [24,25]. Veterinary potassium gluconate preparations are commonly used because they are powders that are easily added to the food and are palatable. Potassium citrate, bicarbonate, and acetate preparations also are available, but one must monitor the serum chloride concentration if these products are used chronically. In cats, one typically administers potassium at a dosage of 2 to 5 mEq twice a day [19]. After the crisis has passed, the serum potassium concentration is monitored as the dosage is adjusted until the correct dosage for that patient is determined. Unfortunately, many patients that are hypokalemic because of other causes are vomiting, making the oral route unreliable. If the patient can be relied on to eat and not to vomit, however, oral supplementation is an excellent way to administer potassium chronically. The dosage for oral potassium in the dog is variable and ranges from 2 to greater than 40 mEq/d. Again, one must titrate the dosage for each dog.

Conventional thinking has long suggested that parenteral administration of potassium should be limited to a maximum rate of 0.5 mEq/kg/h so as to avoid cardiotoxicity. This limit is no longer as definitive as was once thought. People (especially diabetic patients being aggressively treated for ketoacidosis) have been treated at nearly double that rate without problems [26]. As long as there is careful electrocardiographic (ECG) monitoring to detect cardiotoxicity, it is acceptable to use faster rates of administration. One should avoid fluids with potassium chloride at a rate greater than 60 mEq/L for intravenous administration, however, to prevent phlebitis from occurring at the catheter site [27]. If giving potassium-containing fluids subcutaneously, one should not exceed 35 to 40 mEq/L. Some patients with hypokalemia, especially diabetic patients, have concurrent phosphorous deficiencies. In such cases, K_2PO_4/KH_2PO_4 can be used in conjunction with potassium chloride as a fluid additive.

MAGNESIUM

Hypermagnesemia seems primarily to be associated with renal dysfunction. There has not been an obvious need to lower chronically high serum magnesium concentrations in dogs and cats.

Hypomagnesemia is common in small animals [28]. It is most commonly caused by renal losses, although gastrointestinal losses also may occur. At this time, it is not clear how clinically relevant hypomagnesemia is in dogs and cats; therefore, the value of chronic magnesium supplementation is uncertain. Chronic hypomagnesemia generally is treated only when the serum magnesium concentration is extremely low or when it is thought to be contributing to other electrolyte disorders (eg, hypokalemia [29,30], hypocalcemia [31]). In severely hypomagnesemic patients, one may administer $MgSO_4$ or $MgCl_2$

intravenously. In both cases, the magnesium is mixed in 5% dextrose in water and administered as a constant rate infusion at 0.3 to 0.5 mEq/kg/d for routine replacement or at twice that rate for fast replacement [32]. Blood magnesium concentration is monitored until it is sufficiently close to normal. Oral administration then can be provided for patients that seem to be chronically losing magnesium through their urinary or gastrointestinal tract. MgSO$_4$ often is avoided in such cases because it acts as a laxative, something that is best avoided in such patients. Magnesium oxide can be administered orally with minimal laxative effects. The dosage is uncertain, but 1 to 2 mEq/kg/d is a reasonable place to start. The dosage then is adjusted based on periodic monitoring.

SUMMARY

In summary, clinically relevant abnormalities of sodium concentrations must be altered slowly, whereas abnormalities of potassium serum concentration typically are altered more quickly. Oral potassium supplementation tends to be easy and effective. The need for magnesium supplementation is less certain, and time will tell if symptomatic therapy of hypomagnesemia is commonly warranted.

References

[1] DiBartola SP. Disorders of sodium and water: hypernatremia and hyponatremia. In: DiBartola SP, editor. Fluid, electrolyte and acid-base disorders in small animal practice. 3rd edition. St. Louis (MO): Saunders Elsevier; 2006. p. 47–79.

[2] Bagley RS. Adipsia and the nervous system. Compendium of Continuing Education for the Veterinary Practitioner 1995;17:311–8.

[3] DiBartola SP, Johnson SE, Johnson GC, et al. Hypodipsic hypernatremia in a dog with defective osmoregulation of antidiuretic hormone. J Am Vet Med Assoc 1994;204(6): 922–5.

[4] Sullivan SA, Harmon BG, Purinton PT, et al. Lobar holoprosencephaly in a miniature schnauzer with hypodipsic hypernatremia. J Am Vet Med Assoc 2003;223:1783–7.

[5] Bagley RS, de Lahunta A, Randolph JF, et al. Hypernatremia, adipsia, and diabetes insipidus in a dog with hypothalamic dysplasia. J Am Anim Hosp Assoc 1993;29:267–71.

[6] Hanselman B, Kruth S, Poma R, et al. Hypernatremia and hyperlipidemia in a dog with central nervous system lymphosarcoma. J Vet Intern Med 2006;20:1029–32.

[7] Hawks D, Giger U, Miselis R, et al. Essential hypernatremia in a young dog. J Small Anim Pract 1991;32:420–4.

[8] Hardy RM. Hypernatremia. Vet Clin North Am Small Anim Pract 1989;19:231–40.

[9] Khanna C, Boermans HJ, Wilcock B. Fatal hypernatremia in a dog from salt ingestion. J Am Anim Hosp Assoc 1997;33:113–7.

[10] Brady CA, Vite CH, Drobatz KJ. Severe neurologic sequelae in a dog after treatment of hypoadrenal crisis. J Am Vet Med Assoc 1999;215:222–5.

[11] Churcher RK, Watson ADJ, Eaton A. Suspected myelinolysis following rapid correction of hyponatremia in a dog. J Am Anim Hosp Assoc 1999;35:493–7.

[12] O'Brien DP, Kroll RA, Johnson GC, et al. Myelinolysis after correction of hyponatremia in two dogs. J Vet Intern Med 1994;8:40–8.

[13] Brofman PJ, Knostman KAB, DiBartola SP. Granulomatous amebic meningoencephalitis causing the syndrome of inappropriate secretion of antidiuretic hormone in a dog. J Vet Intern Med 2003;17:230–4.

[14] DiBartola SP, de Morais HA. Disorders of potassium: hypokalemia and hyperkalemia. In: DiBartola SP, editor. Fluid, electrolyte, and acid-base disorders in small animal practice. 3rd edition. St. Louis (MO): Saunders Elsevier; 2006. p. 91–121.

[15] Schaer M. Disorders of potassium metabolism. Vet Clin North Am Small Anim Pract 1982;12(3):399–409.

[16] Willard MD. Disorders of potassium homeostasis. Vet Clin North Am Small Anim Pract 1989;19(2):241–63.

[17] Jezyk PF. Hyperkalemic periodic paralysis in a dog. J Am Anim Hosp Assoc 1982;18: 977–80.

[18] Gerstman BB, Kirkman K, Platt R. Intestinal necrosis associated with postoperative orally administered sodium polystyrene sulfonate in sorbitol. Am J Kidney Dis 1992:159–61.

[19] Dow SW, Fettman MJ, Curtis CR, et al. Hypokalemia in cats: 186 cases (1984–1987). J Am Vet Med Assoc 1989;194(11):1604–8.

[20] Mason KV. A hereditary disease in Burmese cats manifesting as an episodic weakness with head nodding and neck ventroflexion. J Am Anim Hosp Assoc 1988;24:481.

[21] Stolze M, Lund C, Kresken J, et al. Periodische hypokaliamische polymyopathie bei der burmakatze. Kleintierpraxis 2001;5:257–320.

[22] Dow SW, Fettman MJ, LeCouteur RA, et al. Potassium depletion in cats: renal and dietary influences. J Am Vet Med Assoc 1987;191(12):1569–75.

[23] Fournier G, Pfaff-Poulard C, Methani K. Rapid correction of hypokalaemia via the oral route. Lancet 1987;2:163.

[24] Pemberton J. Oesophageal obstruction and ulceration caused by oral potassium therapy. Br Heart J 1970;32:267–8.

[25] Trechot P, Moore N, Bresler L, et al. Potassium chloride tablets and small bowel stenoses and perforations: two studies in the French pharmacovigilance system. Am J Gastroenterol 1994;89:1268.

[26] Hamill RJ, Robinson LM, Wexler HR, et al. Efficacy and safety of potassium infusion therapy in hypokalemic critically ill patients. Crit Care Med 1991;19:694–9.

[27] Rose BD. Hypokalemia. In: Rose BD, editor. Clinical physiology of acid-base and electrolyte disorders. New York: McGraw Hill; 2000. p. 836–87.

[28] Khanna C, Lund EM, Raffe M, et al. Hypomagnesemia in 188 dogs: a hospital population-based prevalence study. J Vet Intern Med 1998;12:304–9.

[29] Whang R. Refractory potassium repletion due to magnesium deficiency. Arch Intern Med 1992;152:2346.

[30] Cohn JN, Kowey PR, Whelton PK, et al. New guidelines for potassium replacement in clinical practice. Arch Intern Med 2000;160:2429–36.

[31] Bush WW, Kimmel SE, Wosar MA, et al. Secondary hypoparathyroidism attributed to hypomagnesemia in a dog with protein-losing enteropathy. J Am Vet Med Assoc 2001;219:1732–4.

[32] Bateman S. Disorders of magnesium: magnesium deficit and excess. In: DiBartola SP, editor. Fluid, electrolyte, and acid-base disorders in small animal practice. 3rd edition. St. Louis (MO): Saunders Elsevier; 2006. p. 210–26.

Making Sense of Blood Gas Results

Shane W. Bateman, DVM, DVSc

Department of Veterinary Clinical Sciences, The Ohio State University,
601 Vernon L. Tharp Street, Columbus, OH 43210-1089, USA

Recent technologic advances have allowed the production and marketing of cage-side blood gas analyzers to private practitioners. Rapid expansion of emergency and critical care medicine as a specialty and increased numbers of veterinary emergency and veterinary specialty practices have occurred concurrently with the availability of blood gas analyzers that are affordable for private practitioners. As a result, evaluation of blood gas results is no longer an activity confined to academic institutions and has become a daily part of many practicing veterinarians' activities.

Numerous physiologic processes are optimized at or near a pH of 7.4. Organisms have evolved with multiple systems that act somewhat interdependently to achieve the ideal pH of 7.4. The study of acid-base balance is a complex and imperfect science. Numerous theoretic approaches have been developed for assessment of acid-base status. Reviews outlining the historical development of competing theories and comparing the accuracy and use of various approaches are available and continue to be debated in academic circles [1–5]. The goal of this article is to provide a practical approach to evaluation of blood gas results without explanation of the theoretic approach. The approach used incorporates numerous theories and methods.

WHAT ARE THE NUMBERS?

Depending on the blood gas analyzer in use, more or fewer numbers will form the "results." It is important to understand the various components of each of these numbers. Only a few of the numbers are measured by the analyzer. The remainder is calculated from various formulas or nomograms that are programmed into the analyzer. Some of the calculated values are derived using values that are appropriate and accurate for human plasma but not for veterinary patients. These variables may differ from analyzer to analyzer. Table 1 contains a listing of the common variables found on a blood gas analysis.

ACID-BASE OR RESPIRATORY FUNCTION

Blood gas analysis can be performed to obtain information about the acid-base status of a patient and about gas exchange in the lungs. If information about the

E-mail address: bateman.36@osu.edu

0195-5616/08/$ – see front matter
doi:10.1016/j.cvsm.2008.01.002

Table 1
Variables that commonly form the results of a blood gas analysis

Variable	Definition	Measured or calculated
pH	The pH of the sample	Measured
pCO_2	The partial pressure of carbon dioxide in the sample	Measured
pO_2	The partial pressure of oxygen in the sample	Measured
sO_2	The percent of hemoglobin saturated with oxygen	Measured/ calculated
HCO_3^-	The concentration of bicarbonate in the sample	Calculated
BE	The base excess	Calculated
SBE or BE_{ecf}	The standard base excess	Calculated

acid-base status of the patient is desired, a venous sample is most informative. Venous blood contains cellular waste products and provides a more accurate reflection of acid-base state at the cellular level. If evaluation of respiratory gas exchange is the goal, then an arterial sample is desired. Arterial blood has been through the lungs (unless there is a shunt present) but has not been exposed to any cellular uptake or waste, which allows a view of how effectively the lungs have been able to load oxygen into blood and remove carbon dioxide.

SAMPLING METHODS

Appropriate sampling methods should be used when analyzing blood gases to ensure that no preanalytical errors are introduced. Numerous vendors manufacture blood-gas–specific syringes. Features of such syringes typically include lyophilized lithium heparin as an anticoagulant and an arterial self-filling function. Because of the self-filling feature for arterial samples, such syringes cannot be used to aspirate blood from a venous site. The dry lithium heparin is used to minimize errors in ionized calcium that can result from the use of liquid sodium heparin. (If the analyzer in use does not measure ionized calcium, this is less important.) If such a syringe type is to be used for venous blood gas analysis, the sample should be drawn using a normal plastic syringe and needle and then the blood gas syringe can be filled by inserting the needle and syringe with the non-anticoagulated blood sample through the hub of the blood gas syringe and slowly filling the syringe barrel chamber.

Alternatively, a regular 3-mL plastic syringe can be heparinized before sample collection. The quantity of heparin used is crucial to ensure that no preanalytical errors are introduced. A recent study showed that the following heparinization technique produced the most accurate results: (1) fill a 3-mL syringe to the 3-mL mark using liquid heparin and a 22-gauge needle, (2) depress the plunger to expel all of the heparin from the syringe, (3) aspirate 3 mL of air back into the syringe and rapidly expel the contents of the syringe, (4) repeat the air aspiration and expulsion two additional times, and (5) fill the syringe with 1 mL of arterial or venous blood [6].

After collection of the sample, the expected time to analysis determines whether the sample should be stored anaerobically and on ice to ensure the most accurate results. If the sample is being analyzed immediately, as would be expected with most bedside analyzers, then "corking" the sample to store it as an anaerobic sample between the time of collection and analysis is not necessary. It is advisable to be sure all air bubbles are expelled within 30 seconds of collection of the sample. If the sample will not be analyzed immediately after collection, then it should be stored anaerobically on ice before analysis. Some increase in oxygen tension in the sample can be expected after 30 minutes to 2 hours (depending on sample volume) when the sample is stored in a plastic syringe [7].

PHYSIOLOGY

At least two organs are responsible for maintaining normal acid-base physiology or compensating for acid-base disturbances. The lungs are responsible for regulating the carbon dioxide concentration of blood. More carbon dioxide in the bloodstream results in a more acidic pH. Disturbances that cause increased or decreased carbon dioxide concentrations are termed respiratory acid-base alterations, which are generally a result of neurologic, respiratory musculoskeletal, or extrarespiratory system dysfunction. For example, a patient with a high cervical spinal cord lesion may have decreased intercostal muscle function and be unable to breathe deeply enough to remove adequate amounts of carbon dioxide from the body's metabolism, resulting in increased partial pressure of carbon dioxide in the blood. On the other hand, a patient with severe acute anemia may have increased respiratory rate, increased depth of respiration, or both to try to compensate for decreased oxygen delivery to the tissues and have decreased partial pressure of carbon dioxide in the blood.

The kidney is the site of numerous regulatory mechanisms controlling the amount of acid or base that is excreted in urine. The gastrointestinal tract may be the source of increased loss of acid or base through vomiting or diarrhea. Cellular metabolism, ingestion of toxins with acidic or basic characteristics, and liver dysfunction that alters normal metabolism could result in increases or decreases of acids or bases in the body. Collectively, these alternations in physiologic function can be said to represent the nonrespiratory (or metabolic) acid-base disturbances. The many possible causes for nonrespiratory acid-base disturbances can confound the clinician's ability to identify the cause in a given situation.

In general, the respiratory system attempts to compensate for derangements in the nonrespiratory system and vice versa. Because of the volatile nature of carbon dioxide and the fact that it can be exhaled from the body rapidly, the respiratory system is able to compensate quickly for nonrespiratory disturbances. The kidney is generally the organ responsible for altering acid or base excretion from the body. It is slower to compensate for respiratory disturbances, but if given sufficient time, it can be efficient. If a single acid-base disturbance is present, the unaffected system begins compensating in an attempt to mitigate any severe alteration in blood pH that could impair cellular enzymatic function. In severely ill patients, however, dysfunction may be present in multiple systems, and compensation may be inadequate or absent, resulting in complex or mixed acid-base disturbances.

Advanced understanding of acid-base physiology attempts to explain what substances play roles as acids or bases and what strength they may have on influencing acid-base balance. When all of the individual "players" can be identified, numerous physical and chemical principles govern their activity. Some investigators have spent considerable time attempting to understand the complex interactions and simplify them into a unifying theory or set of principles.

ACIDEMIA OR ALKALEMIA?

The first step in determining the acid-base status of the patient is to determine if the patient's pH is less than or more than 7.4 (or the sample site appropriate reference point) (Table 2). In other words, the beginning step is to determine if acidemia or alkalemia is present. One or more processes may have caused the pH to change. These processes are termed acidosis or alkalosis and may be summative if there is a complex or mixed acid-base disorder present.

RESPIRATORY OR NONRESPIRATORY?

The next step in analyzing blood gas data is to parse out the individual derangements. The partial pressure of carbon dioxide always reflects the respiratory component. As mentioned previously, the bicarbonate and base excess are calculated and not measured variables. Both reflect the nonrespiratory acid-base derangement that is occurring. Different schools of thought offer arguments as to why one may be superior to the other when assessing the nonrespiratory contribution [8–11].

Before results can be labeled increased or decreased, a reference point of comparison must be established. For most chemistry and hematology variables that are analyzed in veterinary species, a reference interval is established from a representative sample of the normal population. For the purposes of blood gas analysis, it is simpler to choose a single reference point for comparison (ie, the carbon dioxide is higher or lower than the normal reference point). Some general reference points, which are the midpoints of the reference interval for the analytes in

Table 2
Reference points for blood gas analytes

	Canine venous	Canine arterial	Feline venous	Feline arterial
pH	7.397	7.407	7.343	7.386
pCO_2 (mm Hg)	37.4	36.8	38.7	31.0
HCO_3 (mEq/L)	22.5	22.2	22.6	18.0
Anion gap (mEq/L)	12–24		13–27	
Sodium (mEq/L)	147		150	
Chloride (mEq/L)	111		117	

Abbreviations: pH, blood pH; pCO_2, partial pressure of carbon dioxide; HCO_3, bicarbonate concentration.

question, are presented in Table 2. These reference points may change depending on the instrument used and the population sampled. When interpreting acid-base balance, the normal reference interval and corresponding reference points that have been established for the instrument in use should be used.

The next step is to determine the effect of increases or decreases in the respiratory and nonrespiratory components. For example, if the pH of a canine venous sample indicates that acidemia is present and the bicarbonate concentration and carbon dioxide tension both are decreased, then a nonrespiratory acidosis is present. To explain, a decrease in bicarbonate concentration has an acidifying effect, thus a nonrespiratory acidosis is contributing to the acidemia. A decrease in carbon dioxide concentration has an alkalinizing effect and could not cause acidemia. It is a logical assumption at this stage that the patient has a respiratory compensation for a primary nonrespiratory acidosis. Further analysis is needed to determine if the respiratory compensation is appropriate for the magnitude of the nonrespiratory acidosis.

If the bicarbonate concentration and carbon dioxide tension are both increased or decreased, it is safe to assume (at least at this stage of analysis) that a simple acid-base disturbance with compensation is present. If these analytes are moving in opposite directions (one is increased, the other decreased) then they will have additive effects on the pH, and a mixed acid-base disturbance can be diagnosed. In other words, if the blood is alkalemic (ie, high pH), the bicarbonate is increased (nonrespiratory alkalosis), and the carbon dioxide decreased (respiratory alkalosis), there is no compensatory response present to attempt to modulate the pH. The resulting pH derangement is likely to be much more clinically relevant, and evaluation of the patient should reveal derangements in the respiratory and nonrespiratory systems. Table 3 lists the six possible acid-base disturbances.

COMPENSATED OR NOT?

For the four simple acid-base disturbances listed in Table 3, the next step is to determine the magnitude of the compensatory response to determine if it is

Table 3
Primary (with compensation) and mixed acid-base disturbance patterns

	Primary non-respiratory alkalosis ± compensation	Primary respiratory alkalosis ± compensation	Not possible	Mixed alkalosis	If pH > 7.4 use this row ⇐
CO_2	⇑	⇓	⇑	⇓	
HCO_3	⇑	⇓	⇓	⇑	
	Primary respiratory acidosis ± compensation	Primary non-respiratory alkalosis ± compensation	Mixed acidosis	Not possible	If pH < 7.4 use this row ⇐

Abbreviations: CO_2, partial pressure of carbon dioxide; HCO_3, bicarbonate.

appropriate. If compensation is adequate, dysfunction in the compensatory system can be ruled out and a simple acid-base disturbance is present. Predicted compensatory responses were derived from laboratory models of healthy dogs [12]. Compensatory responses in cats have not been determined, and in most cases their response is assumed to be similar to dogs. As mentioned previously, the kidney gains efficiency in its compensatory response to a primary respiratory acid-base disturbance over several days. As a result, the nonrespiratory compensatory response can be divided into acute and chronic phases. The rule of thumb is that if the primary respiratory disturbance lasts longer than 24 hours, then the chronic compensatory response should be used for calculation. The magnitude of the compensatory response can be predicted using Table 4. For example, if a canine venous blood gas sample indicates that a nonrespiratory acidosis is present (pH 7.25; HCO_3 12.5 mEq/L; pCO_2 30.4 mm Hg), appropriate compensation can be determined in the following manner: Because the primary disturbance is a nonrespiratory acidosis, for every 1 mEq/L decrease in bicarbonate, a corresponding decrease of 0.7 mm Hg of carbon dioxide can be expected. In this example, the patient's bicarbonate has decreased by 10 mEq/L (22.5–12.5 mEq/L), so we can expect a 7 mm Hg (10×0.7 mm Hg/mEq HCO_3) decrease in carbon dioxide. The patient's actual value is exactly the same as what would be predicted. Effective compensation can be said to have taken place if the actual value is within 1 to 2 mEq/L or 1 to 2 mm Hg of the expected or predicted value. Overcompensation is not thought to occur. If the actual value in the example were to be considerably higher than the predicted value, dysfunction within both systems (respiratory and nonrespiratory) should be suspected and the patient can be diagnosed with a mixed acid-base disturbance. Fig. 1 demonstrates the appropriate diagnostic language to apply to the compensating analyte's response.

BASE EXCESS

Although North Americans typically use the bicarbonate approach when assessing nonrespiratory acid-base disturbances, the base excess (or deficit) also can be used. In the approach presented in this article, the base excess or base deficit should be evaluated to determine the magnitude of the nonrespiratory contribution in any acid-base disturbance. It can serve to double-check

Table 4
Predicted compensatory responses to primary acid-base disturbances

Disorder	Change in primary analyte	Predicted change in compensatory analyte
Nonrespiratory acidosis/alkalosis	⇧⇩ 1 mEq HCO_3	Δ pCO_2 0.7 mm Hg
Acute respiratory acidosis	⇧ 1 mm Hg pCO_2	Δ HCO_3 0.15 mEq/L
Chronic respiratory acidosis	⇧ 1 mm Hg pCO_2	Δ HCO_3 0.35 mEq/L
Acute respiratory alkalosis	⇩ 1 mm Hg pCO_2	Δ HCO_3 0.25 mEq/L
Chronic respiratory alkalosis	⇩ 1 mm Hg pCO_2	Δ HCO_3 0.55 mEq/L

Abbreviations: pCO_2, partial pressure of carbon dioxide; HCO_3, bicarbonate concentration.

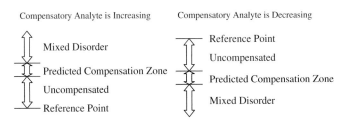

Fig. 1. Nomenclature to describe compensatory analyte's predicted/actual response.

the mathematical evaluation presented previously. In other words, an error of assessment has been made if the diagnosis reached using the previous approach is nonrespiratory alkalosis and the base excess is negative (ie, a base deficit is present).

Base excess is a concept that was developed by European physiologists. It is defined as the amount of strong acid or alkali required to titrate 1 L of blood to pH 7.40 at 37°C while the partial pressure of carbon dioxide is held constant at 40 mm Hg. In essence, the blood sample no longer has any respiratory acid-base disturbance, and the amount of acid or base required to titrate to a pH of 7.4 is representative of the summation of all nonrespiratory acid-base disturbances. The concept of standard base excess was developed because the buffering capacity of a blood sample outside of the patient is not representative of what might take place in vivo. The standard base excess evaluates the acid or base that would be required to titrate the extracellular fluid space back to a pH of 7.4. Some analyzers may report these calculated values. These values are also often used in calculating the amount of buffer (usually in the form of sodium bicarbonate) to administer to a patient with a severe acidosis.

PARSING OUT CAUSES OF NONRESPIRATORY DISTURBANCES

Once the diagnosis of the acid-base disturbance has been made, the next step is to determine if the diagnosis fits the patient's clinical condition. The underlying clinical cause of primary respiratory disorders should be obvious in most cases. As mentioned previously, nonrespiratory disorders may be more challenging to assess. Numerous factors can contribute to nonrespiratory acid-base disturbances. Debate has continued for years regarding what is the most accurate approach to take. The theories of Stewart and other approaches derived from his initial theories are generally thought to be the most accurate in terms of deciphering all of the nonrespiratory contributions relevant to a particular acid-base disturbance [1,3–5]. These methods are commonly criticized as being excessively complex and far too involved for routine clinical use. They may be helpful, however, when complex disorders are present.

One simplified approach that helps in understanding the contributory causes of nonrespiratory acid-base disturbances is the use of the Gamblegram [13], which is a graphical representation of the principles of Stewart and others. It does not allow quantification of the specific contributing causes to a nonrespiratory acid-base disturbance, but it does allow the principles to be evaluated and understood. A Gamblegram is constructed by placing the clinically relevant cations that may contribute to acid-base balance in one column according to their relative concentrations. The second column is constructed using all of the clinically relevant anions that may contribute to acid-base balance (Fig. 2). The fundamental rule of thumb when evaluating a Gamblegram is the law of electroneutrality. In other words, anions must equal cations. Several ions (eg, potassium) are omitted from the Gamblegram because they are not considered clinically relevant. In other words, for potassium to have a clinically relevant effect on acid-base disturbances, its concentration would exceed that thought to be compatible with life.

The simplest approach to using a Gamblegram is to think of all of the contributing anions and cations except bicarbonate as independent variables. In other words, each of them has an independent effect on acid-base status. Bicarbonate is the only dependent variable. It increases or decreases as a result of the summative effect of all of the independent variables. We can parse out the individual contributions by evaluating how individual anion or cation changes affect the bicarbonate concentration. For example, an increase in sodium concentration would have to be balanced by an increase in bicarbonate concentration in order for anions and cations to be equal. Hypernatremia (typically the result of a free water deficit) has an alkalinizing effect. If we evaluate the effect of hypochloremia (eg, as a consequence of pyloric obstruction), the bicarbonate concentration must increase to satisfy the law of electroneutrality. Hypochloremia causes a nonrespiratory alkalosis. Table 5 lists the influence of each

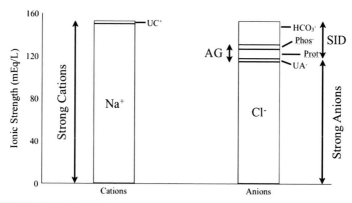

Fig. 2. Gamblegram used to assist in determining the contributing causes of nonrespiratory acid-base disturbances. UC^+, unmeasured strong cations; AG, anion gap; UA^-, unmeasured strong anions; $Phos^-$, phosphorus; $Prot^-$, protein; Na^+, sodium; Cl^-, chloride, SID, strong ion difference. (*Adapted from* de Morais HA, Constable PD. Strong ion approach to acid-base disorders. In: DiBartola SP, editor. Fluid, electrolyte, and acid-base disorders in small animal practice. 3rd edition. St. Louis: Saunders Elsevier; 2006. p. 311; with permission.)

Table 5
Nonrespiratory acid-base alterations

Nonrespiratory acidoses	Nonrespiratory alkaloses
Hyponatremia (or free water excess)	Hypernatremia (or free water deficit)
Hyperchloremia	Hypochloremia
Hyperproteinemia	Hypoproteinemia
Hyperphosphatemia	Increased unmeasured strong cations (rare)
Increased unmeasured strong anions (eg, lactate, ketoacids, ethylene glycol)	

independent variable on the nonrespiratory acid-base status. Note that some of the independent variables cannot exert bidirectional influences. For example, a decrease in phosphorus is not thought to have a sufficiently strong alkalinizing effect to cause a clinically relevant nonrespiratory alkalosis.

Unmeasured strong anions are much more commonly encountered clinically when compared with unmeasured strong cations. In the past, one approach in attempting to determine if unmeasured strong anions were influencing acid-base status was to evaluate the anion gap (ie, the difference between the sum of chloride and bicarbonate concentrations and the sodium concentration or sum of the sodium and potassium concentrations). If the total protein and phosphorus concentrations are within normal limits, then they are considered constants and dropped from the anion gap calculation. In this way, the anion gap can be said to represent the unmeasured strong anions in the patient's plasma (assuming there are no unmeasured strong cations in the solution). Thus, the anion gap can be a useful tool to identify common clinical situations in which increased unmeasured strong anions are present, such as an increase in lactate or ketoacids. Obviously, if protein or phosphorus concentrations are abnormal, then the anion gap is much less useful. For example, in critically ill patients, hypoproteinemia is commonly encountered at the same time as increased lactate concentration. Often these two disorders cancel each other out, and the anion gap remains within expected normal intervals. General reference intervals for anion gap can be found in Table 2. Reference intervals specific to the instrumentation in use in each practice should be developed.

Similar to the anion gap, the strong ion difference is another approach to considering the major effect of a clinically relevant difference between the strong cations and the strong anions (see Fig. 2). The unmeasured strong cations and the unmeasured strong anions are difficult to quantify; the clinical use of this measure has been troublesome. Persons seeking an advanced understanding of these concepts are referred to the work of Constable [1,3], who has attempted to adapt these principles for many veterinary species.

ASSESSMENT OF RESPIRATORY FUNCTION

Excellent reviews of respiratory physiology and gas exchange are available for interested readers. The aim of this article is not to explore these concepts in depth. Rather, the aim is to distill some of the concepts into a practical approach to evaluation of respiratory function by analyzing the respiratory gas measurements on a blood gas analysis.

One of the most important functions of the lung is to remove carbon dioxide from the blood and exhale it to the environment. The partial pressure of carbon dioxide in the blood is directly proportional to the minute ventilation—the volume of air that washes through the lungs each minute. As described earlier, an increase in carbon dioxide in the blood is generally a direct result of hypoventilation or decreased minute volume. Numerous causes are possible. In severe forms of pulmonary injury, the respiratory epithelium of the alveoli or the matching of ventilation to perfusion may be so damaged as to prevent carbon dioxide escape from the blood despite a substantial increase in respiratory rate or tidal volume. Hypocarbia is generally an indicator of good pulmonary function because the increased minute volume is removing more carbon dioxide than necessary. A cause of the hypocarbia typically is found outside of the respiratory system.

The loading of oxygen into the blood is a complex and highly evolved process. Hypoxia can have several causes: (1) decreased inspired concentration of oxygen, (2) intrapulmonary or cardiac shunting, (3) ventilation/perfusion mismatching, (4) hypoventilation, and (5) diffusion impairment. The most challenging aspect of evaluating oxygenation from blood gas data is the change imposed on that process by changes in altitude and barometric pressure. At increasing altitudes, changes in the barometric pressure decrease the effective concentration of oxygen in the atmosphere and consequently in the alveoli, and as a result, decrease the amount of oxygen that is carried in the blood. The normal or expected partial pressure of oxygen in the bloodstream changes with changes in altitude, which makes assessment of normal oxygenation challenging.

Two formulas are useful when attempting to determine the effectiveness of oxygen loading by the lungs into the bloodstream. The simpler of the two is the PaO_2/FiO_2 ratio (sometimes referred to as the P/F ratio). It can be calculated when the PaO_2 (partial pressure of oxygen in an arterial blood sample) and the FiO_2 (fraction of inspired oxygen) are both known. The FiO_2 is easily measured using a relatively inexpensive hand-held oximeter that has been calibrated against a gas sample with a known or standardized oxygen concentration. At sea level and lower altitudes, the FiO_2 can be safely assumed to be 0.21 (or 21%). At higher altitudes, it should be measured. If the P/F ratio is more than 400, pulmonary function should be considered normal. As the P/F ratio decreases from 400 and approaches 200, respiratory function can be said to be progressively decreased. A P/F ratio less than 200 indicates severe pulmonary dysfunction and is commonly used as a criterion for the diagnosis of acute respiratory distress syndrome in humans.

A second, more cumbersome formula commonly used is the alveolar-arterial oxygen gradient equation or A-a gradient. The formula aims to determine the difference between the predicted partial pressure of oxygen in the alveolus based on gas physics laws and known physiologic principles and the known amount of oxygen in the arterial blood. Large differences between these values (or a large A-a gradient) are predictive of a clinically relevant defect in oxygen loading into the blood. If the A-a gradient is within the normal range in a hypoxemic patient, the assumption is that the hypoxemia is caused by extrarespiratory causes or hypoventilation. The accuracy of the A-a gradient is limited when the FiO_2 is more than 0.21, thus the A-a gradient always should be calculated using room air [14]. One of the criticisms of this approach is that patients who are oxygen dependent may be compromised by attempts to measure the A-a gradient in this way. Determining when the patient who has been receiving supplemental oxygen has reached a new steady state when breathing room air also can be complicated. In room air, the A-a gradient should be less than 15 mm Hg. It is calculated using the following formula:

$$\text{A-a gradient} = (FiO_2[P_b - P_{H_2O}] - [PaCO_2/R]) - PaO_2$$

where FiO_2 is fraction of inspired oxygen expressed as a decimal, P_b is barometric pressure in mm Hg, P_{H_2O} is partial pressure of water vapor in humidified gas, $PaCO_2$ is the partial pressure of CO_2 in an arterial blood sample, R is the respiratory quotient (assumed to be 8 in animals), and PaO_2 is the partial pressure of oxygen in an arterial blood sample.

The respiratory quotient can vary slightly among animal species with varying diets and has even been reported to be different depending on the recumbent position of the patient [15,16]. The A-a gradient also can vary with age in humans and when positive pressure ventilation is in use [17,18].

SUMMARY

With patience and steady practice, anyone can become adept at interpreting blood gas results. The complexity of blood gas analysis can be likened to layers of onion skin. As you peel back each layer, you expose a deeper understanding of the complex physiologic and physical principles that govern acid-base balance. The widespread use of cage-side portable blood gas analyzers in veterinary practices has increased the need to develop the basic skills of blood gas analysis as part of the tool kit for practicing veterinarians.

APPENDIX 1. CLINICAL EXAMPLES OF BLOOD GAS ANALYSIS

Case One

A 2-year-old male Rottweiler presents moribund and in decompensated shock after vomiting and having diarrhea all night. A partial listing of the venous blood gas results is as follows:

pH, 7.165
pCO_2, 32.3 mm Hg
HCO_3, 11.1 mEq/L
pO_2, 45.3 mm Hg
BE (base excess), −16.6 mEq/L

To begin the analysis, note that the pH < 7.4 indicates that the dog has an acidemia that must be explained. To determine if it is primarily respiratory or nonrespiratory in origin, note that the pCO_2 is less than 37.4 mm Hg and the HCO_3 is less than 22.5 mEq/L. Using Table 3, we find that this measurement indicates that the patient has a primary metabolic acidosis that may be—or at first glance seems to be—compensated. This requires an assessment of the appropriateness of the compensatory attempt. The patient's decrease in bicarbonate is 11.4 mEq/L (normal − actual or 22.5 − 11.1 = 11.4 mEq/L). If we multiply by the expected compensatory factor of 0.7 mm Hg for each mEq/L of bicarbonate, we find the expected decrease in pCO_2 is 8 mm Hg (11.4 × 0.7 = 8). The expected pCO_2 for this patient is 29.4 mm Hg (normal − expected change or 37.4 − 8). Finally, for compensation to have occurred we expect the actual to be within 1 to 2 of the expected or predicted value. In this case, as the pCO_2 begins to decline from normal of 37.4 mm Hg, the actual pCO_2 of 32.3 mm Hg is 2.9 mm Hg shy of the expected value of 29.4 mm Hg. This value is in the uncompensated range (although clearly close to being compensated), as indicated in Fig. 1. The base deficit in this case confirms that there is a substantial nonrespiratory acidosis present. Review of the patient's problems would indicate that likely sources of the nonrespiratory acidosis might include lactic acidosis from poor perfusion and loss of bicarbonate in diarrhea. Further evaluation of the nonrespiratory acidosis could be accomplished by using a Gamblegram. In this patient, the failure of the respiratory system to compensate effectively may be caused by the advanced state of the patient's disease. The advanced shock state and low pH may contribute to poor respiratory muscle function.

Case Two

A 3-year-old castrated male domestic shorthair cat presents for treatment of urethral obstruction of 18 hours' duration. A venous blood gas analysis reveals the following results:

pH, 6.96
pCO_2, 52.0 mm Hg
HCO_3, 11.0 mEq/L
pO_2, 47.1 mm Hg
BE, −22 mEq/L

The results indicate that the cat has severe acidemia. The HCO_3 is markedly decreased, which is consistent with a nonrespiratory acidosis. The pCO_2 is also markedly increased, consistent with a respiratory acidosis. No compensatory response is occurring, and the patient has a mixed acidosis. The base deficit confirms our original diagnosis of a nonrespiratory acidosis. A Gamblegram analysis would be needed to parse out the potential causes of the nonrespiratory acidosis; however, postrenal azotemia, combined with the possibility of decreased perfusion and lactic acidosis, would be a logical source of the nonrespiratory acidosis. The respiratory component could be explained by severe hypokalemia, hypothermia, and severe acidosis, which would all have a summative negative impact on respiratory function. As the respiratory function and ability to compensate for the nonrespiratory acidosis decrease, the pH may rapidly worsen along with the patient's condition.

Case Three

A 9-year-old castrated male dog is diagnosed with gastrointestinal lymphoma, and a perforation with peritonitis is suspected. Arterial blood gas analysis in room air at sea level reveals

pH, 7.376
pCO_2, 12.6 mm Hg
HCO_3, 7.4 mEq/L
pO_2, 116.0 mm Hg
BE, 15.0 mEq/L
Lactate, 8.8 mmol/L

The patient's pH less than 7.4 indicates that acidemia is present. The patient's pCO_2 is less than 36.8 mm Hg and the HCO_3 is less than 22.2 mEq/L, which indicates that a compensatory nonrespiratory acidosis may be present. Evaluation of the compensatory response indicates that a decrease of 10.4 mm Hg in pCO_2 is expected ($22.2 - 7.4 = 14.8 \times 0.7 = 10.4$). The expected pCO_2 should be 26.4 mm Hg ($36.8 - 10.4$). The actual pCO_2 value of 12.6 mm Hg is 13.8 mm Hg more than the expected value, which indicates that a mixed disorder consisting of a nonrespiratory acidosis and respiratory alkalosis is present. A large base deficit is consistent with our diagnosis of nonrespiratory acidosis. Possible explanations include nonrespiratory acidosis caused by increased lactate concentration and respiratory alkalosis from pain or stress. The nonrespiratory acidosis could be evaluated more completely using a Gamblegram. Because this is an arterial sample, a PaO_2/FiO_2 ratio can be calculated ($116/0.21 = 552$) and is found to be in the normal range. We could also see that the PaO_2 value is more than five times the FiO_2 and indicates no abnormal respiratory function without calculating the P/F ratio. Because this is normal, an A-a gradient calculation also seems unnecessarily complex.

Case Four

A 12-year-old castrated male domestic shorthair cat presents for evaluation of hemorrhagic pleural effusion (likely neoplastic in origin). A venous blood gas analysis reveals

pH, 7.36
pCO_2, 39 mm Hg
HCO_3, 21.7 mEq/L
BE, −3 mEq/L
Sodium, 136 mEq/L
Potassium, 4 mEq/L
Chloride, 98 mEq/L
Phosphorus, 7.2 mg/dL
Total protein, 3.8 g/dL

At first glance, evaluation of the results indicates that a mild compensated nonrespiratory acidosis is present. The base deficit also indicates that there is a mild nonrespiratory acidosis. Calculation of the anion gap also indicates nothing abnormal (20.4 mEq/L), and there is no suspicion of any unmeasured anions. There would be a temptation not to evaluate this situation further. Evaluation of this patient using a Gamblegram approach, however, shows a moderate acidosis attributed to the hyponatremia (ie, gain of free water), a moderate alkalosis that could be attributed to the hypochloremia, and a marked decrease in protein that would contribute to an alkalosis. It seems that some additional acidosis must be present to explain the minimal decrease in bicarbonate. Unmeasured strong anions (eg, lactate or ketoacids) may be present, and the patient should be assessed appropriately to screen for this potential. In this case, the marked hypoproteinemia obscures the ability of the anion gap to successfully identify the increased unmeasured strong anions, which makes use of the Gamblegram approach more important in cases with derangements of protein and phosphorus.

References

[1] Constable P. Clinical assessment of acid-base status: comparison of the Henderson-Hasselbalch and strong ion approaches. Vet Clin Pathol 2000;29(4):115–28.

[2] Corey H. Bench-to-bedside review: fundamental principles of acid-base physiology. Crit Care 2005;9(2):184–92.

[3] Constable P. Clinical assessment of acid-base status: strong ion difference theory. Vet Clin North Am Food Anim Pract 1999;15(3):447–71.

[4] Story D. Bench-to-bedside review: a brief history of clinical acid-base. Crit Care 2004;8(4): 253–8.

[5] Severinghaus J, Astrup P. History of blood gas analysis. II. Ph and acid-base balance measurements. J Clin Monit 1985;1(4):259–77.

[6] Hopper K, Rezende M, Haskins S. Assessment of the effect of dilution of blood samples with sodium heparin on blood gas, electrolyte, and lactate measurements in dogs. Am J Vet Res 2005;66(4):656–60.

[7] Rezende M, Haskins S, Hopper K. The effects of ice-water storage on blood gas and acid-base measurements. Journal of Veterinary Emergency & Critical Care 2007;17(1):67–71.

[8] Schwartz W, Relman A. A critique of the parameters used in the evaluation of acid-base disorders: "whole-blood buffer base" and "standard bicarbonate" compared with blood pH and plasma bicarbonate concentration. N Engl J Med 1963;268:1382–8.

[9] Severinghaus J. Siggaard-Andersen and the "Great trans-Atlantic acid-base debate." Scand J Clin Lab Invest Suppl 1993;214:99–104.

[10] Severinghaus J. Acid-base balance nomogram: a Boston-Copenhagen detente. Anesthesiology 1976;45(5):539–41.

[11] Severinghaus J. Acid-base balance controversy: case for standard-base excess as the measure of nonrespiratory acid-base imbalance. J Clin Monit 1991;7(3):276–7.

[12] deMorais H, DiBartola S. Ventilatory and metabolic compensation in dogs with acid-base disturbances. Journal of Veterinary Emergency & Critical Care 1991;1:39–49.

[13] MacDonald R. The gamblegram as an aid to electrolyte study. J Mich State Med Soc 1956;55(5):538–41.

[14] Gilbert R, Keighley J. The arterial-alveolar oxygen tension ratio: an index of gas exchange applicable to varying inspired oxygen concentrations. Am Rev Respir Dis 1974;109(1): 142–5.

[15] Bornscheuer A, Mahr K, Bötel C, et al. Cardiopulmonary effects of lying position in anesthetized and mechanically ventilated dogs. J Exp Anim Sci 1996;38(1):20–7.
[16] Ogilvie G, Walters L, Fettman M, et al. Energy expenditure in dogs with lymphoma fed two specialized diets. Cancer 1993;71(10):3146–52.
[17] Harris E, Kenyon A, Nisbet H, et al. The normal alveolar-arterial oxygen-tension gradient in man. Clin Sci Mol Med 1974;46(1):89–104.
[18] Carroll G. Misapplication of alveolar gas equation. N Engl J Med 1985;312(9):586.

Metabolic Acid-Base Disorders in the Critical Care Unit

Helio Autran de Morais, DVM, Phd[a],*, Jonathan F. Bach, DVM[b], Stephen P. DiBartola, DVM[c]

[a]Department of Medical Sciences, University of Wisconsin–Madison, 2015 Linden Drive, Madison, WI 53706, USA
[b]Department of Medical Science, School of Veterinary Medicine, University of Wisconsin, Madison, WI 53706, USA
[c]Department of Veterinary Clinical Sciences, The Ohio State University, 601 Vernon L. Tharp Street, Columbus, OH 43210, USA

The recognition and management of acid-base disorders is a commonplace activity in the critical care unit. Adequate evaluation of the acid-base status requires a routine electrolyte panel, albumin or total protein concentration, and arterial blood gas analysis because of the interrelation between electrolytes (as strong ions), proteins (weak acids), and acid-base changes [1]. Metabolic acid-base disorders are caused by alteration in the strong ion difference (SID) or total weak acid concentration. A decrease in the SID is associated with metabolic acidosis, whereas an increase in the SID is associated with metabolic alkalosis. Care must be taken when using different analyzers to measure electrolytes, however. Direct potentiometry is commonly used in blood gas analyzers and point-of-care electrolyte analyzers, whereas indirect potentiometry is commonly used in the large chemistry analyzers located in the central laboratory [2]. Significant differences between a point-of-care analysis and the central laboratory in detecting sodium and chloride values have been found [3,4] and may be worse in hypoalbuminemic patients [5]. These differences ultimately affect quantitative acid-base measurements, because differences in results may be based on technology rather than on pathophysiology.

The criticalist benefits from classifying acid-base disorders into three groups: a fixed feature of a preexisting disease process (eg, chronic renal failure, hypoalbuminemia), a labile feature of an evolving disease process (ie, lactic acidosis from hemorrhage, hypochloremic alkalosis from vomiting), or iatrogenically induced (ie, hyperchloremic metabolic acidosis from saline administration, hypochloremic alkalosis from loop diuretic administration) [6]. The therapy for, and the outcome from, each of these three categories may be distinctly different.

*Corresponding author. E-mail address: demorais@vetmed.wisc.edu (H. Autran de Morais).

0195-5616/08/$ – see front matter
doi:10.1016/j.cvsm.2008.02.003

WEAK ACIDS AND ACID-BASE DISORDERS

Albumin, globulins, and inorganic phosphate are nonvolatile weak acids. Consequently, changes in their concentrations directly change pH. Hypoalbuminemia is associated with a decrease in pH, whereas hyperphosphatemia leads to metabolic acidosis.

Hypoalbuminemia

In vitro, a 1-g/dL decrease in albumin concentration is associated with an increase in pH of 0.093 in cats [7] and 0.047 in dogs [8]. The anion gap (AG) in healthy dogs and cats essentially reflects the total protein concentration. Thus, hypoalbuminemia also decreases the AG. At a plasma pH of 7.4 in dogs, each decrease of 1 g/dL in albumin concentration is associated with a decrease of 4.1 mEq/L in the AG, whereas each decrease of 1 g/dL in total protein concentration is associated with a decrease of 2.5 mEq/L in the AG [8]. Similar data are not available for cats.

Hyperphosphatemia

At a pH of 7.4, a 1-mg/dL increase in phosphate concentration is associated with a 0.58-mEq/L decrease in HCO_3^- concentration. Although the contribution of serum phosphate concentration to the AG is negligible in normal dogs and cats, hyperphosphatemia can increase the AG in the absence of an increase in strong unmeasured anions. The AG can be adjusted for an increase in phosphate concentration by multiplying the phosphate concentration (in mg/dL) by 0.58 [1].

STRONG IONS AND ACID BASE-DISORDERS

Strong ions are fully dissociated at physiologic pH, and therefore exert no buffering effect. Strong ions do exert an electrical effect, however, because the sum of completely dissociated cations does not equal the sum of completely dissociated anions. Stewart [9] called this difference the SID. Because strong ions do not participate in chemical reactions in plasma at physiologic pH, they act as a collective positive unit of charge (SID). Neither hydrogen nor hydroxyl ions are strong ions, because water is not a strong electrolyte; in fact, it is a weak one. Bicarbonate is also not a strong electrolyte because it can combine with numerous other chemical species, such as hydrogen ions. The quantitatively most important strong ions in plasma are Na^+, K^+, Ca^{2+}, Mg^{2+}, Cl^-, lactate, β-hydroxybutyrate, acetoacetate, and SO_4^{2-}. The influence of strong ions on pH and on HCO_3^- concentration can always be summarized in terms of the SID [9]. Changes in SID of a magnitude capable of altering acid-base balance usually occur as a result of increasing concentrations of Na^+, Cl^-, SO_4^{2-}, or organic anions or decreasing concentrations of Na^+ or Cl^-. An increase in SID (by decreasing Cl^- or increasing Na^+) causes a strong ion (metabolic) alkalosis, whereas a decrease in SID (by decreasing Na^+ or increasing Cl^-, SO_4^{2-}, or organic anions) causes a strong ion (metabolic) acidosis.

METABOLIC ALKALOSIS

Metabolic alkalosis may develop secondary to hypoalbuminemia (hypoalbuminemic alkalosis) or corrected hypochloremia (hypochloremic alkalosis) (Box 1) [1]. Metabolic alkalosis is not common in dogs and cats in a critical care setting. In human medicine, however, metabolic alkalosis accounted for more than half of all acid-base disorders in an intensive care setting and was also associated with high mortality rates [10–12]. Because mortality is especially high when a pH in excess of 7.6 develops, intervention at a pH of 7.55 or greater has been recommended in human patients [13]. In dogs, however, alkalemia is rare unless there is concomitant respiratory alkalosis [14].

Increase of blood pH may predispose to cardiac arrhythmia [15], cause alteration of consciousness, increase seizure activity, decrease oxygen release to tissue from hemoglobin, cause tetany secondary to hypocalcemia, increase ammonia generation by the kidney, and, in some instances, depress the respiratory drive [13,16].

Box 1: Common causes of metabolic alkalosis in critically ill patients

Preexisting disease process
  Hypoalbuminemic alkalosis
    Liver failure
    Protein-losing enteropathy
    Protein-losing nephropathy
  Hypochloremic alkalosis
    Diuretic therapy
    Vomiting of stomach contents
Labile feature of an evolving process
  Hypoalbuminemic alkalosis
    Vasculitis
    Third space losses
  Hypochloremic alkalosis
    Vomiting of stomach contents
    After correction of chronic respiratory acidosis
Iatrogenic
  Hypochloremic alkalosis
    Bicarbonate administration
    Diuretic therapy
    Stomach draining

Hypoalbuminemic Alkalosis

Hypoalbuminemic alkalosis is common in critically ill patients [17]. The presence of hypoalbuminemia complicates identification of increased unmeasured anions (eg, lactate, ketoanions), because hypoproteinemia not only increases pH but decreases the AG [18–20]. Thus, the severity of the underlying disease leading to metabolic acidosis may be underestimated if the effects of hypoalbuminemia on the pH, HCO_3^- concentration, and AG are not considered. Treatment for hypoalbuminemic alkalosis should be directed at the underlying cause and the decreased colloid oncotic pressure.

Hypochloremic Alkalosis

Hypochloremic alkalosis usually occurs secondary to vomiting of stomach contents or excessive administration of loop diuretics or sodium bicarbonate (see Box 1). Clinical signs associated with gastrointestinal disorders were preponderant in 13 alkalemic dogs with metabolic alkalosis, whereas overzealous administration of sodium bicarbonate or diuretics may have contributed to metabolic alkalosis in 8 of the dogs [14].

Treatment of hypochloremic alkalosis has been relatively constant for decades. If there is evidence of volume depletion, the deficit should be repaired with a chloride-containing fluid. From the perspective of physical chemistry, any hypochloremic alkalosis is "saline responsive," provided that sufficient saline (or any fluid with an SID of 0) can be administered [21]. Unfortunately, in the absence of hypovolemia, the amount of saline required introduces a risk for overload [21]. If the metabolic alkalosis is associated with hypokalemia and total body potassium deficits, correcting the deficit with potassium chloride (KCl) is a particularly effective way to reverse the alkalosis. From the Stewart perspective, this practice has similarities to infusing hydrogen chloride (HCl) minus the pH disadvantages of a negative SID. This is because potassium and potassium deficits are predominantly intracellular; thus, all but a small fraction of retained potassium ends up within the cells during correction. The net effect of KCl administration is that the retained strong anion (Cl^-) stays extracellular, whereas most of the retained strong cation disappears into the intracellular space. This is a potent stimulus for reducing plasma and extracellular SID [21]. Acetazolamide decreases SID and can be used as adjunct therapy for the correction of metabolic alkalosis in critical care patients [22].

METABOLIC ACIDOSIS

Metabolic acidosis may develop secondary to hyperphosphatemia (hyperphosphatemic acidosis), corrected hyperchloremia (hyperchloremic acidosis), and accumulation of metabolically produced strong anions (strong ion gap or high-AG acidosis) (Box 2) [1]. Metabolic acidosis, especially lactic acidosis, uremic acidosis, and diabetic ketoacidosis (DKA), occurs commonly in critically ill patients. In one study, metabolic acidosis was the most common acid-base disorder in dogs and cats [23].

Box 2: Common causes of metabolic acidosis in critically ill patients

Preexisting disease process
  Hyperphosphatemic acidosis
    Renal failure
  Hyperchloremic acidosis
    Renal tubular acidosis
    Renal failure
    Diarrhea
  High-AG acidosis
    Diabetes mellitus
    Renal failure

Labile feature of an evolving process
  Hyperphosphatemic acidosis
    Phosphate-containing enemas
    Acute renal failure
  Hyperchloremic acidosis
    Diarrhea
    After correction of chronic respiratory alkalosis
  High-AG acidosis
    DKA
    Uremic acidosis
    Lactic acidosis
    Toxicities (eg, ethylene glycol, salicylates)

Iatrogenic
  Hyperphosphatemic acidosis
    Intravenous phosphate administration
  Hyperchloremic acidosis
    0.9% sodium chloride administration
    KCl administration
    Total parenteral nutrition
  High-AG acidosis
    Propylene glycol as drug vehicle (eg, nitroglycerin, diazepam)
    Gelatin administration (increases AG without causing acidosis)

The effects of metabolic acidosis are multiple. The severity and reversibility of dysfunction, however, largely depend on the underlying cause and magnitude of the derangement. Despite the existence of many studies examining the effects of acidosis on isolated cells and perfused organs, the effects of changes in pH on whole-body physiology are largely unknown [24]. Although it intuitively makes sense that severe acidosis should adversely affect cell function, evidence clearly supporting this supposition is difficult to find. Severe acidosis has serious detrimental effects on cardiovascular function, including decreased cardiac output, decreased arterial blood pressure, and decreased hepatic and renal blood flow [25]. Myocardial contractility is decreased when blood pH decreases to less than 7.20 [26,27]. Impaired contractility may result from a decrease in myocardial intracellular pH and displacement of calcium ions from critical binding sites on contractile proteins. Acidosis may predispose the heart to ventricular arrhythmias or ventricular fibrillation. Acidosis has a direct arterial vasodilating effect that is offset by increased release of endogenous catecholamines. The inotropic response to catecholamines, however, is impaired, and this may be associated with a reduction in the number of β–adrenergic receptors [28]. Acidosis has a direct vasoconstrictive effect on the venous side of the circulation, which tends to centralize blood volume and predisposes to pulmonary congestion. Acidosis shifts the oxygen–hemoglobin dissociation curve to the right, thus enhancing oxygen release from hemoglobin, but this effect is offset by a decrease in red blood cell 2,3–diphosphoglycerate, which develops after 6 to 8 hours of acidosis and shifts the curve back to the left [26].

Acidemia produces insulin resistance that impairs peripheral uptake of glucose and inhibits anaerobic glycolysis by inhibiting phosphofructokinase [25]. During severe acidosis, the liver may be converted from a consumer to a producer of lactate [29]. Severe acidosis also impairs the ability of the brain to regulate its volume, leading to obtundation and coma. Acute mineral acidosis causes hyperkalemia by a transcellular shifting of potassium from intracellular fluid to extracellular fluid (ECF) in exchange for hydrogen ions. This effect causes a variable change in serum potassium concentration and is not observed with organic acidosis [30]. Acute reduction in blood pH causes displacement of calcium ions from negatively charged binding sites (eg, COO^- groups) on proteins (primarily albumin), because these sites become protonated and an increase in ionized serum calcium concentration results. Chronic metabolic acidosis leads to release of buffer (mainly calcium carbonate) from bone, and osteodystrophy and hypercalciuria result.

Hyperphosphatemic Acidosis

Hyperphosphatemia, especially if severe, can cause metabolic acidosis. The most important cause of hyperphosphatemic acidosis is renal failure. Metabolic acidosis in patients that have renal failure is multifactorial but is mostly caused by hyperphosphatemia and increases in unmeasured strong anions [31,32]. Hyperphosphatemic acidosis also has been observed after hypertonic sodium phosphate enema administration in cats [33] and in a cat that received a phosphate-containing urinary acidifier [34].

In a study of prevalence and outcome of different types of metabolic acidosis in a human critical care unit, hyperphosphatemia was associated with mortality [35]. One possible explanation was that the presence of hyperphosphatemia was only a marker of renal failure. Even after exclusion of patients with a phosphate concentration of greater than 5 mg/dL, however, the association between phosphate and mortality remained just as strong [35].

Treatment for hyperphosphatemic acidosis should be directed at re-establishing renal function and correcting the underlying cause of the hyperphosphatemia. Sodium bicarbonate [36] and glucose solutions [37] administered intravenously shift phosphate inside cells and may be used as adjunctive therapy in patients that have hyperphosphatemic acidosis [1].

Hyperchloremic Acidosis

Hyperchloremic acidosis may be caused by chloride retention (eg, early renal failure, renal tubular acidosis), by excessive loss of sodium relative to chloride (eg, diarrhea), or by administration of substances containing more chloride than sodium as compared with normal ECF composition (eg, administration of KCl, 0.9% sodium chloride [NaCl]). Even though many causes of metabolic acidosis may be unavoidable, the source of hyperchloremic acidosis is often iatrogenic. In critically ill patients, a common cause is related to the volume of saline infused during resuscitation from shock. It is a common cause of hyperchloremic acidosis in hospitalized patients [38] and is the classic example of strong ion acidosis [39]. In this setting, the genesis of hyperchloremic metabolic acidosis stems from excess chloride administration relative to sodium, commonly as 0.9% normal saline solution, 0.45% normal saline solution, and even lactated Ringer's solution in large quantities [40,41]. Treatment of hyperchloremic acidosis should be directed at correction of the underlying disease process. In patients that have severe hyperchloremic metabolic acidosis from diarrhea or renal tubular acidosis, the administration of sodium bicarbonate is reasonable. Whether a patient is likely to benefit from this therapy is difficult to predict and probably depends on the clinical circumstance [42].

Uremic Acidosis

Metabolic acidosis in critically ill human patients who have acute renal failure is multifactorial [31]. Compared with other critical care patients matched by Acute Physiological Assessment and Chronic Health Evaluation (APACHE) II score, patients who had acute renal failure had a lower pH with increased strong ion gap (organic acidosis), decreased albumin (hypoalbuminemic alkalosis), and increased phosphate (hyperphosphatemic acidosis). The anions responsible for the increase in strong ion gap were not identified, but lactate was similar in both groups. Potential culprits include sulfate, urate, hydroxypropionate, hippurate, oxalate, and furanpropionate [43].

In human patients who had chronic renal failure (mean creatinine concentration of 3.06 mg/dL) compared with normal subjects [44], there was mild SID acidosis attributable to a combination of hyponatremia and hyperchloremia. Unmeasured strong ions had a minimal role in the genesis of metabolic acidosis in these patients. There was a significant difference in phosphate concentration, but it was small (mean of 0.54 mg/dL or 0.31 mEq/L). Hyperphosphatemic acidosis was a contributor to the metabolic acidosis in chronic renal failure, however [45]. When 25 dogs with chronic renal failure and metabolic acidosis were compared with a group of healthy dogs, they showed an increase in the AG, decrease in albumin, and increase in phosphate concentration [46]. Unfortunately, data for sodium and chloride were not provided. The mean difference in the AG was 10 mEq/L. Correction of the AG for the decrease in albumin would raise the differences in the AG between the groups to 13 mEq/L. An increase in phosphate concentration in patients that had renal failure accounted for 55% (7.1 of 13 mEq/L) of the increase in the AG. This suggests that this population of dogs that had renal failure had a combination of hypoalbuminemic alkalosis with a more severe hyperphosphatemic acidosis. The AG suggests that other unmeasured strong anions were also increased in these dogs that had chronic renal failure.

In cats that had severe chronic renal failure, deterioration of renal function was associated with metabolic acidosis [47]. In those patients, there was a combination of hypochloremic alkalosis (decrease in corrected chloride of 7 mEq/L) and an increase in the AG of 6.6 mEq/L. Phosphate and albumin concentrations were not reported, and their contribution to the AG and to changes in acid-base balance cannot be estimated. The AG would have been higher in the absence of hypochloremic alkalosis, however. Severe hyperphosphatemia (mean of 9 mEq/L) has been previously identified in cats that had chronic renal failure before undergoing hemodialysis [48]. The role of hyperphosphatemia in the genesis of metabolic acidosis may help to explain why uremic acidosis is one of the few high-AG acidoses that responds to bicarbonate therapy [24]. Sodium bicarbonate administered intravenously shifts phosphate inside cells and may be used as adjunctive therapy in patients that have hyperphosphatemic acidosis [36].

Toxin-Induced Acidosis

Ingestions of various toxins can cause severe metabolic acidosis with an increased AG and should always be suspected in these cases. Ethylene glycol (EG), a sweet liquid found in antifreeze, is metabolized by alcohol dehydrogenase into glycolic acid and, subsequently, oxalic acid. In dogs, a severe high-AG metabolic acidosis occurs within 3 hours of EG ingestion and persists for at least 24 hours [49–52]. Serum hyperosmolality and the osmolal gap peak 1 to 6 hours after ingestion and persist for 12 to 24 hours, but the osmolal gap may be normal in animals presented later in the course of the disease. Calcium oxalate dihydrate crystals ("Maltese cross" or "envelope" form) may be observed in the urine, but calcium oxalate monohydrate crystals ("picket fence" or "dumbbell" form) are observed more commonly. Other laboratory findings include azotemia, isosthenuria, hypocalcemia, hyperphosphatemia, and hyperglycemia [50]. Hyperphosphatemia observed early in the course of EG intoxication (3–12 hours after ingestion) is probably attributable to the high phosphorus content of rust–retardant antifreeze preparations [52,53].

The response to treatment depends on the amount of EG ingested and the amount of time that elapses before treatment. Treatment consists of inducing vomiting with apomorphine or performing gastric lavage with activated charcoal if ingestion has been recent (<8 hours before presentation). Severe hypocalcemia is corrected with calcium gluconate, and $NaHCO_3$ is administered to combat metabolic acidosis. A dose of $NaHCO_3$ of 1 to 2 mEq/kg may be used empirically. Calcium gluconate and $NaHCO_3$ must not be given simultaneously, because calcium carbonate crystals form and the solution becomes turbid. Alcohol dehydrogenase has greater affinity for ethanol than for EG. For this reason, 20% ethanol has been administered intravenously to affected dogs and cats. This treatment is unlikely to be of benefit if longer than 12 to 24 hours has elapsed, because of ingestion of EG. 4–Methylpyrazole is a pharmacologic inhibitor of alcohol dehydrogenase that has become available to treat dogs that have EG toxicosis [52,54]. Unfortunately, 4–methylpyrazole is not efficacious in EG–intoxicated cats unless administered at the same time that the EG is consumed.

Diabetic Ketoacidosis

Overproduction of acetoacetate ($pK_a' = 3.58$) and β–hydroxybutyrate ($pK_a' = 4.70$) by the liver occurs in diabetes mellitus because of a deficiency of insulin and relative excess of glucagon. Acetone is formed by the nonenzymatic decarboxylation of acetoacetate and does not contribute additional fixed acid. Metabolic acidosis is common in dogs and cats that have DKA [55,56]. Although classically considered a high-AG acidosis, the AG is elevated in less than half of dogs that have DKA [55]. In one study of dogs that had diabetes mellitus, the mean plasma HCO_3^- concentration was 13.7 mEq/L in eight survivors (range: 9.3–21.0 mEq/L) and 18.1 mEq/L in five nonsurvivors (range: 13.4–30.2 mEq/L) [57]. Venous pH and base deficit (but not AG) were associated with survival [56]. In another study of dogs that had DKA, mean arterial pH and HCO_3^- concentrations were 7.201 (range: 6.986–7.395) and 11.1 mEq/L (range: 4.1–19.7 mEq/L) before treatment and 7.407 ± 0.053 and 18.2 ± 0.7 mEq/L 24 hours after treatment [58]. Only three dogs (those with a pH <7.1) received sodium bicarbonate treatment. Metabolic acidosis with a median pH of 7.14 (range: 7.04–7.24) and HCO_3^- concentration of 10 mEq/L (range: 6–15 mEq/L) was found in 25 of 33 cats evaluated by venous blood gas analysis in a survey of cats that had DKA [59]. Cats with HCO_3^- concentrations less than 14 mEq/L received bicarbonate supplementation of their fluids. In another series of diabetic cats, the median total carbon dioxide was 13 mEq/L in cats that had DKA and 15 mEq/L in cats that did not have DKA [60].

To some extent, the anions of these ketoanions are excreted in the urine, along with sodium and potassium, for electroneutrality. The extent of impairment in renal function may determine whether patients that have DKA have an increased AG metabolic acidosis or hyperchloremic metabolic acidosis at the time of presentation. Patients with severe volume depletion have an increased AG gap because of retention of ketoanions, whereas those without volume depletion have hyperchloremia as a result of increased urinary excretion of the sodium and potassium salts of ketoanions and retention of chloride [61,62]. Volume-depleted patients may develop lactic acidosis associated with decreased tissue perfusion or impaired lactate use caused by decreased insulin activity. In this circumstance, lactic acidosis promotes conversion of acetoacetate to β-hydroxybutyrate, which does not react with nitroprusside in the urinalysis dipstrip reagent pad, thereby masking the ketoacidosis [63]. It has been suggested that adding a few drops of hydrogen peroxide to the urine specimen would nonenzymatically convert β-hydroxybutyrate to acetoacetate, which would then be detected by the nitroprusside reagent [64]. This method has been shown to be ineffective in converting β-hydroxybutyrate to acetoacetate in dogs, however [65]. Patients that have diabetes mellitus may have a mixed high-AG and hyperchloremic acidosis because of development of diarrhea or in the resolving phase of the ketoacidotic crisis [66,67]. Hyperchloremia in the recovery phase develops for at least three reasons: (1) large volumes of saline are administered; (2) KCl is infused in large doses; and (3) ketones are lost in the urine, and NaCl is reabsorbed by the kidneys [63].

The treatment of DKA consists of three parts: fluid resuscitation, insulin administration, and correction of potassium deficits. Patients that have DKA often have profound deficits of volume and free water. Hypovolemia, as demonstrated by cardiovascular compromise, should always be treated first [24]. Regular insulin should be administered after fluid resuscitation is well underway. If insulin is given precipitously, the rapid uptake by the cells of glucose can cause water to follow osmotically, resulting in cardiovascular collapse. Insulin administration allows glucose use by skeletal muscle and adipose tissue, decreases hepatic glucose production, prevents lipolysis and ketogenesis, and permits peripheral metabolism of ketoacids. Most patients that have DKA have total body potassium depletion. Despite this, their serum potassium may be normal to high because of a shift from out of the cells caused by the profound insulinopenia. When insulin is restored, extracellular potassium is rapidly taken up and severe serum hypokalemia may result. Thus, supplementation of potassium is needed as soon as potassium concentration is less than 5 mEq/L.

The use of $NaHCO_3$ to treat DKA is highly controversial, and clear benefits of its use have not been demonstrated in human patients. For example, there was no difference in recovery (based on the rate of decrease of blood glucose and ketone concentrations and the rate of increase of blood or cerebrospinal fluid [CSF] pH or HCO_3^- concentration) when $NaHCO_3$ was or was not administered to human patients who had DKA and presented with blood pH values in the range 6.90 to 7.14 [68]. In another study, treatment with $NaHCO_3$ actually delayed resolution of ketosis in DKA [69]. Possible deleterious effects of bicarbonate administration may occur even in patients with a serum pH less than 7.0 [67]. Because the acidosis is rapidly improved with appropriate management, administration of sodium bicarbonate to patients that have DKA cannot be recommended at any pH [24].

Lactic Acidosis

Lactic acidosis is characterized by an accumulation of lactate in body fluids and a plasma lactate concentration greater than 5 mEq/L. The pK_a' of lactic acid is

3.86, and it is completely dissociated at the normal pH of ECF (7.40). Lactic acidosis is a final common feature of a variety of processes that engender hypoperfusion, including DKA, septic shock, cardiogenic shock, and a variety of intoxications. An early approach to the broad classification of elevated lactate concentration was based on the presence (type A) or absence (type B) of hypoperfusion (Box 3). Although heuristically pleasing, most cases of type A lactic acidosis are likely not secondary to hypoxemia. Contemporary

---

Box 3: Causes of L-lactic acidosis

Hypoxic patients (lactic acidosis is not likely a result of hypoxia)
Increased oxygen demand
    Severe exercise
    Convulsions
Decreased oxygen availability
    Reduced tissue perfusion
        Cardiac arrest, cardiopulmonary resuscitation
        Shock
        Hypovolemia
        Left ventricular failure
        Low cardiac output
        Acute pulmonary edema
    Reduced arterial oxygen content
        Hypoxemia ($PO_2 \leq 30$ mm Hg)
        Extremely severe anemia (packed cell volume <10%)

Nonhypoxic patients
Drugs and toxins
    Salicylates
    EG
    Propylene glycol
Diabetes mellitus
Liver failure
Neoplasia (eg, lymphosarcoma)
Sepsis
Renal failure
Hypoglycemia
Hereditary defects

Adapted from DiBartola SP. Metabolic acid-base disorders. In: DiBartola SP, editor. Fluid, electrolyte, and acid-base disorders. 3rd edition. St. Louis (MO): Elsevier; 2006. p. 264.

understanding of the complexity of lactate production and metabolism in critical illness has practically relegated this classification system to that of a historical one [2,70,71]. The improved understanding of the complexities of lactate metabolism has fueled the controversy regarding lactate's role in the care of critically ill patients [2,72]. Aside from hypoperfusion leading to cellular dysoxia, elevated lactate has been associated with several common cellular processes that are present in critical illness. These include increased activity of Na^+/K^+-ATPase in normoxia [73], increased pyruvate and lactate as a result of increased aerobic glycolysis [74], and decreased lactate clearance [75].

In the traditional classification, type A (hypoxic) lactic acidosis was associated with normal mitochondrial function but inadequate oxygen delivery to tissues, whereas in type B, (nonhypoxic) lactic acidosis, there was adequate oxygen delivery to tissues but defective mitochondrial oxidative function and abnormal carbohydrate metabolism. There is now evidence that hyperlactatemia after injury and sepsis may result from an adrenaline surge that stimulates sarcolemmal Na^+-K^+-ATPase activity and coupled aerobic glycolysis [73,76]. Persistent hyperlactatemia in the face of hemodynamic stability may reflect adrenaline-stimulated aerobic glycolysis rather than tissue hypoxia [73]. Na^+-K^+-ATPase activity is also activated during exercise [77,78]. Evidence now suggests that the increase in lactate production and hyperlactemia as a result of anoxia or dysoxia is the exception rather than the rule [70,72].

Lactic acidosis may occur in several clinical settings, especially those in which poor perfusion and tissue hypoxia (eg, cardiac arrest and cardiopulmonary resuscitation, shock, left ventricular failure) may be present. Even knowing that hypoxia is likely not the cause of hyperlactatemia in those settings, the clinician should strongly consider the possibility of concomitant lactic acidosis. Usually, lactic acidosis results from accumulation of the L isomer of lactate. Lactic acidosis should be suspected whenever there is an unexplained increase in unmeasured anions (ie, an unexplained increase in the AG). Confirmation requires measurement of plasma lactate concentration. Care should be taken to avoid vascular stasis when collecting venous blood for lactate determinations, and blood samples should be centrifuged immediately after collection to avoid a spurious increase in lactate concentration related to anaerobic glycolysis by red blood cells.

The treatment of lactic acidosis is fraught with controversy. Clinicians universally agree that the most important step in the treatment of lactic acidosis is to treat the underlying cause [24]. Tissue perfusion and oxygen delivery should be improved by aggressive fluid therapy to expand the ECF volume. Ventilation with oxygen should be considered if the patient's spontaneous ventilation is inadequate. Infections should be treated with appropriate antimicrobial agents, and cardiac output should be improved, if necessary, by administration of inotropic agents. If the underlying disease cannot be corrected, the prognosis for patients that have lactic acidosis is poor. If the underlying disease can be corrected, the accumulated lactate is metabolized, yielding an equivalent amount of HCO_3^-, and the acidosis is reversed.

Intravenous sodium bicarbonate may increase blood pH when ventilation is not limited, but its effect on intracellular pH is unclear. Perhaps more importantly, no clinical benefit from sodium bicarbonate has been demonstrated in the setting of lactic acidosis [42]. Administration of sodium bicarbonate to patients that have lactic acidosis is not recommended, regardless of the pH. This includes lactic acidosis caused by hypoperfusion, sepsis, mitochondrial dysfunction, or liver failure [42]. Although not universally endorsed [79], use of sodium bicarbonate has been suggested if serum bicarbonate decreases to less than 5 mEq/L, because at this concentration, even a small decrease in serum bicarbonate can have a large effect on serum pH [24]. Limited data exist for other buffer agents, such as Carbicarb and tromethamine, or for drugs that stimulate pyruvate kinase (eg, dichloroacetate) [42].

References

[1] de Morais HA, Constable PD. Strong ion approach to acid-base disorders. In: DiBartola SP, editor. Fluid, electrolyte, and acid-base disorders. St. Louis (MO): Elsevier; 2006. p. 310–21.

[2] Gunnerson KJ. Clinical review: the meaning of acid-base abnormalities in the intensive care unit part I—epidemiology. Crit Care 2005;9(5):508–16.

[3] Morimatsu H, Rocktaschel J, Bellomo R, et al. Comparison of point-of-care versus central laboratory measurement of electrolyte concentrations on calculations of the anion gap and the strong ion difference. Anesthesiology 2003;98(5):1077–84.

[4] Loughrey CM, Hanna EV, McDonnell M, et al. Sodium measurement: effects of differing sampling and analytical methods. Ann Clin Biochem 2006;43(Pt 6):488–93.

[5] Story DA, Morimatsu H, Egi M, et al. The effect of albumin concentration on plasma sodium and chloride measurements in critically ill patients. Anesth Analg 2007;104(4):893–7.

[6] Kaplan LJ, Frangos S. Clinical review: acid-base abnormalities in the intensive care unit—part II. Crit Care 2005;9(2):198–203.

[7] McCullough SM, Constable PD. Calculation of the total plasma concentration of nonvolatile weak acids and the effective dissociation constant of nonvolatile buffers in plasma for use in the strong ion approach to acid-base balance in cats. Am J Vet Res 2003;64(8):1047–51.

[8] Constable PD, Stampfli HR. Experimental determination of net protein charge and A(tot) and K(a) of nonvolatile buffers in canine plasma. J Vet Intern Med 2005;19(4):507–14.

[9] Stewart PA. Independent and dependent variables of acid-base control. Resp Physiol 1978;33:9–26.

[10] Hodgkin JE, Soeprono FF, Chan DM. Incidence of metabolic alkalemia in hospitalized patients. Crit Care Med 1980;8(12):725–8.

[11] Wilson RF, Gibson D, Percinel AK, et al. Severe alkalosis in critically ill surgical patients. Arch Surg 1972;105(2):197–203.

[12] Anderson LE, Henrich WL. Alkalemia-associated morbidity and mortality in medical and surgical patients. South Med J 1987;80(6):729–33.

[13] Laski ME, Sabatini S. Metabolic alkalosis, bedside and bench. Semin Nephrol 2006;26(6):404–21.

[14] Robinson EP, Hardy RM. Clinical signs, diagnosis, and treatment of alkalemia in dogs: 20 cases (1982–1984). J Am Vet Med Assoc 1988;7(1):943–9.

[15] McKinney TD, Burg MB. Bicarbonate transport by rabbit cortical collecting tubules. Effect of acid and alkali loads in vivo on transport in vitro. J Clin Invest 1977;60(3):766–8.

[16] Laski ME, Kurtzman NA. Acid-base disorders in medicine. Dis Mon 1996;42(2):51–125.

[17] Fencl V, Jabor A, Kazda A, et al. Diagnosis of metabolic acid-base disturbances in critically ill patients. Am J Respir Crit Care Med 2000;162(6):2246–51.

[18] Figge J, Jabor A, Kazda A, et al. Anion gap and hypoalbuminemia. Crit Care Med 1998;26(11):1807–10.

[19] Hatherill M, Waggie Z, Purves L, et al. Correction of the anion gap for albumin in order to detect occult tissue anions in shock. Arch Dis Child 2002;87(6):526–9.

[20] Durward A, Mayer A, Skellett S, et al. Hypoalbuminaemia in critically ill children: incidence, prognosis, and influence on the anion gap. Arch Dis Child 2003;88(5):419–22.

[21] Morgan TJ. The meaning of acid-base abnormalities in the intensive care unit: part III—effects of fluid administration. Crit Care 2005;9(2):204–11.

[22] Moviat M, Pickkers P, van der Voort PH, et al. Acetazolamide-mediated decrease in strong ion difference accounts for the correction of metabolic alkalosis in critically ill patients. Crit Care 2006;10(1):R14.

[23] Cornelius LM, Rawlings CA. Arterial blood gas and acid-base values in dogs with various diseases and signs of disease. J Am Vet Med Assoc 1981;178(9):992–5.

[24] Gauthier PM, Szerlip HM. Metabolic acidosis in the intensive care unit. Crit Care Clin 2002;18(2):289–308.

[25] Adrogue HJ, Madias NE. Management of life-threatening acid-base disorders. First of two parts. N Engl J Med 1998;338(1):26–34.

[26] Mitchell JH, Wildenthal K, Johnson RL Jr. The effects of acid-base disturbances on cardiovascular and pulmonary function. Kidney Int 1972;1(5):375–89.

[27] Orchard CH, Kentish JC. Effects of changes of pH on the contractile function of cardiac muscle. Am J Physiol 1990;258(6 Pt 1):C967–81.

[28] Marsh JD, Margolis TI, Kim D. Mechanism of diminished contractile response to catecholamines during acidosis. Am J Physiol 1988;254(1 Pt 2):H20–7.

[29] Madias NE. Lactic acidosis. Kidney Int 1986;29:752–74.

[30] Adrogué JH, Madias NE. Changes in plasma potassium concentration during acute acid-base disturbances. Am J Med 1981;71:456–71.

[31] Rocktaeschel J, Morimatsu H, Uchino S, et al. Acid-base status of critically ill patients with acute renal failure: analysis based on Stewart-Figge methodology. Crit Care 2003;7(4): R60–6.

[32] Naka T, Bellomo R. Bench-to-bedside review: treating acid-base abnormalities in the intensive care unit—the role of renal replacement therapy. Crit Care 2004;8(2):108–14.

[33] Atkins CE, Tyler R, Greenlee P. Clinical, biochemical, acid-base, and electrolyte abnormalities in cats after hypertonic sodium phosphate enema administration. Am J Vet Res 1985;46(4):980–8.

[34] Fulton R, Fruechte L. Poisoning induced by administration of a phosphate-containing urinary acidifier in a cat. J Am Vet Med Assoc 1991;198(5):883–5.

[35] Gunnerson KJ, Saul M, He S, et al. Lactate versus non-lactate metabolic acidosis: a retrospective outcome evaluation of critically ill patients. Crit Care 2006;10(1):R22.

[36] Barsotti G, Lazzeri M, Cristofano C, et al. The role of metabolic acidosis in causing uremic hyperphosphatemia. Miner Electrolyte Metab 1986;12(2):103–6.

[37] Biarent D, Brumagne C, Steppe M, et al. Acute phosphate intoxication in seven infants under parenteral nutrition. JPEN J Parenter Enteral Nutr 1992;16(6):558–60.

[38] de Morais HSA. Chloride ion in small animal practice: the forgotten ion. Journal of Veterinary Emergency and Critical Care 1992;2(1):11–24.

[39] Constable PD. Hyperchloremic acidosis: the classic example of strong ion acidosis. Anesth Analg 2003;96(4):919–22.

[40] Moviat M, van Haren F, van der Hoeven H. Conventional or physicochemical approach in intensive care unit patients with metabolic acidosis. Crit Care 2003;7(3):R41–5.

[41] Scheingraber S, Rehm M, Sehmisch C, et al. Rapid saline infusion produces hyperchloremic acidosis in patients undergoing gynecologic surgery. Anesthesiology 1999;90(5): 1265–70.

[42] Gehlbach BK, Schmidt GA. Bench-to-bedside review: treating acid-base abnormalities in the intensive care unit—the role of buffers. Crit Care 2004;8(4):259–65.

[43] Niwa T, Asada H, Maeda K, et al. Profiling of organic acids and polyols in nerves of uraemic and non-uraemic patients. J Chromatogr 1986;377:15–22.

[44] Story DA, Tosolini A, Bellomo R, et al. Plasma acid-base changes in chronic renal failure: a Stewart analysis. Int J Artif Organs 2005;28(10):961–5.

[45] Bellomo R, Ronco C. New ideas in science and medicine and the renal control of acid-base balance. Int J Artif Organs 2005;28(10):957–60.

[46] Kogika MM, Lustoza MD, Notomi MK, et al. Serum ionized calcium in dogs with chronic renal failure and metabolic acidosis. Vet Clin Pathol 2006;35(4):441–5.

[47] Elliott J, Syme HM, Markwell PJ. Acid-base balance of cats with chronic renal failure: effect of deterioration in renal function. J Small Anim Pract 2003;44(6):261–8.

[48] Langston CE, Cowgill LD, Spano JA. Applications and outcome of hemodialysis in cats: a review of 29 cases. J Vet Intern Med 1997;11(6):348–55.

[49] Grauer GF, Thrall MA, Henre BA, et al. Early clinicopathologic findings in dogs ingesting ethylene glycol. Am J Vet Res 1984;45(11):2299–303.

[50] Thrall MA, Grauer GF, Mero KN. Clinicopathologic findings in dogs and cats with ethylene glycol intoxication. J Am Vet Med Assoc 1984;184(1):37–41.

[51] Dial SM, Thrall MA, Hamar DW. Comparison of ethanol and 4-methylpyrazole as treatments for ethylene glycol intoxication in cats. Am J Vet Res 1994;55(12):1771–82.

[52] Dial SM, Thrall MA, Hamar DW. Efficacy of 4-methylpyrazole for treatment of ethylene glycol intoxication in dogs. Am J Vet Res 1994;55(12):1762–70.

[53] Connally HE, Thrall MA, Forney SD, et al. Safety and efficacy of 4-methylpyrazole for treatment of suspected or confirmed ethylene glycol intoxication in dogs: 107 cases (1983–1995). J Am Vet Med Assoc 1996;209(11):1880–3.

[54] Dial SM, Thrall MA, Hamar DW. 4-Methylpyrazole as treatment for naturally acquired ethylene glycol intoxication in dogs. J Am Vet Med Assoc 1989;195(1):73–6.

[55] Duarte R, Simoes DM, Franchini ML, et al. Accuracy of serum beta-hydroxybutyrate measurements for the diagnosis of diabetic ketoacidosis in 116 dogs. J Vet Intern Med 2002;16(4):411–7.

[56] Hume DZ, Drobatz KJ, Hess RS. Outcome of dogs with diabetic ketoacidosis: 127 dogs (1993–2003). J Vet Intern Med 2006;20(3):547–55.

[57] Ling GV, Lowenstine LJ, Pulley LT, et al. Diabetes mellitus in dogs: a review of initial evaluation, immediate and long-term management, and outcome. J Am Vet Med Assoc 1977;170(5):521–30.

[58] Macintire DK. Treatment of diabetic ketoacidosis in dogs by continuous low-dose intravenous infusion of insulin. J Am Vet Med Assoc 1993;202(8):1266–72.

[59] Bruskiewicz KA, Nelson RW, Feldman EC, et al. Diabetic ketosis and ketoacidosis in cats: 42 cases (1980–1995). J Am Vet Med Assoc 1997;211(2):188–92.

[60] Crenshaw KL, Peterson ME. Pretreatment clinical and laboratory evaluation of cats with diabetes mellitus: 104 cases (1992–1994). J Am Vet Med Assoc 1996;209(5):943–9.

[61] Adrogué HJ, Wilson H, Boyd AE III, et al. Plasma acid-base patterns in diabetic ketoacidosis. N Engl J Med 1982;307:1603–10.

[62] Adrogue HJ, Eknoyan G, Suki WK. Diabetic ketoacidosis: role of the kidney in the acid-base homeostasis re-evaluated. Kidney Int 1984;25(4):591–8.

[63] Narins RG, Emmett M. Simple and mixed acid-base disorders: a practical approach. Medicine 1980;59(3):161–87.

[64] Narins RG, Jones ER, Stom MC, et al. Diagnostic strategies in disorders of fluid, electrolyte and acid-base homeostasis. Am J Med 1982;72:496–506.

[65] Christopher MM, Pereira JL, Brigmon RL. Adaptation of an automated assay for determination of beta-hydroxybutyrate in dogs using a random access analyzer. Vet Clin Pathol 1992;21(1):3–8.

[66] Ray S, Piraino B, Chong TK, et al. Acid excretion and serum electrolyte patterns in patients with advanced chronic renal failure. Miner Electrolyte Metab 1990;16:355–61.

[67] Viallon A, Zeni F, Lafond P, et al. Does bicarbonate therapy improve the management of severe diabetic ketoacidosis? Crit Care Med 1999;27(12):2690–3.

[68] Morris LR, Murphy MB, Kitabchi AE. Bicarbonate therapy in severe diabetic ketoacidosis. Ann Intern Med 1986;105(6):836–40.

[69] Okuda Y, Adrogue HJ, Field JB, et al. Counterproductive effects of sodium bicarbonate in diabetic ketoacidosis. J Clin Endocrinol Metab 1996;81(1):314–20.

[70] Gladden LB. Lactate metabolism: a new paradigm for the third millennium. J Physiol 2004;558(Pt 1):5–30.

[71] Philp A, Macdonald AL, Watt PW. Lactate—a signal coordinating cell and systemic function. J Exp Biol 2005;208(Pt 24):4561–75.

[72] Levy B. Lactate and shock state: the metabolic view. Curr Opin Crit Care 2006;12(4): 315–21.

[73] James JH, Fang CH, Schrantz SJ, et al. Linkage of aerobic glycolysis to sodium-potassium transport in rat skeletal muscle. Implications for increased muscle lactate production in sepsis. J Clin Invest 1996;98(10):2388–97.

[74] Gore DC, Jahoor F, Hibbert JM, et al. Lactic acidosis during sepsis is related to increased pyruvate production, not deficits in tissue oxygen availability. Ann Surg 1996;224(1): 97–102.

[75] Levraut J, Ciebiera JP, Chave S, et al. Mild hyperlactatemia in stable septic patients is due to impaired lactate clearance rather than overproduction. Am J Respir Crit Care Med 1998;157(4 Pt 1):1021–6.

[76] James JH, Luchette FA, McCarter FD, et al. Lactate is an unreliable indicator of tissue hypoxia in injury or sepsis. Lancet 1999;354(9177):505–8.

[77] Cairns SP. Lactic acid and exercise performance: culprit or friend? Sports Med 2006;36(4): 279–91.

[78] Nielsen OB, Clausen T. The Na+/K(+)-pump protects muscle excitability and contractility during exercise. Exerc Sport Sci Rev 2000;28(4):159–64.

[79] Forsythe SM, Schmidt GA. Sodium bicarbonate for the treatment of lactic acidosis. Chest 2000;117(1):260–7.

Fluid Therapy: Options and Rational Administration

Steven Mensack, VMD*

Pet Emergency Clinic, Inc., 2301 S. Victoria Avenue, Ventura, CA 93003, USA

F luid support is a basic treatment for many hospitalized patients and some outpatients. Proper use of fluids can be beneficial and even life saving. Fluids represent medication, however, and just as with any other medication, their inappropriate or injudicious use can lead to detrimental or even tragic outcomes. Fluid therapy is a complex topic, and this review is not meant to be all-encompassing. Rather, it provides general guidelines for effective fluid administration in juvenile and adult small animal patients. There are many exceptions to the basic tenets discussed here, including fluid therapy in neonatal small animal patients.

PHYSIOLOGY OF BODY FLUIDS

To administer fluid therapy properly, a general understanding of where fluids reside within the body and how they are lost during normal and abnormal physiologic states is necessary. Sixty percent of the body in the average nonobese dog or cat is made up of water. This amount may vary slightly based on the age of the patient, species, or body composition (overweight patients have a higher water content). Of this 60%, approximately two thirds resides within the intracellular space (40% of body weight [BW]). The remaining one third of total body water comprises the interstitial and vascular fluid spaces. Of this 20% of total BW, 5% of total body fluid resides in the intravascular space and 15% of total body fluid resides in the interstitial space [1].

Water and small dissolved solutes move among the fluid spaces in the body based on their concentration gradients and the osmotic effects of larger less diffusible macromolecules. The barriers for fluid movement among the different compartments vary; thus, different amounts of water and solutes are able to move across these barriers. For example, the capillary walls are permeable to electrolytes and water, thus enabling water and small dissolved solutes to move readily between the intravascular and interstitial fluid spaces. The movement of these fluids and electrolytes is governed by hydrostatic and oncotic forces (ie, Starling forces). The cellular membrane is freely permeable only to water and select small solutes, such as urea (serum urea nitrogen [BUN])

*202 Ashford Street, Brighton, MI 48114. *E-mail address:* criticalcarevet@comcast.net

0195-5616/08/$ – see front matter
doi:10.1016/j.cvsm.2008.01.028

and potassium, however. The movement of solutes other than urea and potassium into or out of the cell is a process of active transport. Water, urea, and potassium move between the intracellular and interstitial spaces by means of osmosis based on the gradient of less diffusible solutes across the cell membrane according to each compartment's effective osmolality. Because urea and potassium move by passive mechanisms, these molecules contribute little to effective osmolality. The effective extracellular fluid osmolality can thus be calculated by the formula:

$$2 \times Na^+ + \frac{Glucose}{18}$$

Because of the different permeability properties of membranes (capillary and other cellular membranes), clinical signs of volume loss can vary depending on the type and volume of fluid lost from the body. Loss of water in excess of solute (hypotonic fluid loss) causes water to shift from the intracellular space into the extracellular space, and ultimately into the intravascular space. The most extreme types of hypotonic fluid loss include diabetes insipidus, excessive panting, fever, and inadvertent water restriction. The most common causes of this type of fluid loss include vomiting, diarrhea, and third space loss of fluids into body cavities. With this type of fluid loss, signs of dehydration predominate. These signs include tacky or dry mucous membranes and decreased skin turgor with mild to moderate fluid losses. With loss of solute in excess of water (hypertonic fluid loss), water moves out of the intravascular and interstitial spaces into the cells by means of an osmotic gradient. With this type of fluid loss, signs of decreased perfusion and hypovolemia predominate. The most common cause of this type of fluid loss is a secretory diarrhea commonly encountered in hemorrhagic gastroenteritis. Signs may include pale mucous membranes, bounding or hypodynamic pulses, and increases in heart rate and respiratory rate. Losses of water and solute in the same proportions as those found within the extracellular space (isotonic fluid losses) produce effects on the intracellular and extracellular spaces in proportion to the total body fluid volume. In these cases, signs of dehydration and intravascular hypovolemia can be observed, although larger volumes of loss are needed to produce clinical signs. Finally, with loss of large volumes of intravascular fluid because of hemorrhage, signs of intravascular hypovolemia are noted (as described for hypertonic fluid losses).

TYPES OF FLUIDS

Five basic categories of fluid currently are available for intravenous use in small animal patients: crystalloids, colloids, hemoglobin-based oxygen-carrying solutions, blood products, and intravenous nutrition. Each of these fluid types has specific indications for its use.

Crystalloid fluids are the mainstay of fluid therapy. Crystalloid fluids consist primarily of water with a sodium or glucose base, plus the addition of other electrolytes or buffers. The variable concentration of these different solutes dictates the use of a particular crystalloid in various clinical situations. Within the crystalloid group, there are four different types of fluids: replacement solutions, maintenance solutions, hypertonic solutions, and dextrose in water. Replacement crystalloid solutions contain dissolved solutes that approximate the solute concentrations found in plasma water. These solutions are indicated for the rapid replacement of intravascular volume and electrolytes, as seen with shock and hemorrhage or severe volume depletion secondary to losses associated with vomiting, diarrhea, third body space loss of fluid, or excessive diuresis. When using replacement crystalloid fluids, only 20% to 25% of the infused volume of fluid remains within the intravascular space 1 hour after infusion [2]. Therefore, large volumes of replacement crystalloids must be administered to replace intravascular volume. The commonly available replacement solutions include normal saline (0.9% sodium chloride [NaCl]) and balanced electrolyte solutions, such as Ringer's solution (with lactate or acetate), Normosol R (Hospira, Inc., Lake Forest, Illinois), and Plasmalyte A (Baxter Healthcare Corp., Deerfield, Illinois). Each type of replacement fluid listed here has a different electrolyte composition and absence (ie, 0.9% NaCl) or presence of different types of buffers (eg, lactate, acetate, gluconate) that makes its use in certain situations preferential, although not absolute [3].

Maintenance solutions also are composed of dissolved solutes that approximate the solute concentration found in extracellular fluid. The difference in these solutions compared with replacement solutions is that maintenance solutions are designed to fulfill the electrolyte requirements of patients with normal daily electrolyte losses that are unable to maintain adequate fluid and electrolyte intake [3]. Because these solutions are hypotonic, less than 10% of the infused volume remains within the vascular space 1 hour after infusion. Therefore, they rarely are infused at rates greater than necessary to meet the patient's maintenance needs. Commercially available maintenance fluid solutions include half-strength saline (0.45% NaCl), half-strength saline and 2.5% dextrose, half-strength lactated Ringer's solution and 2.5% dextrose, Normosol M (Hospira, Inc., Lake Forest, Illinois), and Plasmalyte 56 (Baxter Healthcare Corp., Deerfield, Illinois). Commonly, maintenance solutions are supplemented with potassium to balance them further for the patient's electrolyte requirements.

Hypertonic saline (7.2%–23% NaCl) is used to increase intravascular volume rapidly. This effect is accomplished because of the high sodium content of the fluid. When hypertonic saline is infused, the increase in intravascular sodium causes fluid to shift from the interstitial space into the intravascular space in an attempt to normalize the intravascular sodium concentration. Most commonly, hypertonic saline is used when severe hypovolemia is present and may lead to impending death, when low-volume resuscitation is appropriate (eg, cerebral trauma Refs. [4,5]), or when large volumes of crystalloids cannot be infused fast enough to have the desired rapid effect (eg, gastric dilatation-volvulus). Doses of 4 to 7 mL/kg (dogs) [6] or 2 to 4 mL/kg (cats) [7] of a 7% solution infused at a rate of 1 mL/kg/min of hypertonic saline produce a hemodynamic effect similar to infusion of 60 to 90 mL/kg of a replacement crystalloid solution. Administration of hypertonic saline too rapidly has been associated with vagally mediated hypotension and bradycardia. Because of rapid diffusion of sodium back out of the vasculature, the effect of hypertonic saline is transient and only lasts up to 30 minutes [3]. To prolong this effect, hypertonic saline often is combined with a colloid to help keep fluid in the vascular space. Replacement crystalloid fluids should be administered after hypertonic saline to replace the fluid that was translocated into the vasculature. Contraindications for hypertonic saline include patients that are dehydrated (ie, inadequate interstitial fluid to draw into intravascular space), hyperosmolar patients, hypokalemic patients, those that may develop problems with hypervolemia (ie, preexisting heart or lung disease), and those that have uncontrolled hemorrhage (eg, intracranial hemorrhage, intra-abdominal hemorrhage, pulmonary contusion) [8].

Five percent dextrose in water (D5W) is not commonly used in veterinary medicine. Once the dextrose is metabolized, this fluid contains no active solute; therefore, it readily redistributes throughout the body. The most common indications for D5W are as a vehicle for infusion of other medications and to provide free water in severe hypernatremic states. Infusion of large volumes of D5W can lead to dilution of serum electrolytes or development of edema.

Colloids are high-molecular-weight compounds that do not readily leave the intravascular space. They exert their effect of expanding intravascular volume by holding and potentially drawing water into the vasculature [9,10]. Colloidal fluid solutions are indicated for rapid intravascular volume expansion in the treatment of hypovolemia; volume replacement for surgical blood loss; and low-volume resuscitation protocols, such as those advocated in patients that have cerebral trauma [4]. These solutions also are used to improve colloid osmotic (oncotic) pressure in patients with low serum albumin concentration from protein loss secondary to renal or gastroenteric disease or burns and in conditions in which proteins may leak into the interstitial spaces because of an inflammatory response (eg, vasculitis, pancreatitis, sepsis). Colloid solutions include plasma; human serum albumin (5% and 25%); and synthetic compounds, such as hetastarch, dextrans, modified gelatin solutions, and stroma-free hemoglobin-based oxygen-carrying solutions (Oxyglobin, Biopure Corp., Cambridge, Massachusetts). Plasma use for strictly colloidal effects is relatively ineffective: a patient requires plasma at a rate of approximately 50 to 100 mL/kg to raise serum albumin concentration by 1 g/dL [11,12]. Therefore, synthetic compounds are a better choice for colloidal support. Contraindications and complications for the use of colloidal fluids include coagulopathies, potential for volume overload (eg, heart disease, pulmonary disease, oliguric renal failure), and anaphylactic reactions.

Stroma-free, hemoglobin-based, oxygen-carrying solutions (Oxyglobin) are colloidal solutions made of cross-linked bovine hemoglobin molecules. These fluids have the added benefit of allowing oxygen to be carried in the plasma, allowing transport of oxygen to areas in which red blood cells may be restricted (eg, traumatized tissue), and they do not depend on 2,3-diphosphoglycerate for oxygen unloading [13]. Indications for their use include volume resuscitation in shock or hypovolemic states and treatment of anemia. Hemoglobin-based oxygen-carrying solutions also have been used in an extralabel manner in the treatment of trauma, burns, severe wounds, sepsis, and other conditions. The greatest advantage of Oxyglobin is its ability to carry oxygen to the tissues and offload oxygen more effectively because it is not limited by red blood cell flow. Other advantages of Oxyglobin are that it is a colloid; as such, it provides intravascular volume support. No blood typing or cross-matching is required before infusion; it also has been shown to improve microvascular perfusion, thus improving oxygen tension in injured tissues. Also, because it is a synthetic compound, it has a long shelf life and does not require special storage procedures. Disadvantages of Oxyglobin are that certain clinical chemistry variables are invalidated by its presence, laboratory monitoring of its effect requires a hemoglobinometer, and its colloidal effect can lead to fluid overload and pulmonary edema if not monitored carefully (especially in cats). At this time, Oxyglobin is not approved for use in cats. According to the package insert, Oxyglobin has a flexible dosage range of 10 to 30 mL/kg, which allows the clinician to tailor therapy to the approximate duration of needed effect.

Blood products are indicated to replace red blood cells, plasma proteins, platelets, or coagulation factors. Blood products are available as whole blood or components. The type of product needed is based on the component of patient blood that needs to be replaced. For more specific information regarding the proper selection and administration of blood products, consult one of the many excellent review articles on the subject [14–17].

Parenteral nutrition is considered for short- or long-term treatment in patients whose clinical condition dictates that enteral nutrition is not feasible or when enteral nutrition may not provide sufficient nutrient intake to assist recovery. Some of these conditions include severe pancreatitis, protracted vomiting or regurgitation, extremely painful conditions, burns, sepsis, multiple trauma, or intestinal malabsorption. Parenteral nutrition can be provided through a peripheral or central vein. Elemental formulations of amino acids, lipids, carbohydrates, vitamins, and trace minerals are formulated for each patient based on BW, type of injury or illness, duration of parenteral nutritional supplementation, and type of nutrition being administered. There are several different formulations of parenteral nutrition available. The most basic is a supplement consisting of a solution of amino acids and electrolytes in glycerol. This solution may be delivered through a peripheral vein and can supply up to 25% of basal metabolic needs [18]. Partial or peripheral parenteral nutrition (PPN) is delivered through a peripheral vein and can supply up to 50% of basal metabolic needs [19]. Total parenteral nutrition (TPN) is delivered through a central vein and provides 100% of a patient's basal nutritional needs [20].

REASONS FOR FLUID THERAPY

When choosing a fluid type for the patient, an important question to ask is: "What am I trying to accomplish?" The most common reasons for administration of supplemental fluid therapy include replacing intravascular volume deficits to improve tissue perfusion; replacing tissue interstitial volume deficits (dehydration); meeting maintenance fluid needs in patients that are not consuming sufficient quantities of fluid; and replacing ongoing losses attributable to vomiting, diarrhea, pneumonia, burns, severe wounds, and third body space fluid accumulation. In most of these situations, crystalloid fluid therapy is all that is required, although colloids or Oxyglobin can be beneficial in providing intravascular volume.

At certain times, fluid diuresis is required, such as with renal disease or to hasten elimination of toxins that are excreted by the kidneys. In these situations, replacement crystalloid fluids are indicated. Rates required to induce adequate diuresis can be as high as 2.5 to 4.0 times a patient's maintenance requirements; however, ideally, the rate should be matched to urine output.

Fluid therapy also is indicated for patients undergoing anesthesia and surgery. Anesthetics commonly decrease vascular tone, cardiac output, or both. When this occurs, blood flow to the tissues is decreased (ie, poor perfusion). Fluid therapy increases vascular volume, thereby improving perfusion. Also, many surgical procedures cause enough blood loss to decrease intravascular volume further. Commonly suggested replacement crystalloid fluid administration rates for normovolemic patients undergoing anesthesia are 5 mL/kg/h for procedures in which minimal blood loss is anticipated (eg, orthopedic surgery, uncomplicated soft tissue surgery) and 10 to 15 mL/kg/h for procedures in which moderate blood loss is anticipated (eg, soft tissue procedures, such as liver and splenic surgery) [21]. In surgical procedures in which the patient is unstable or may lose large volumes of blood, crystalloid fluids, colloid fluids, blood products, Oxyglobin, or some combination of these may be required at rates higher than those listed previously.

Fluid therapy also is appropriate when there is need for a specialized fluid. In situations in which the patient is anemic, whole blood (fresh or stored), packed red blood cells, or Oxyglobin can be administered to provide oxygen-carrying molecules. In situations in which the patient has a coagulopathy, regularly frozen plasma, fresh-frozen plasma, or cryoprecipitate can provide certain clotting factors. Fresh-frozen plasma provides all clotting factors, and regularly frozen plasma provides all clotting factors except the most labile (ie, factors V and VIII). When a patient has low plasma protein concentration, such as may occur in protein-losing renal or intestinal disease, prolonged starvation, or vasculitis, fluids with large osmotically active particles, such as colloids, Oxyglobin, or plasma (fresh-frozen or regularly frozen), should be administered for oncotic support. Finally, intravenous nutritional solutions are indicated when the patient is not able to consume sufficient food for a prolonged period.

HOW TO ADMINISTER FLUIDS

Parenteral fluid therapy is commonly administered as subcutaneous therapy, as a rapid intravenous bolus, or as an intravenous constant rate infusion. Fluid therapy also can be administered by the intraosseous route in small patients in which venous access cannot be obtained or by the intraperitoneal route. Subcutaneous fluid therapy is indicated for the replacement of deficits, for maintenance needs, or to counteract ongoing losses. It is usually used on an outpatient basis, because intravenous fluid therapy has been proved more effective in the hospital setting. Because only a limited amount of fluid can be administered subcutaneously, this route cannot meet the daily fluid needs of most patients. It is best used in patients that are mildly dehydrated or mildly hypovolemic Contraindications for subcutaneous fluid therapy include patients that are severely volume depleted because of dehydration or hypovolemia and hypothermic patients. In these situations, blood is shunted away from the subcutaneous vasculature, leading to poor and inconsistent absorption of administered fluids.

In the hospitalized setting, intravenous administration is the preferred route of fluid therapy. Although convenient, determination of fluid therapy as a multiple of "maintenance needs" is inappropriate, because most patients do not lose or require fluid in simple multiples of maintenance; at best, this approach provides only a crude estimate of actual patient fluid requirements. Fluids may be administered as a bolus or as a constant rate infusion. Bolus fluid therapy is indicated in severely volume-depleted and dehydrated patients. In the patient with intravascular volume depletion, the volume of the bolus is determined based on resolution of clinical signs (eg, slower heart rate and respirations, improved pulse quality, improved mucous membrane color, improved capillary refill time) or improvement in other indicators of perfusion, such as acid-base status, serum lactate concentration, or gastric mucosal pH. Therefore, frequent reassessment of the volume-depleted patient is required. Crystalloid fluid rates up to 90 mL/kg/h in dogs and 60 mL/kg/h in cats or higher may be required. Colloids also can be administered as boluses. Colloids are administered in boluses of 5 to 40 mL/kg [22]. The patient should be reassessed after each bolus of crystalloid or colloid to determine if the bolus has been effective in resolving volume depletion or if additional boluses are needed. Crystalloid fluids often are administered along with colloids to augment their vascular volume-expanding effect. Smaller doses of crystalloids than those listed previously are necessary with the concomitant use of colloid. In the dehydrated patient, the quantity of a fluid bolus is based on the estimated degree of dehydration. The dehydration deficit can be calculated as: BW (kg) × Estimated Degree of Dehydration (%) × 100 = mL of Fluid Required. One half of the dehydration deficit should be administered as a bolus, and the remainder should be replaced as a constant rate infusion over 12 to 24 hours.

Constant rate fluid administration is indicated in several situations. As described previously, it is used to replace dehydration deficits. It is also necessary to account for a patient's maintenance fluid requirements if the patient is not consuming sufficient quantities of fluid on its own. Daily maintenance needs for patients varies based on the age and size of the patient. Maintenance crystalloid fluid needs traditionally have been considered to be 54 to 66 mL/kg/d (with the lower end of the range applying to large dogs and the higher end to small dogs and cats) [23]. In the pediatric patient, fluid requirements may be as high as 180 mL/kg/d [24]. Veterinarians may be overestimating our patients' maintenance fluid needs, however. Several studies have evaluated basal metabolic rate and used indirect calorimetry with limited success in an attempt to determine actual fluid requirements [25,26]. Based on these studies, the daily maintenance fluid requirement for a healthy cat or dog weighing between 2 and 70 kg is as follows: (30 × BW [kg]) + 70 (Figs. 1 and 2) [25]. Using 6% hydroxyethyl starch (hetastarch) colloid fluid therapy, infusions of 20 mL/kg/d (dog) [15,18] or 10 to 40 mL/kg/d (cat) [22] have been used to provide continuous intravascular volume support. With the infusion of colloids, lower infusion rates of crystalloids are necessary. If a patient has ongoing losses attributable to vomiting, diarrhea, third space fluid accumulation (eg, ascites, pleural effusion), or diuresis (eg, postobstructive diuresis; glucosuria; diseases that cause polyuria, such as hyperadrenocorticism or renal failure), these losses should be replaced with 2 mL of crystalloid per 1 mL of fluid lost [27].

Administration of specialized fluids, such as natural and synthetic colloids, blood products, and intravenous nutrition, is covered in other excellent review articles [14–17,19,28–33]. Because blood products and nutrition are provided intravenously and there is a higher potential for complications compared with other forms of fluid therapy, patients receiving blood products or parenteral nutrition require hospitalization and extensive monitoring.

MONITORING FLUID THERAPY

As with any other medication, monitoring for the desired effect and for potential adverse effects is necessary during fluid administration. Proper monitoring

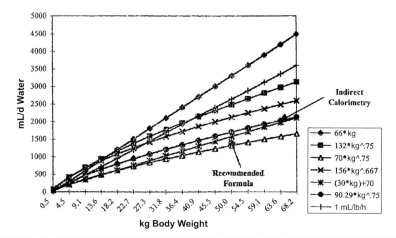

Fig. 1. Daily water requirements for the dog. The recommended formula is as follows: (30 × kg BW) + 70. This formula closely approximates findings of indirect calorimetry (90.29 × kg$^{0.75}$) in the dog. (*From* Wingfield WE, Raffe MR. The veterinary ICU book. Jackson (WY): Teton NewMedia; 2002. p. 176; with permission.)

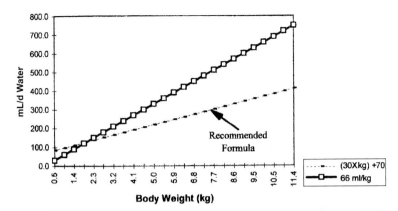

Fig. 2. Estimating fluid requirements for the cat. The recommended formula is as follows: (30 × kg BW) + 70. (*From* Wingfield WE, Raffe MR. The veterinary ICU Book. Jackson (WY): Teton NewMedia; 2002. p. 177; with permission.)

of the patient receiving fluids is a "hands-on" endeavor. Much of the necessary information is gained by serial examination of the patient. No single evaluated variable can provide all the information required to guide fluid therapy properly. Physical examination findings that should be evaluated include the patient's weight, physical appearance, mentation, skin turgor, pulse rate and quality, respiratory rate and effort, serial lung auscultation for crackles, mucous membrane color, and capillary refill time. Skin turgor allows for gross assessment of hydration status. Skin turgor is notably prolonged with 6% to 8% dehydration and markedly prolonged with greater than 8% dehydration. Body condition can limit the effectiveness of skin turgor assessment, because obesity can mask decreases in skin turgor and emaciation may artifactually worsen skin turgor. If an indwelling urinary catheter is in place, serial evaluation of fluid input and urine output can provide useful information about whether too little or too much fluid has been administered.

Cage-side testing and conventional laboratory testing should be used in combination with assessment of vital parameters. Renal function parameters (eg, BUN and serum creatinine concentrations, urine specific gravity) provide additional useful information. Increased BUN and serum creatinine concentrations, in conjunction with increased urine specific gravity (ie, prerenal azotemia), may indicate that a patient is receiving insufficient amounts of fluid. Blood gas analysis or measurement of serum lactate concentration [34] can provide information about tissue perfusion. Metabolic acidosis or increased serum lactate concentration may indicate that tissues are not receiving adequate oxygen for metabolism and instead are relying on anaerobic metabolism to provide energy. The clinical standard in veterinary medicine for evaluating adequacy of fluid therapy is serial central venous pressure (CVP) measurement, which approximates the ability of the right side of the heart to pump blood forward. This method allows the clinician to make adjustments to fluid type and rate based on the ability of the patient's heart to handle the infused volume [35]. Performing CVP measurement is well covered in many review articles on fluid therapy monitoring [36,37]. Monitoring of the patient receiving intravenous fluid therapy should involve a combination of these tests to ensure adequate volume status and to help prevent inadequate resuscitation or volume overload.

CONTRAINDICATIONS FOR FLUID THERAPY

In some situations, fluid therapy is not necessarily in the best interest of the patient. The most common situation is the patient that has congestive heart failure. In this situation, the patient develops congestion because the heart is not able to pump the volume it currently has presented to it effectively. Heart disease is not an absolute contraindication to fluid therapy, however. In some situations, there may be concomitant dehydration or a need for medications infused by constant rate infusion to treat the heart disease, and judicious use of fluid therapy may be warranted. In these patients, hypotonic maintenance crystalloids or, less commonly, D5W is indicated. Meticulous monitoring of vital parameters, urine output, and CVP is necessary for successful use of fluid therapy in patients that have congestive heart failure.

The other situation when fluid therapy may not be necessary is when the patient is already consuming adequate volumes of water and is normally hydrated. In this situation, fluid therapy may lead to dilution of blood compartment constituents, renal medullary solute washout, or development of pulmonary edema if occult heart disease is present. Even in this situation, however, fluid therapy may be warranted if diuresis is indicated because of ingestion of a toxin or if a medication must be administered by constant rate infusion.

DISCONTINUATION OF FLUID THERAPY

Discontinuing fluid therapy is as important as initiating fluid therapy. In most instances, fluid therapy should not be abruptly discontinued, especially if the patient is receiving high flow rates. During fluid therapy, the solute gradient in the kidneys may be changed as a result of fluid therapy (ie, renal medullary solute washout). If fluid therapy is abruptly discontinued, the patient may not be able to concentrate urine well and may continue to lose excessive fluid in the urine for several days. This can be a serious problem if the patient is not ingesting adequate amounts of water and may lead to dehydration. The patient should be gradually weaned from fluid therapy. In the ideal situation, fluid therapy should be tapered to lower than maintenance for at least 24 hours before discontinuation of fluid therapy. This approach is not always possible, however. If fluid therapy must be abruptly discontinued, the patient should have access to adequate quantities of water and the owner should be informed of the patient's increased water requirements over the next several days.

As stated throughout, the overview presented here is not meant to be comprehensive and exceptions to many of the "rules of thumb" presented here do exist. The most important caveat is that there is no set formula for fluid administration, and the clinician must tailor fluid composition and rate of administration to the patient's needs as required by its clinical condition and results of parameters that are monitored. Careful monitoring of patients receiving fluid therapy is required to ensure a successful outcome.

References

[1] Wellman ML, DiBartola SP, Kohn CW. Applied physiology of body fluids in dogs and cats. In: DiBartola SP, editor. Fluid, electrolyte, and acid-base disorders in small animal practice. 3rd edition. St. Louis (MO): Saunders Elsevier; 2006. p. 3–26.
[2] Griffel MI, Kaufman BS. Pharmacology of colloids and crystalloids. Crit Care Clin 1992;8(2):235–53.
[3] Mathews KA. The various types of parenteral fluids and their indications. Vet Clin North Am Small Anim Pract 1998;28(3):483–513.
[4] Ducey JP, Mozingo DW, Lamiell JM, et al. A comparison of the cerebral and cardiovascular effects of complete resuscitation with isotonic and hypertonic saline, hetastarch, and whole blood following hemorrhage. J Trauma 1989;29(11):1510–8.
[5] Dewey CW, Budsberg SC, Oliver JE. Principles of head trauma management in dogs and cats—part II. Compendium of Continuing Education for the Practicing Veterinarian 1993;15(2):177–93.
[6] Schertel ER, Allen DA, Muir WW, et al. Evaluation of a hypertonic saline-dextran solution for treatment of dogs with shock induced by gastric dilatation-volvulus. J Am Vet Med Assoc 1997;210:226–30.
[7] Muir WW, Sally J. Small-volume resuscitation with hypertonic saline solution in hypovolemic cats. Am J Vet Res 1989;50(11):1883–8.
[8] Krausz MM. Controversies in shock research: hypertonic resuscitation—pros and cons. Shock 1995;3(1):69–72.
[9] Thompson WL, Fukushima T, Rutherford RB, et al. Intravascular persistence, tissue storage, and excretion of hydroxyethyl starch. Surg Gynecol Obstet 1970;131(5):965–72.
[10] Khosropur R, Lackner F, Steinbereithner K, et al. Comparison of the effect of pre- and intra-operative administration of medium molecular weight hydroxyethyl starch (HES 200/0.5) and dextran 40(60) in vascular surgery. Anaesthesist 1980;29(11):616–22.
[11] Mazzaferro EM, Rudloff E, Kirby R. The role of albumin replacement in the critically ill veterinary patient. Journal of Veterinary Emergency Care 2002;12(2):113–24.
[12] Logan JC, Callan MB, Drew K, et al. Clinical indications for the use of fresh frozen plasma in dogs: 74 dogs (October through December 1999. J Am Vet Med Assoc 2001;218(9):1449–54.
[13] Fronticelli C, Bucci E, Orth C. Solvent regulation of oxygen affinity in hemoglobin. Sensitivity of bovine hemoglobin to chloride ions. J Biol Chem 1984;259:10841–4.
[14] Haldane S, Roberts J, Marks SL, et al. Transfusion medicine. Compendium of Continuing Education for the Practicing Veterinarian 2004;26(7):502–18.
[15] Hughes D, Boag A. Fluid therapy with macromolecular plasma volume expanders. In: DiBartola SP, editor. Fluid, electrolyte, and acid-base disorders in small animal practice. 3rd edition. St. Louis (MO): Saunders Elsevier; 2006. p. 621–34.
[16] Griot-Wenk ME, Giger U. Feline transfusion medicine. Vet Clin North Am Small Anim Pract 1995;25(6):1305–22.
[17] Kristensen AT, Feldman BF. General principles of small animal blood component administration. Vet Clin North Am Small Anim Pract 1995;25(6):1277–90.
[18] Freeman JB, Fairful-Smith R, Rodman GH, et al. Safety and efficacy of a new peripheral intravenously administered amino acid solution containing glycerol and electrolytes. Surg Gynecol Obstet 1983;156(5):625–31.
[19] Zsombor-Murray E, Freeman LM. Peripheral parenteral nutrition. Compendium of Continuing Education for the Practicing Veterinarian 1999;21(6):512–23.
[20] Remillard RL, Thatcher CD. Parenteral nutritional support in the small animal patient. Vet Clin North Am Small Anim Pract 1989;19(6):1287–306.

[21] Kudnig ST, Mama K. Guidelines for perioperative fluid therapy. Compendium of Continuing Education for the Practicing Veterinarian 2003;25(2):102–11.

[22] Rudloff E, Kirby R. Colloids: current recommendations. In: Bonagura JD, editor. Current veterinary therapy XIII. Philadelphia: WB Saunders; 2000. p. 131–6.

[23] Garvey MS. Fluid and electrolyte balance in critical patients. Vet Clin North Am Small Anim Pract 1989;19(6):1021–57.

[24] Mosier JE. Canine pediatrics—the neonate. Journal of the American Animal Hospital Association 1981;48:339–47.

[25] Wingfield W. Fluid and electrolyte therapy. In: Wingfield W, editor. The veterinary ICU book. Jackson (WY): Teton NewMedia; 2002. p. 166–88.

[26] Olgilvie GK, Salman MD, Kessel ML, et al. Effect of anesthesia and surgery on energy expenditure determined by indirect calorimetry in dogs with malignant and nonmalignant conditions. Am J Vet Res 1996;57(9):1321–6.

[27] Greco DS. The distribution of body water and general approach to the patient. Vet Clin North Am Small Anim Pract 1998;28(3):473–82.

[28] Day TK. Current development and use of hemoglobin-based oxygen-carrying (HBOC) solutions. Journal of Veterinary Emergency Care 2003;13(2):77–93.

[29] Kerl ME, Cohn LA. Albumin in health and disease: causes and treatment of hypoalbuminemia. Compendium of Continuing Education for the Practicing Veterinarian 2004;26(12): 940–8.

[30] Martin L. Human albumin solutions in the critical patient. Proceedings of the International Veterinary Emergency and Critical Care Society 2004;274–8.

[31] Mathews KA, Barry M. The use of 25% human serum albumin: outcome and efficacy in raising serum albumin and systemic blood pressure in critically ill dogs and cats. Journal of Veterinary Emergency Care 2005;15(2):110–8.

[32] Rudloff E, Kirby R. The critical need for colloids: selecting the right colloid. Compendium of Continuing Education for the Practicing Veterinarian 1997;19(7):811–25.

[33] Rudloff E, Kirby R. The critical need for colloids: administering colloids effectively. Compendium of Continuing Education for the Practicing Veterinarian 1998;20(1):27–43.

[34] Karagiannis MH, Reniker AN, Kerl ME, et al. Lactate measurement as an indicator of perfusion. Compendium of Continuing Education for the Practicing Veterinarian 2006;28(4):287–98.

[35] Jennings PB, Anderson RW, Martin AM. Central venous pressure monitoring: a guide to blood volume replacement in the dog. J Am Vet Med Assoc 1967;151(10):1283–93.

[36] Hansen BD. Technical aspects of fluid therapy. In: DiBartola SP, editor. Fluid, electrolyte, and acid-base disorders in small animal practice. 3rd edition. St. Louis (MO): Saunders Elsevier; 2006. p. 344–76.

[37] Oakley RE, Olivier B, Eyester GE, et al. Experimental evaluation of central venous pressure monitoring in the dog. J Am Anim Hosp Assoc 1997;33(1):77–82.

Colloids: Current Recommendations

Daniel L. Chan, DVM, MRCVS

Department of Veterinary Clinical Sciences, The Royal Veterinary College,
University of London, Hawkshead Lane, North Mymms, Hertfordshire, AL9 7TA, UK

Fluid administration remains the cornerstone of critical care medicine and is the standard therapy used to maintain or restore intravascular volume. The optimal choice of fluid for resuscitation likely will remain one of the most enduring controversies in medicine. Advantages of crystalloid resuscitation include the fact that crystalloids replace interstitial and intravascular fluid losses, minimally impair the coagulation system, do not cause allergic reactions, are inexpensive, and are widely available. Proponents of crystalloid fluid therapy also cite the various meta-analyses that suggest that colloid use is associated with greater mortality rates, although these studies may have been underpowered to truly demonstrate such associations [1–3]. The main disadvantages associated with crystalloid use include limited duration of intravascular volume expansion and greater propensity for formation of tissue edema by lowering plasma colloid osmotic pressure (COP), which may contribute to impaired gas exchange in the lungs, increased bacterial translocation in the gut, and negative impact on wound healing [3]. Advantages of colloid use include longer intravascular effect, smaller volume requirements to achieve comparable intravascular expansion, and decreased risk of tissue edema formation by provision of oncotic support. Disadvantages attributed to colloids that have been well described in people include allergic reactions (particularly with gelatins), possible renal impairment (dextrans, hetastarches), impairment of coagulation (dextrans, hetastarches), and substantially higher costs. The purported benefits colloids have led to widespread use of colloids in critical care patients, however.

Concerns over the apparent association between colloid use and increased risk of morbidity and mortality have prompted researchers to develop newer and better synthetic colloids that produce less serious complications. As these newer colloids become more widely available, guidelines for their effective use are needed. Renewed interest in natural colloids, such as concentrated human albumin, has added a new dilemma for practitioners in the selection of the most appropriate fluid type for treatment of various conditions. Recommendations for the use of colloids in veterinary patients must take into consideration issues such as physiologic rationale, available efficacy data, and patient safety

E-mail address: dchan@rvc.ac.uk

0195-5616/08/$ – see front matter
doi:10.1016/j.cvsm.2008.01.006

concerns. Veterinary-specific data on colloids are limited, and extrapolations from other species continue to form the basis of many current recommendations for colloid fluid therapy in veterinary patients.

ESTABLISHMENT OF GUIDELINES

As with all emerging therapies, the use of colloids has evolved over time. Major influences shaping how colloids are used include better understanding of physiologic processes governing fluid dynamics, greater awareness of complications associated with colloid use, and greater clinical experience. The widespread use of synthetic colloids in veterinary practice can be attributed to several factors. The primary reason for seeking an alternative to crystalloids may have been the consequences that occur when large quantities of crystalloids are administered. With increasing amounts of crystalloid administration, there is a decrease in plasma COP and a concomitant increase in hydrostatic pressure. As the hydrostatic pressure gradient between the intravascular and interstitial compartments increases and the oncotic gradient between those compartments decreases, interstitial edema may result [4–6]. Although a decrease in plasma or intravascular COP alone is often blamed for the formation of peripheral edema, this may be an oversimplified description of the processes involved. The formation of tissue edema involves several other factors, including impairment of tissue safety factors, alterations of hormones that regulate sodium and water retention, changes in interstitial pressures, and failure of lymphatic clearance [7–10]. Because colloids may generate oncotic pressure greater than that achieved with crystalloids or the patient's own plasma or blood, colloids are deemed preferable when the administration of large quantities of fluids is required or when the patient is at risk or already manifesting signs of tissue edema. Because the various colloids themselves generate different oncotic pressures (Table 1), one colloid may be chosen over another partly based on this property, although other properties of the colloid also should be considered.

Although colloid administration could positively impact a patient's COP, only limited data are available to quantify this effect in clinically affected veterinary patients [11–13]. Based on these small studies, the actual impact on COP with natural and synthetic colloids is modest [11–13]. Most dosage recommendations for colloid administration are not based on actual effects on plasma COP or optimal volume expansion but on extrapolations from safety guidelines for people. Various veterinary references cite a 20- to 30-mL/kg/d maximum dosage for synthetic colloids [4,14–16]. Such recommendations stem from concerns that higher dosages adversely impact the coagulation system, and any change to these recommendations must take these safety issues into consideration [2,17–20].

Specific effects of synthetic colloids on coagulation include decreased circulating factor VIII and von Willebrand factor concentrations (beyond what would be expected from dilutional effects alone), impairment of platelet function, and interference with fibrin clot stabilization increasing its vulnerability to fibrinolytic degradation [2,16–23]. Although many studies document only in vitro

Table 1
Physiochemical properties and recommended dosages of commercially available synthetic colloids

Fluid	Mean MW (KDa)	Molar substitution	COP (mm Hg)	Recommended maximal dose (mL/kg/d)	Other effects
Dextran 70	70	N/A	61.7 ± 0.5	20	Impairs primary and secondary hemostasis; may negatively impact renal function
4% succinylated fluid gelatin: Gelofusine	30	N/A	N/A	N/A	Anaphylactoid reactions
3.5% urea cross-linked gelatin: Haemaccel	35	N/A	15.2 ± 0.3	N/A	Anaphylactoid reactions
6% hetastarch in 0.9% NaCl	600	0.7	32.7 ± 0.2	20	Impairs primary and secondary hemostasis; may negatively impact renal function
6% hetastach in balanced electrolyte solution: Hextend	670	0.75	37.9 ± 0.1	20	Impairs coagulation to a lesser degree compared with other hetastarches
10% pentastarch	200	0.5	32.0 ± 1.4	33	Minimal effects on coagulation
6% tetrastarch: Voluven	130	0.4	37.1 ± 0.8	50	Minimal effects of coagulation; may attenuate inflammatory mediators and decrease capillary permeability
HBOC—Oxyglobin	200	N/A	43.3 ± 0.1	N/A	Vasoconstriction

Abbreviation: HBOC, hemoglobin-based oxygen carrier.
Data from Chan DL, Freeman LM, Rozanski EA, et al. Colloid osmotic pressure of parenteral nutrition components and intravenous fluids. J Vet Emerg Crit Care 2001;11(4):269–73; and Humm K, Chan DL. Colloid osmotic pressure of synthetic colloids available in veterinary clinical practice [abstract]. J Vet Intern Med 2007; 21(3):656.

or marginal (but statistically significant) abnormalities in clotting times, the major concern is that critically ill patients generally are at risk for coagulation disturbances, and the additional detrimental effects of colloids on coagulation may become unacceptable [16,24]. With respect to clotting times, activated partial thromboplastin times are more sensitive to the effects of synthetic colloids than other coagulation tests [16,24]. Studies demonstrating poorer outcomes with colloid use suggest that clinically relevant bleeding may have resulted from the effects of colloids on coagulation [1,2,23].

DEVELOPMENT OF NEW SYNTHETIC COLLOIDS

The adverse effects of synthetic colloids, including those on the coagulation system, are the major driving forces behind development of newer synthetic colloids. To understand some of the progress in manufacturing newer colloids, a brief overview of their chemical properties may be helpful. Dextrans are composed of naturally occurring glucose polymers. Gelatins are derived from hydrolysis of bovine collagen followed by being either succinylated or linked to urea. Hemoglobin-based oxygen carriers, such as Oxyglobin, are stroma-free ultrapurified hemoglobin glutamers. Bovine hemoglobin is highly polymerized to delay its clearance by the kidneys. Hydroxyethyl starches (HES) are modified polymers of amylopectin that vary substantially in molecular weight (MW) and other chemical features that affect their pharmacokinetics and metabolism. In general, colloids are polydisperse solutions with molecules that range in size from a few thousand to several million Daltons. The quoted MW for a specific product represents the weight average MW of the molecules in that solution. Solutions with high MW have a longer plasma half-life because they have delayed renal clearance. The MW of the colloid is particularly important to note because the detrimental effects of colloids on coagulation are partly related to the presence of the higher MW polymers (see Table 1).

This article focuses primarily on HES because they are the most commonly used colloids in practice. A key modification in the molecular structure of the amylopectin molecule is the substitution of some hydroxyl groups on the glucose units with hydroxyethyl groups, which stabilize the polymer and interfere with plasma amylase activity, thereby prolonging the colloid's effect. A higher degree of hydroxyethylation (ie, molar substitution) correlates with slower degradation of HES by amylase and longer persistence in plasma. Unfortunately, higher degrees of molar substitution also impact coagulation. There are several types of HES, which are grouped by their degree of substitution. The term "hetastarch" should not be considered synonymous with "HES" but rather is used to describe a type of HES with a high degree of substitution (between 0.6 and 0.7). Pentastarches and tetrastarches have degrees of substitution of 0.5 and 0.4, respectively. Hydroxyethyl groups usually are added at the C2, C3, and C6 carbon positions of the constituent glucose molecules. The degree of substitution is not the only way to prolong persistence in plasma, however. Higher substitution on position C2 in relation to C6 (expressed as the

C2:C6 ratio) also imparts greater resistance to amylase degradation without compromising coagulation.

Newer HES solutions have been developed to address the problems associated with coagulation. These colloids are widely available in Europe and generally have smaller mean MW and are hydroxyethylated to a lesser degree. To compensate for the reduction in plasma half-life incurred by these alterations, there is an increase in C2:C6 ratio, which improves amylase resistance. By manipulation of these characteristics, these newer colloids can be administered at higher dosages without affecting clotting times. For example, the maximal dosage of HES 130/0.4 (mean MW of 130 kDa and molar ratio of 0.4) is 50 mL/kg as compared with the typical dosage of 20 mL/kg for HES 450/0.7, which is more commonly found in the United States.

Because most colloids are suspended in sodium chloride solutions, an additional complication associated with their use is development of hyperchloremic metabolic acidosis [25]. This effect has been a particular problem in people treated with saline-based colloids, but there is limited information about this problem in animals. Newer HES solutions suspended in balanced electrolyte solutions (eg, Hextend) have been developed to decrease the risk of this complication. The inclusion of calcium in such solutions has been proposed to ameliorate some of the effects of the colloid on coagulation, particularly effects on platelet function [22,26]. The effects on coagulation, however, cannot be corrected completely by calcium supplementation alone, which suggests that other features of the balanced electrolyte colloid solutions may confer these benefits [27,28]. Recent studies also have yielded conflicting results with regard to differences in coagulation parameters between sodium-based and balanced electrolyte colloid solutions, emphasizing the need for additional studies [22,23,26–28].

Another intriguing effect of synthetic colloids, which is only beginning to be exploited, is their potential to modulate inflammation [29–33]. Although some authors originally hypothesized that colloids acted by physically sealing the barrier defects created by injury [34], only recently have the actual mechanisms for attenuation of capillary leakage and the anti-inflammatory effects of colloids been more clearly understood [30,32,33,35]. It is becoming increasingly clear that certain colloids can decrease capillary permeability, down-regulate the expression of adhesion molecules, inhibit neutrophil recruitment, and decrease cytokine production [30,32,33,35]. Colloids with lower MW (< 200 kDa) and molar substitution (< 0.4) seem to be superior in this respect. In the setting of critical illness, in which inflammation is a major component of most disorders, colloids with lower MW and lower degree of substitution may be the preferred type of colloid. As these newer colloids become more widely available, future studies evaluating their efficacy in clinical patients are warranted.

SUMMARY

Colloids are increasingly becoming considered indispensable in the management of critically ill patients, especially patients that require administration of large quantities of fluid and demonstrate signs of tissue edema. Current guidelines for the use of colloids in veterinary patients balance the benefits of superior and longer-lasting volume expansion with the risks of developing complications, such as volume overload and coagulation disturbances. Recent studies substantiate the negative effects of the most commonly available HES preparations (450/0.7 and 670/0.75) on the coagulation system, and maximum safe dosages for these products are approximately 20 mL/kg/d, although dosages of 30 to 40 mL/kg/d have been used in clinical patients. In animals with pre-existing coagulopathies, lower dosages should be used, and such patients may require fresh frozen plasma transfusions if synthetic colloid therapy is necessary. Newer preparations of synthetic colloids with decreased impact on the coagulation system may have maximal safe dosages approaching 50 mL/kg/d. Other advantages of these newer colloids include anti-inflammatory properties, which could prove to be particularly useful in the management of critically ill patients. Although the debate over which fluid type is optimal for fluid resuscitation will continue, acquiring a better understanding of how different fluids influence the host response may enable us to target disturbances other than volume deficits.

References

[1] Choi PT, Yip G, Quinonez LG, et al. Crystalloids vs colloids in fluid resuscitation: a systematic review. Crit Care Med 1999;27(1):200–10.

[2] Barron ME, Wilkes MM, Navickis RJ. A systematic review of the comparative safety of colloids. Arch Surg 2004;139(5):552–63.

[3] Soreide E, Deakin CD. Pre-hospital fluid therapy in the critically injured patient: a clinical update. Injury 2005;36(9):1001–10.

[4] Hughes D, Boag AK. Fluid therapy with macromolecular plasma volume expanders. In: DiBartola SP, editor. Fluid, electrolyte, and acid-base disorders in small animal practice. 3rd edition. St. Louis (MO): Saunders Elsevier; 2006. p. 621–34.

[5] Chan DL, Rozanski EA, Freeman LM, et al. Colloid osmotic pressure in health and disease. Compend Contin Educ Pract Vet 2001;23(10):896–904.

[6] Concannon KT. Colloid osmotic pressure and the clinical use of colloidal solutions. Journal of Veterinary Emergency and Critical Care 1993;3(2):49–62.

[7] Guyton AC, Granger HJ, Taylor AE. Interstitial fluid pressure. Physiol Rev 1971;51(3): 527–63.

[8] Bandt C, Rozanski EA, Chan DL, et al. Characterization of fluid retention in critically ill dogs with peripheral edema. Journal of Veterinary Emergency and Critical Care 2005;15(3):S2.

[9] Taylor AE. The lymphatic edema safety factor: the role of edema dependent lymphatic factors (EDLF). Lymphology 1990;23(3):111–23.

[10] Lund T, Onarheim H, Wiig H, et al. Mechanisms behind increased dermal imbibition pressure in acute burn edema. Am J Physiol 1989;256(4 Pt 2):H940–8.

[11] Moore LE, Garvey MS. The effect of hetastarch on serum colloid osmotic pressure in hypoalbuminemic dogs. J Vet Intern Med 1996;10(5):300–3.

[12] Smiley LE, Garvey MS. The use of hetastarch as adjunct therapy in 26 dogs with hypoalbuminemia: a phase two clinical trial. J Vet Intern Med 1994;8(3):195–202.

[13] Chan DL, Rozanksi EA, Freeman LM, et al. Retrospective evaluation of human albumin use in critically ill dogs [abstract]. Journal of Veterinary Emergency and Critical Care 2004; 14(S1):S8.

[14] Driessen B, Brainard B. Fluid therapy for the traumatized patient. Journal of Veterinary Emergency and Critical Care 2006;16(4):276–99.

[15] Kudnig ST, Mama K. Perioperative fluid therapy. J Am Vet Med Assoc 2002;221(8): 1112–21.

[16] Concannon KT, Haskins SC, Feldman BF. Hemostatic defects associated with two infusion rates of dextran 70 in dogs. Am J Vet Res 1992;53(8):1369–75.

[17] Dieterich HJ. Recent developments in European colloid solutions. J Trauma 2003;54(Suppl): S26–30.

[18] Glowaski MM, Moon-Massat PF, Erb HN, et al. Effects of oxypogelatin and dextran 70 on hemostatic variables in dogs. Vet Anaesth Analg 2003;30(4):202–10.

[19] Treib J, Barron JF, Grauer MT, et al. An international view of hydroxyethyl starches. Intensive Care Med 1999;25(3):258–68.

[20] Strauss RG, Stump DC, Henriksen RA, et al. Effects of hydroxyethyl starch on fibrinogen, fibrin clot formation, and fibrinolysis. Transfusion 1985;25(3):230–4.

[21] Wierenga JR, Jandrey KE, Haskins SC, et al. In vitro comparison of the effects of two forms of hydroxyethyl starch solutions on platelet function in dogs. Am J Vet Res 2007;68(6):605–9.

[22] Franz A, Braunlich P, Gamsjager T, et al. The effects of hydroxyethyl starches of varying molecular weights on platelet function. Anesth Analg 2001;92(6):1402–7.

[23] Brummel-Ziedins K, Whelihan MF, Ziedins EG, et al. The resuscitative fluid you choose may potentiate bleeding. J Trauma 2006;61(6):1350–8.

[24] Chan DL, Freeman LM, Rozanski EA, et al. Dilutional effects of saline, hetastarch, and fresh frozen plasma on clotting times [abstract]. Journal of Veterinary Emergency and Critical Care 2002;12(3):195.

[25] Wilkes NJ, Woolf R, Mutch M, et al. The effects of balanced versus saline-based hetastarch and crystalloid solutions on acid-base and electrolyte status and gastric mucosal perfusion in elderly surgical patients. Anesth Analg 2001;93(4):811–6.

[26] Deusch E, Thaler U, Kozek-Langenecker SA. The effects of high molecular weight hydroxyethyl starch solutions on platelets. Anesth Analg 2004;99(3):665–8.

[27] Roche AM, James MF, Bennett-Guerrero E, et al. Calcium supplementation of saline-based colloids does not produce equivalent coagulation profiles to similarly balanced salt preparations. J Cardiothorac Vasc Anesth 2006;20(6):807–11.

[28] Roche AM, James MF, Bennet-Guerrero E, et al. A head-to-head comparison of the in vitro coagulation effects of saline-based and balanced electrolyte crystalloid and colloid intravenous solutions. Anesth Analg 2006;102(4):1274–9.

[29] Marx G, Pedder S, Smith L, et al. Attenuation of capillary leakage by hydroxyethyl starch (130/0.42) in a porcine model of septic shock. Crit Care Med 2006;34(12):3005–10.

[30] Tian J, Lin X, Guan R, et al. The effects of hydroxyethyl starch on lung capillary permeability in endotoxic rats and possible mechanisms. Anesth Analg 2004;98(3):768–74.

[31] Feng X, Ren B, Xie W, et al. Influence of hydroxyethyl starch 130/0.4 in pulmonary neutrophil recruitment and acute lung injury during polymicrobial sepsis in rats. Acta Anaesthesiol Scand 2006;50(9):1081–8.

[32] Lv R, Zhou ZQ, Wu HW, et al. Hydroxyethyl starch exhibits anti-inflammatory effects in the intestines of endotoxemic rats. Anesth Analg 2006;103(1):149–55.

[33] Di Filippo A, Ciapetti M, Prencipe D, et al. Experimentally-induced acute lung injury: the protective effect of hydroethyl starch. Ann Clin Lab Sci 2006;36(3):345–52.

[34] Zikria BA, King TC, Standford J, et al. A biophysical approach to capillary permeability. Surgery 1989;105:625–31.

[35] Feng X, Liu J, Yu M, et al. Hydroxyethyl starch, but not modified fluid gelatin, affects inflammatory response in a rat model of polymicrobial sepsis with capillary leakage. Anesth Analg 2007;104(3):624–30.

The Therapeutic Use of 25% Human Serum Albumin in Critically Ill Dogs and Cats

Karol A. Mathews, DVM, DVSc

Department of Clinical Studies, Emergency and Critical Care Medicine,
Ontario Veterinary College, University of Guelph, Guelph, Ontario N1H 6H8, Canada

Albumin is the most abundant protein in the body. It is produced by the liver and is thought to have arisen from a common ancestral molecule of hemoglobin and myoglobin. This theory is supported by the highly conserved amino acid sequence of albumin among species [1,2]. The serum half-life of albumin in normal dogs is 8.2 days, with hepatic synthesis at 33% of maximum capacity [3]. Of the total body albumin, 40% is within the intravascular space, whereas 60% is in the interstitium. Albumin normally moves out of the intravascular space into the interstitium and circulates within the lymphatic system.

Albumin serves many diverse functions in health and illness [4]. Of major importance is albumin's role in the maintenance of colloid osmotic pressure (COP) and overall endothelial integrity. The albumin molecules exert 75% to 80% of normal COP [5], reduce microvascular permeability, and inhibit endothelial cell apoptosis [6,7]. Should a reduction in albumin occur, fewer molecules are available to maintain the integrity of the endothelium. At a critical point, the endothelium may become more permeable, potentially resulting in even greater albumin loss ("hypoalbuminemia begets hypoalbuminemia"). With capillary leak, such as that seen with inflammation, albumin loss is even greater.

Many critical illnesses, such as sepsis, pancreatitis, immune-mediated diseases, pneumonia, and others, are associated with an inflammatory response that results in endothelial cell injury or dysfunction [8]. During states of metabolic stress, especially in the systemic inflammatory response syndrome (SIRS), albumin becomes a negative acute-phase protein. There is a reduction in albumin formation as cytokines shunt amino acids away from albumin production to increase synthesis of acute-phase proteins important to the inflammatory process [9]. With decreased production, increased use associated with the catabolic state, and increased loss (eg, peritonitis, inflammatory bowel

E-mail address: kmathews@uoguelph.ca

0195-5616/08/$ – see front matter
doi:10.1016/j.cvsm.2008.02.004

disease) of albumin, a reduction in oncotic pressure may occur as illness progresses [10]. The reduction in oncotic pressure associated with endothelial or alveolar epithelial cell injury leads to plasma leak from capillaries into the interstitium and the alveolar space [8]. The consequence is edema of multiple organs, which results in organ dysfunction, respiratory distress, and, potentially, death [11,12]. Extravascular lung water (pulmonary edema) has been correlated directly with survival, and increased values are an independent predictor of mortality in critically ill human patients across all diagnostic groups [13]. In these settings, a small volume of a colloid solution in combination with a crystalloid solution may be required for adequate organ perfusion and to maintain fluid within the intravascular space. Synthetic colloids are recommended for treatment in low-oncotic states in veterinary medicine [14–20]. The potential for capillary leakage with these products may be a concern in inflammatory states, however, because of some of their smaller sized molecules (10,000 d) [21,22].

Albumin is a carrier protein for many drugs and endogenous substances, has metabolic and acid-base functions, and has anticoagulant effects (decreased platelet aggregation and augmentation of antithrombin concentration) [23,24]. Albumin also has antioxidant properties [25–27]; is a direct scavenger of reactive oxygen species; and can bind iron, preventing iron-dependent oxidizing events, such as lipid peroxidation [28]. As such, albumin may confer protection against ischemia and reperfusion injury [29]. Most of these specific properties do not exist with the synthetic colloids; therefore, albumin may have additional benefits in managing animals with SIRS and capillary leak disorders associated with marked hypoalbuminemia. The concentration of administered albumin also seems to be important. In a hemorrhagic shock rat model, 25% human serum albumin (25% HSA; but not 5% HSA) has exerted anti-inflammatory and protective effects by means of marked inhibition of macrophage activation against lung injury [5]. Interestingly, CD18 adhesion molecule expression and oxidative burst were greater when neutrophils were incubated with Ringer's lactate solution or 5% HSA than with 25% HSA [5,30]. The protective effect was not attributed to osmolarity of the solution.

Despite all these positive attributes, it is interesting to note that the use of albumin in human medicine is still controversial. Benefits and controversies from several studies reviewed in 1944 [31] are still heavily debated today. A Cochrane meta-analysis based on many heterogeneous studies indicated that colloid administration (4% or 5% albumin) may cause harm. No explanation as to potential risks was given to support the statement, however [32]. In fact, in a retrospective study investigating the safety of human albumin based on spontaneously reported serious adverse events linked to albumin use in people, only 123 serious adverse events occurred in 95 million 40-g doses administered [33]. Subsequent reviews found fault with the Cochrane analysis [34–37]. This prompted further studies investigating the use of albumin in human patients. The Saline versus Albumin Fluid Evaluation (SAFE) study was designed to identify benefits or risks for fluid resuscitation with normal saline or 4%

albumin (a common resuscitative fluid in Australia and New Zealand) of patients admitted to the intensive care unit (ICU), regardless of the cause for
admission or albumin levels, [38]. A further review by the Cochrane Group
on the use of albumin concluded that there was no overall evidence that albumin increased mortality. Nevertheless, albumin might be beneficial for some
subgroups, with sepsis being one, but may increase mortality in patients who
have hypoalbuminemia, burns, or traumatic brain injury [39,40]. There defi-
nitely seems to be two camps on the opinion of benefits of albumin administration, because other studies and meta-analyses support the use of albumin,
showing potential benefits from albumin administration [36,41,42].

Potentially, the lack of clear-cut benefits of the use of albumin in these
human studies is attributable to the concentration of albumin (4% or 5%
versus 25%) used and the indications for its administration. It would
seem to be intuitive that these two important factors should be considered
before any recommendations are made. Unfortunately, only a few studies
have targeted specific medical problems and selection of a 4%, 5%, or
25% solution of albumin. As a product, HSA is manufactured from pooled
human plasma that is ultrafiltrated and heat sterilized. Two concentrations
are available: the iso-oncotic 5% at 308 mOsm (COP = 20 mm Hg) and
the hyperoncotic 25% at 1500 mOsm (COP = 200 mm Hg). As a comparison, the COP of 6% hetastarch is 30 to 45 mm Hg, whereas that of dextran 70 is 60 mm Hg (normal canine plasma COP ~20 mm Hg). An
infusion of the 25% solution increases intravascular volume by as much
as four to five times the infused volume as a result of the van't Hoff and
Gibbs-Donnan effect. In laboratory studies, the 5% HSA solution did not
confer any advantage over Ringer's lactate when compared with 25%
HSA [5,30]. Because a 25% HSA solution may be more beneficial in the
clinical setting than the 4% or 5% solution, the routine supplemental administration of 25% HSA to patients with an albumin concentration less than
30 g/L was studied [43]. No advantage of 25% HSA for treatment of patients in the surgical ICU was detected, however [43].

A more recent study investigating the outcome of patients in a medical/sur-
gical ICU with an albumin concentration less than 31 g/L (3.1 g/dL) receiving
20% HSA showed that organ function improved more in the group receiving
albumin than in the control group [44]. The investigators concluded that albumin administration may improve organ function in hypoalbuminemic critically
ill patients because it results in a less positive fluid balance and a better tolerance to enteral feeding [44].

These two studies illustrate the controversial aspect of albumin infusion
when broad entrance criteria are used.

As with human patients, critically ill veterinary patients may need supplementation with albumin to improve outcome. Plasma transfusions are frequently recommended for critically ill animals to maintain albumin
between 15 and 20 g/L (1.5–2.0 g/dL) with clinical manifestations of hypoalbuminemia [45] or greater than 20 g/L (2.0 g/dL) [16–19,24]. Species-specific

albumin is only available as plasma in veterinary medicine. One liter of canine plasma contains albumin, on average, at a rate of 25 to 30 g (equal to 25% HSA, 100 mL), requiring large volumes to supply a conservative amount of albumin at recommended volumes [20,46,47]. Consequently, a large volume of "fluid" accompanies the albumin transfusion as plasma, which contributes to increased hydrostatic pressure. Because no canine or feline concentrated albumin solutions are commercially available, no veterinary clinical studies exist to compare with human studies. Two retrospective analyses on the use of 25% HSA prescribed for a range of clinical problems in critically ill veterinary patients have been published, however [48,49]. The study by Chan and colleagues [48] is only available as an abstract, and details of patient diagnosis are not provided. Diseases incorporated in the study by Mathews and Barry [49] included severe hemorrhagic pancreatitis, fractured pelvis with hemorrhage, urethral tear with urine peritonitis, postoperative jejunal dehiscence, retained fetus with uterine rupture, thrombosis of splenic and hepatic veins, duodenal or jejunal perforation, bile duct rupture, gastric dilation-volvulus necrosis, and inflammatory bowel disease with protein-losing enteropathy and surgical biopsy [49]. Serum albumin and total solids in these patients increased significantly greater than pretransfusion concentrations. At discharge, the increase in serum albumin in most patients was up to 45% greater than preinfusion concentrations, with a continuous increase after transfusion. The increase in albumin concentration in dogs with protein-losing enteropathy was short-lived, however, because albumin started to decline at discharge from hospital. This demonstrates that albumin administration is only of short-term value when ongoing losses are not halted. Dogs with pulmonary and subcutaneous edema in this study were also treated with furosemide, and the ongoing fluid therapy dose could be reduced with the addition of 25% HSA. This reduction in crystalloid therapy may also have contributed to resolution and continual improvement in edema. Resolution of pleural and abdominal fluid accumulation was also noted [49]. A similar effect has been demonstrated in cat skeletal muscle, in which infusion of 20% albumin showed a reduced capillary filtration coefficient and dose-dependent absorption of fluid [21]. Several potential reasons for these effects were offered, including the electric charge of the molecule and its size and shape; influence on the endothelium, basement membrane, interstitium, and capillary pores; and high COP. The study also noted no rebound effect of albumin once the infusion was stopped, an effect noted with hetastarch. The rebound effect reflects the degree of interstitial accumulation of the administered colloid and may result in tissue edema in the clinical setting [21,22].

Cost is one of the major negative aspects of albumin administration [32,36,37,41,42]. No pharmacoeconomic studies have been done in human medicine with albumin use in critically ill patients. There is potential for albumin use to be cost-effective if it is associated with a decrease in length of stay in the ICU or with improvement in organ dysfunction [33,43].

INDICATIONS FOR ALBUMIN ADMINISTRATION

Albumin should not be used as a volume replacement strategy or to increase albumin concentration greater than those suggested in veterinary patients (>20 g/L or 2.0 g/dL) [4,19] but to offer an additional therapeutic intervention that may improve oxygen delivery in life-threatening situations that exist in a critically ill patient when standard treatment has failed to do so. It has also been recommended for use based on individual needs [34]. As clinicians, we face this situation on a daily basis, and it has been the author's observation that some animals do respond favorably to 25% HSA administration. Albumin's physiologic role in homeostasis [15–18,33,35] provides reasons for its use in the critically ill patient. A 5-day standardized regimen of 25% HSA and furosemide in hypoalbuminemic human patients that had acute lung injury resulted in improved fluid balance, oxygenation, oxygen delivery, and hemodynamics. It also reduced the number of days on mechanical ventilation and morbidity when compared with the placebo group [24]. A similar combination used in hypoalbuminemic edematous dogs requiring intravascular support resulted in improved fluid balance and recovery [49]. Other medical reports also support its use in the intensive care patient [33,35]. A point to emphasize with respect to hypoalbuminemia is not to assume that broad use of albumin-containing fluids is warranted in all critically ill patients; however, the use of albumin in specific niche populations may prove to have important clinical benefits. The individual animal's response to various illnesses or injuries also differs. Other than treating the underlying problem, it is impossible to establish a definitive protocol for fluid support in each case. Because the albumin debate has existed for approximately 60 years, future studies with a specific focus are required to identify conditions in which albumin administration may be beneficial. When looking at other albumin-containing products, 25% HSA is not considered a replacement for fresh-frozen plasma (FFP), for example, but as an adjunct to that therapy. FFP has other components that are valuable in many of these conditions [26,50] and are quite different from albumin [4,6,7,23–25,29–31]. The author believes that the patient's condition and the clinician's careful judgment dictate the appropriate use of concentrated albumin. An individual animal's response to currently suggested regimens should dictate whether further intervention is indicated. The importance of albumin in critical illness still has to be proved in specific situations; however, advances have been made in our knowledge of the unique and potentially beneficial properties of albumin [23].

SPECIES-SPECIFIC PLASMA

Plasma transfusions are frequently administered to critically ill animals. At the Ontario Veterinary College Veterinary Teaching Hospital (OVC-VTH), recommendations for species-specific transfusion rarely include hypoalbuminemia, but it may be used in patients with clinical manifestations of illness associated with hypoalbuminemia.

Suggested recommendations for plasma transfusion are as follows. The range for normal canine and feline serum albumin concentrations for the author's laboratory is 29 to 43 g/L [2.9 to 4.3 g/dL].

1. Stored plasma (refrigerated as whole blood for 28 days before separation from red blood cells and frozen)
   a. Puppies with severe protein loss attributable to parvovirus diarrhea
   b. In severe hypoalbuminemic patients (albumin <15 g/L [<1.5 g/dL]) requiring volume expansion before surgical intervention
   c. For maintenance of intravascular volume and systemic blood pressure requiring moderate to large volumes of fluids when total solids are less than 40 g/L (<4.0 g/dL)
   d. In capillary leak situations and when an increase in oncotic pressure is required
   e. As component therapy (with packed red blood cells) for whole blood loss
   f. For treatment of warfarin toxicity. Vitamin K–dependent coagulation factors are still effective to a variable degree.
2. FFP
   a. Any inflammatory process or situation with significant cytokine release (ie, sepsis, pancreatitis, major trauma, neoplasia, major surgery) when antithrombin, α-macroglobulins, various anticytokines, antiproteases, and fibronectin are required. Using fresh plasma (or FFP) ensures the maximum concentration of these products.
   b. For coagulation factors, specifically factor VIII and von Willebrand's factor (vWf) and, to a lesser extent, factor V
   c. When any of the situations exist in the recommendations for stored plasma that also require the components of FFP

25% HUMAN SERUM ALBUMIN

25% HSA bottles can be stored at room temperature and have a long shelf life. The suggested recommended uses for concentrated albumin are as follows.

Suggested recommendations for administration of 25% HSA
   a. As in suggested recommendations for stored plasma (1b–d)
   b. For refractory hypotension
   c. Severe hypoalbuminemic patients (albumin <15 g/L [<1.5 g/dL] or <18 g/L [<1.8 g/dL] during dehydration and hypovolemia) with ongoing losses (eg, peritonitis, pleural effusion)
   d. Combined with FFP in hypoalbuminemic septic patients
   e. Patients that have protein-losing enteropathy before surgical biopsy. Although low albumin levels are not considered to influence surgical wound healing [51], they may at extremely low values. An additional potential protective effect of increasing albumin levels before biopsy may be a reduction in edema of the bowel with improved perfusion and oxygen delivery influencing healing rather than having a direct relation to albumin and healing.
   f. Markedly hypoalbuminemic patients that continue to vomit (likely attributable to bowel edema)
   g. Refractory hypotension associated with gastric dilation-volvulus

    h. Markedly hypoalbuminemic patients that have reversible liver failure or insufficiency (eg, portosystemic shunt, acute hepatitis), in which low albumin concentration contributes to mortality

ADMINISTRATION OF 25% HUMAN SERUM ALBUMIN

25% HSA can be administered peripherally or centrally alone or in combination with an established crystalloid intravenous infusion. A vented delivery set is required because the HSA is contained in a bottle. A hypodermic needle cannot be used for continual venting because of the risk for environmental contamination. A blood filter set is not required for HSA administration.

Aseptic technique similar to that used for administration of species-specific transfusions is required. When time permits (nonemergent situation), a test dose of 0.25 mL/kg/h is given over 15 minutes while monitoring heart rate, respiratory rate, and temperature (baseline before transfusion and at end of test dose). Infusion should be discontinued if adverse signs, such as facial swelling, or other signs of anaphylaxis or an anaphylactoid reaction develop. Vital parameters should again be measured on completion of the transfusion.

The maximum volume administered to any dog by the author is 25 mL/kg (6.25 g/kg) administered continuously over 72 hours; the mean volume administered to any dog overall is 5 mL/kg (1.25 g/kg) [49]. The maximum volume given as a slow push or bolus to treat hypotension is 4 mL/kg (1.0 g/kg), with a mean volume of 2 mL/kg (0.5 g/kg) [49]. The range for a continuous rate infusion (CRI) after a bolus administration is 0.1 to 1.7 mL/kg/h (0.025–0.425 g/kg) over 4 to 72 hours. Infusions are empirically selected to meet low normal values. The shorter infusion times are most commonly used for refractory hypotension. It has been shown that continuous administration of albumin at 1 g/kg every 24 hours to human pediatric patients maintains higher serum albumin levels (34% greater than baseline at 24 hours) than the same amount given as a 4-hour infusion (14% greater than baseline at 24 hours) [52]. The bolus infusion of albumin tends to facilitate increased degradation and greater loss in capillary leak states, because the rates of both mass dependent [52].

Once the bottle is opened, the contents must be used or discarded. This does influence the amount administered, because there is a tendency to use all the contents of the bottle rather than discard that remaining after the calculated (empiric) dose.

POTENTIAL ADVERSE EFFECTS OF 25% HUMAN SERUM ALBUMIN

HSA is a foreign antigen and may elicit an immune response. The pet owner should be aware of this and should be counseled on the potential occurrence of immediate or delayed responses. The clinical signs of the delayed responses must be clearly outlined to facilitate early recognition and therapeutic intervention. In a previous study by Mathews and Barry [49], the survival to discharge was 71%, a mortality rate similar to one obtained with use of FFP in 74 critically ill dogs [50]. Immediate reactions, therefore, may be no greater than with other albumin products. Immediate severe reactions have not been noted in any animal at the OVC-VTH after administration of 25% HSA. Facial swelling occurred in two dogs after 2 to 4 hours of transfusion. Potential adverse effects reported included prolonged clotting time, increased respiratory effort, vomiting, and fever in a few cases [48]. Because this information was available only in an abstract, no details were provided on when these potential adverse effects were noted in relation to administration. These complications did not have an impact on the length of hospitalization. Should facial edema occur, diphenhydramine should be given intramuscularly at a dose of 1 to 2 mg/kg and repeated every 8 hours as required. Although anaphylactic shock was not seen in either veterinary report, the clinician should be prepared to treat it should it occur.

Delayed reactions (several days to weeks after administration) may occur. The author has observed immune-mediated complications, such as polyarthritis, vasculitis, or dermatitis, in combination, occur 10 days to 2 months after abdominal surgery, especially complicated intestinal surgery, in dogs receiving and in those not receiving 25% HSA. This may be attributed to an enteropathic etiology, and when albumin is administered, the 25% HSA may act as an adjuvant. Enteropathic polyarthritis is linked to lesions of the intestinal tract in human beings and dogs [53,54]. Foreign albumin alone can cause a severe type III hypersensitivity reaction, however. When 25% HSA was administered at a rate of 2 mL/kg to normal dogs, a severe type III hypersensitivity reaction did occur, which resulted in the death of some dogs [55]. In dogs, 25% bovine serum albumin also is highly immunogenic, potentially causing severe polyarthritis and glomerulonephritis similar to those secondary to 25% HSA administration [56]. The author and his colleagues hypothesized that previous exposure to bovine antigen may occur in dogs, because many vaccines are cultured in calf serum; however, the pathogenesis may be similar to that occurring with 25% HSA. It is unknown why such a profound response occurred in normal dogs; however, severe hypoalbuminemia or illness may have an immunosuppressive effect preventing this response in most ill dogs. The author has used 0.2 mL/kg Tc-99m labelled 25% HSA in six normal dogs with no adverse effects noted over a 4-month observational period or during a following 2-year period after adoption. This suggests that the volume used in normal dogs may also have an impact on immunoreactivity. These studies highlight the importance of evaluating risk versus benefit when considering administration of 25% HSA.

TREATMENT FOR POTENTIAL DELAYED IMMUNE-MEDIATED REACTIONS

Depending on severity, prednisone at a dose of 1 to 2 mg/kg administered every 12 hours on day 1, followed by 1 mg/kg every 12 hours for 2 weeks, and weaning off during the third week. Confirmation of nonseptic polyarthritis should be made before therapy with corticosteroids, especially in areas in which such diseases as ehrlichiosis, anaplasmosis, or Lyme disease are prevalent. The temporal relation to albumin administration, however, would suggest that albumin is responsible for the lesions.

SUMMARY

Twenty-five percent HSA is a foreign protein and can potentially cause immune-mediated reactions. For this reason, the author only recommends 25% HSA use after risk analysis shows that the benefits outweigh the potential risks for adverse events. If it is apparent that a critically ill animal may succumb to its illness because of the problems associated with severe hypoalbuminemia, the benefit outweighs the risk. The veterinarian must inform the owner of potential delayed immune-mediated reactions, describe these lesions, and follow the case weekly to ensure that no reaction has occurred. Although there are many positive attributes to the administration of 25% HSA, there seems to be specific situations in which 25% HSA may be indicated and others in which it may not be indicated. It should not be assumed that "one product fits all" [34–36,38, 40–44,49,57].

References

[1] Brown J. Structural origins of mammalian albumin. Fed Proc 1976;35:2141–4.

[2] Throop JL, Bingaman S, Huxley V. Differences between human and other mammalian albumins raises concerns over the use of human serum albumin in the dog. J Vet Intern Med 2004;18(3):439.

[3] Dixon FJ, Maurer PH, Deichmiller MP. Half-lives of homologous serum albumin in several species. Proc Soc Exp Biol Med 1953;83:287–8.

[4] Mazzaferro EM, Rudloff E, Kirby R. The role of albumin replacement in the critically ill veterinary patient. Journal of Veterinary Emergency and Critical Care 2002;12(2):113–24.

[5] Powers KA, Kapus A, Khadaroo RG, et al. Twenty-five percent albumin prevents lung injury following shock/resuscitation. Crit Care Med 2003;31:2355–63.

[6] Deb S, Sun I, Martin B. Lactated Ringer's solution and hetastarch but not plasma resuscitation after rat hemorrhagic shock is associated with immediate lung apoptosis by the up-regulation of the Bax protein. J Trauma 2000;49:47–53.

[7] Zoellner H, Hou JY, Lovery M. Inhibition of microvascular endothelial apoptosis in tissue explants by serum albumin. Microvasc Res 1999;57:162–73.

[8] Wheeler AP, Bernard GR. Treating patients with sepsis. N Engl J Med 1999;340:207–14.

[9] Rothschild MA, Oratz M, Schreiber SS. Albumin synthesis (second of two parts). N Engl J Med 1972;286(15):816–21.

[10] Guyton AC, Lindsey AW. Effect of elevated left atrial pressure and decreased plasma protein concentration on the development of pulmonary edema. Circ res 1959;7:649–57.

[11] Martin GS, Bernard GR. Airway and lung dysfunction in sepsis. Intensive Care Med 2001;27(Suppl 1):63–79.

[12] Ferguson ND, Meade MO, Hallett DC, et al. High values of the pulmonary artery wedge pressure in patients with acute lung injury and acute respiratory distress syndrome. Intensive Care Med 2002;28:1073–7.

[13] Sakka SG, Klein M, Reinhart K, et al. Prognostic value of extra-vascular lung water in critically ill patients. Chest 2002;122:2080–6.

[14] Smiley LE. The use of hetastarch for plasma expansion. Probl Vet Med 1992;4(4):652–67.

[15] Rudloff E, Kirby R. Hypovolemic shock and resuscitation. Vet Clin North Am Small Anim Pract 1994;24(6):1015–39.

[16] Kirby R, Rudloff E. The critical need for colloids: maintaining fluid balance. Compendium of Continuing Education for Practicing Veterinarians 1997;19:705–18.

[17] Rudloff E, Kirby R. The critical need for colloids: selecting the right colloid. Compendium of Continuing Education for Practicing Veterinarians 1997;19:811–26.

[18] Rudloff E, Kirby R. The critical need for colloids: administering colloids effectively. Compendium of Continuing Education for Practicing Veterinarians 1998;20:27–43.

[19] Rudloff E, Kirby R. Fluid therapy. Crystalloids and colloids. Vet Clin North Am Small Anim Pract 1998;28:297–328.

[20] Weeren FR, Muir WW. Clinical aspects of septic shock and comprehensive approaches to treatment in dogs. J Am Vet Med Assoc 1992;200(12):1859–69.

[21] Holbeck S, Grande P. Effects on capillary fluid permeability and fluid exchange of albumin, dextran, gelatin and hydroxyethyl starch in cat skeletal muscle. Crit Care Med 2000;28(4):1089–95.

[22] Mishler JM. Synthetic plasma volume expanders: their pharmacology, safety and clinical efficacy. Clin Haematol 1984;13:75–92.

[23] Nicholson JP, Wolmarans MR, Park GR. The role of albumin in critical illness. Br J Anaesth 2000;85:599–610.

[24] Hughes D. Fluid therapy with macromolecular plasma volume expanders. In: Di Bartola SP, editor. Fluid therapy in small animal practice. 2nd edition. Philadelphia: WB Saunders; 2000. p. 483–95.

[25] Peters T Jr. Serum albumin. Adv Protein Chem 1985;37:161–245.

[26] Emmerson TE Jr. Unique features of albumin: a brief review. Crit Care Med 1989;17:690–4.

[27] King TP. On the sulfhydryl group of human plasma albumin. J Biol chem 1961;236(2):PC5.

[28] Bourdon E, Blache D. The importance of proteins in defense against oxidation. Antioxid Redox Signal 2001;3:293–311.

[29] Watts JA, Maiorano PC. Trace amounts of albumin protect against ischemia and reperfusion injury in isolated rat hearts. J Mol Cell Cardiol 1999;31:1653–62.

[30] Rhee P, Wang D, Ruff P. Human neutrophil activation and increased adhesion by various resuscitation fluids. Crit Care Med 2000;28:74–8.

[31] Scatchard G, Batchelder AC, Brown A. Chemical, clinical and immunological studies on the products of human plasma fractionation. VI. The osmotic pressure of plasma and of serum albumin. J Clin Invest 1944;23:458–64.

[32] Cochrane Injuries Group Albumin Reviewers. Human albumin administration in critically ill patients: systematic review of randomized controlled trials. BMJ 1998;317:235–40.

[33] Vincent JL. Fluid management: the pharmacoeconomic dimension. Crit Care 2000;4(Suppl 2):S33–5.

[34] Choi PT, Yip G, Quinonez LG, et al. Crystalloids vs colloids in fluid resuscitation: a systematic review. Crit Care Med 1999;27:200–21.

[35] Allison SP, Lobo DN. Debate: albumin administration should not be avoided. Crit Care 2000;4(3):147–50.

[36] Wilkes MM, Navickis RJ. Patient survival after human albumin administration. Ann Intern Med 2001;135:149–64.

[37] Boldt J. The good, the bad and the ugly: should we completely banish human albumin from our intensive care units? Anesth Analg 2000;91:887–95.

[38] The SAFE Study Investigators. A comparison of albumin and saline for fluid resuscitation in the intensive care unit. N Engl J Med 2004;350:2247–56.

[39] Alderson F, Bunn A, Li Wan Po A, et al. Human albumin solution for resuscitation and volume expansion in critically ill patients. Cochrane Database Syst Rev 2004;4:CD001208.

[40] SAFE Study Investigators. Saline or albumin for fluid resuscitation in patients with TBI. N Engl J Med 2007;357:874–84.

[41] Vincent J-L, Dubois M-J, Navickis RJ, et al. Hypoalbuminemia in acute illness: is there a rationale for intervention. A meta-analysis of cohort studies and controlled trials. Ann Surg 2003;
237(3):319–34.

[42] Vincent JL. Fluids for resuscitation. Br J Anaesth 1991;67:185–93.

[43] Golub R, Sorrento JJ Jr, Cantu R Jr, et al. Efficacy of albumin supplementation in the surgical
intensive care unit: a prospective, randomized study. Crit Care Med 1994;22(4):613–9.

[44] Dubois MJ, Orellana-Jimenez C, Melot C, et al. Albumin administration improves organ
function in critically ill hypoalbuminemic patients: a prospective, randomized, controlled,
pilot study. Crit Care Med 2006;34(10):2536–40.

[45] Abram-Ogg ACG. Practical blood transfusion. In: Day MJ, Mackin A, Littlewood JD, editors.
BSAVA manual of canine and feline hematology and transfusion medicine. Gloucester: British Small Animal Veterinary Association; 2000. p. 263–303.

[46] Cotter S. Clinical transfusion medicine. Adv Vet Sci Comp Med 1991;36:187–223.

[47] Kristensen AT. Administration of blood products to animals. In: Bistner SI, Ford RB, editors.
Kirk and Bistner's handbook of veterinary procedures and emergency treatment. Philadelphia: WB Saunders Co.,; 1995. p. 561–73.

[48] Chan DL, Rozanski EA, Freeman LM, et al. Retrospective evaluation of human serum albumin
use in critically ill dogs [abstract]. Journal of Veterinary Emergency and Critical Care
2004;14(Suppl 1):S8.

[49] Mathews KA, Barry M. The use of 25% human serum albumin: outcome and efficacy in
raising serum albumin and systemic blood pressure in critically ill dogs and cats. Journal
of Veterinary Emergency Critical Care 2005;15:110–8.

[50] Logan JC, Callan MB, Drew K, et al. Clinical indications for use of fresh frozen plasma in
dogs: 74 dogs (October through December 1999). J Am Vet Med Assoc 2001;218:
1449–55.

[51] Harvey HJ. Complication of small intestinal biopsy in hypoalbuminemic dogs. Vet Surg
1990;19:289–92.

[52] Greissman A, Silver P, Nimkoff L, et al. Albumin bolus administration vs continuous infusion
in critically ill hypoalbuminemic pediatric patients. Intensive Care Med 1996;22:495–9.

[53] Davidson AP. Immune-mediated joint diseases. In: Slatter DH, editor. Textbook of small animal surgery. 3rd edition. Philadelphia: WB Saunders Company; 2003. p. 2246–50.

[54] Holden W, Orchard T, Wordsworth P. Enteropathic arthritis. Rheum Dis Clin North Am
2003;29:513–30.

[55] Francis A, Martin L, Haldorson GJ, et al. Adverse reactions suggestive of type III hypersensitivity in six healthy dogs given human albumin. J Am Vet Med Assoc 2007;230(6):873–9.

[56] Mosley CA, Mathews KA. The use of concentrated bovine serum albumin in canines. In: Proceedings of the Annual Meeting of the American College of Veterinary Anesthesiologists.
Phoenix, Arizona; 2004. p. 73.

[57] Vincent JL. Resuscitation using albumin in critically ill patients: research in patients at high
risk of complications is now needed. BMJ 2006;333:1029–30.

Complications of Fluid Therapy

Elisa M. Mazzaferro, MS, DVM, PhD

Wheat Ridge Veterinary Specialists, 3695 Kipling Street, Wheat Ridge, CO 80033, USA

The administration of intravenous fluids is one of the most important aspects of patient care in hospitalized animals. Intravenous fluids are administered to replace or prevent dehydration, treat hypovolemic shock and intravascular volume depletion, correct acid-base and electrolyte abnormalities, and maintain vascular access for administration of drugs, blood product components, and parenteral nutrition. Intravenous catheterization also can provide a means of blood sample collection, thus avoiding frequent and uncomfortable venipunctures in critically ill animals. Although the benefits of intravenous catheterization and fluid administration are numerous, there are inherent risks associated with the procedures, and care must be taken to avoid potential complications.

INTRAVENOUS CATHETERIZATION

Avoidance of catheter-induced complications begins with careful assessment of the animal and appropriate selection of the intravenous catheter site. Contamination of the catheter site by the animal's body fluids or excretions (urine or feces) and invasion by nosocomial organisms in the animal's hospital environment are common potential sources of infection. If an animal is vomiting or has epistaxis or ptyalism, forelimb catheters are inappropriate because of the risk of contamination and the frequent need for replacement of the catheter bandage to prevent wicking of bacteria from the environment. Similarly, placement of a medial or lateral saphenous catheter is contraindicated in animals with diarrhea or urinary or fecal incontinence. Elizabethan collars should be placed on inquisitive animals to prevent them from chewing the catheter or intravenous fluid line, which can break sterility and predispose the animal to a catheter-related infection. In animals with coagulopathies, such as disseminated intravascular coagulation or vitamin K antagonist rodenticide intoxication, the use of large-bore central venous catheters should be avoided to prevent excessive hemorrhage from venipuncture sites. Similarly, in animals with hypercoagulable states (eg, immune-mediated hemolytic anemia, hyperadrenocorticism, disseminated intravascular coagulation, protein-losing enteropathy, protein-losing nephropathy), placement of a central venous catheter can induce

E-mail address: emazzaferro@hotmail.com

0195-5616/08/$ – see front matter
doi:10.1016/j.cvsm.2008.01.003

thromboembolism and lead to edema of the site drained by the thrombosed vessel. One report documented cranial vena caval thrombosis from catheterization of the jugular vein in a dog with chylothorax [1].

During placement of an intravenous catheter, careful aseptic technique should be used at all times to decrease the risk of bacterial contamination of the catheter site. Besides the animal itself, one of the most common sources of catheter-induced infection is the hands and equipment of hospital personnel. Hand washing is by far one of the most important tasks that a veterinary technician and veterinarian can perform to prevent catheter-related infections. In one study, the incidence of *Enterobacter* spp bacterial contamination of intravenous catheters decreased significantly when personnel in the critical care unit changed [2]. The authors concluded that lack of hygiene and hand washing between patients contributed greatly to positive bacterial cultures of intravenous catheters.

After carefully clipping and scrubbing the catheter site with an antimicrobial scrub solution, hospital personnel should wear gloves to decrease the risk of sepsis, particularly in immunocompromised animals. The incidence of bacterial contamination of intravenous catheters in puppies with parvoviral enteritis can be as high as 22% [3]. Most bacterial pathogens isolated were from either gastrointestinal or environmental sources and were resistant to multiple antibiotics [3]. Because of the high incidence of bacterial resistance, the environment was thought to be a likely source of contamination, possibly transferred from the environment to the animal by the hands of caretakers. Carefully scrubbing a distal extremity, such as the forelimb, with a 4% chlorhexidine solution followed by a contact time of 1 minute greatly reduces bacterial colonization of skin at intravenous catheter sites [4]. A gauze square 4×4 should be placed over the animal's hair distal to the proposed site of catheterization to prevent dragging the intravenous catheter through contaminated hair. Nonsterile technique during emergency vascular access and vascular cut-down procedures also can predispose an animal to catheter-related infection. Even when strict adherence to aseptic protocols has been used, the catheter site should be evaluated at least once daily for evidence of problems, which may include pain upon injection, erythema, "ropiness" or thickening of the vessel, heat, or any discharge from the catheter site. If any of these abnormalities is noted or if fever develops in a previously afebrile patient, the catheter should be removed, and the tip should be cultured for aerobic bacteria.

Previously it was recommended to empirically change the intravenous catheter every 3 days to avoid catheter-induced infection. A prospective study investigated the risk of bacterial contamination of intravenous catheters left in place for less than 72 hours with those left in place for more than 72 hours. The investigator documented that the risk of bacterial contamination of the catheters was similar in both groups and overall the risk of bacterial contamination was low [5]. Bacteria that were cultured from the catheters included *Enterobacter aerogenes*, *Staphylococcus aureus*, *Pseudomonas aeruginosa*, *Pasteurella multocida*, and *Bacillus* spp. The source of *Bacillus* spp contamination was the gauze sponges used to prepare the catheter sites. Once the source of contamination was found, the incidence of catheter-related bacterial contamination decreased dramatically. This report emphasized the importance of clean technique and clean supplies. The study determined that it is costly and not necessary to change catheters every 72 hours. In another study, the incidence of bacterial contamination of intravenous catheters was not related to the length of time catheters were in place or other catheter complications [2]. Currently, I recommend using a catheter for as long as necessary and for as long as it is functioning properly without any of the complications listed previously. A larger scale observational study of more than 600 intravenous catheters in human patients documented no increased risk of infection, thrombophlebitis, or mechanical complications with prolonged catheterization [6]. As a general rule, once the catheter is no longer needed, it should be removed because it always can be a potential source of infection and thrombophlebitis.

CRYSTALLOID FLUIDS

A wide variety of crystalloid fluids is available for veterinary use. Ideally, the choice of crystalloid fluid is based on the patient's acid-base and electrolyte status. For example, the administration of a fluid that contains bicarbonate precursors as buffers may be inappropriate for an animal with hypochloremic metabolic alkalosis caused by pyloric outflow obstruction. A better fluid choice in this situation would be 0.9% sodium chloride, which contains a high concentration of chloride (154 mEq/L) and no bicarbonate precursors. Administration of 0.9% sodium chloride, however, can cause an additional increase in serum chloride concentration in a patient that already is hyperchloremic. Administration of a solution with no bicarbonate precursors (eg, 0.9% saline, 5% dextrose in water) can exacerbate metabolic acidosis, although in patients with severe hypovolemic shock, administration of these fluids can help restore perfusion and correct lactic acidosis by replacement of intravascular fluid volume alone. Administration of lactated Ringer's solution (which contains calcium) may be inappropriate in an animal with hypercalcemia. Similarly, administration of a potassium-containing fluid to an animal with severe hyperkalemia places that patient at risk for an additional increase in its serum potassium concentration. In many cases, however, administration of intravenous fluids (regardless of composition) improves perfusion and causes dilution of the patient's serum electrolytes. The administration of large volumes of dextrose-containing fluids as a bolus may result in hyperglycemia, which can worsen the prognosis in animals with head trauma [7]. Rapid administration of hypotonic fluids, such as 5% dextrose in water, also potentially can cause intravascular hemolysis. Similarly, overly rapid administration of a hypertonic solution, such as hypertonic saline, can result in crenation of red blood cells if inappropriate volumes are administered too rapidly [8]. Hypertonic saline infusion also can be associated with vagally mediated hypotension and bradycardia and is contraindicated in animals that are hypernatremic or dehydrated [8,9]. Calcium-containing fluids should not be administered concurrently with blood products because of the risk of calcium citrate precipitation in the fluid line.

ACID-BASE AND ELECTROLYTE IMBALANCES

Electrolyte abnormalities are common in a wide variety of illnesses that affect small animal patients. Sodium and potassium are among the most important electrolytes to consider, because imbalances in these electrolytes can dramatically affect neuromuscular function and maintenance of cellular homeostasis. Animals that lose water in excess of solute or animals that have hypothalamic lesions can develop a free water deficit that manifests itself as hypernatremia. Animals that have an aldosterone deficiency cannot reabsorb adequate amounts of sodium and can become profoundly hyponatremic as a result. Abrupt changes in sodium concentration can cause substantial shifts in intracellular or interstitial fluid and lead to cerebral edema or central pontine myelinolysis, particularly in states of severe hyponatremia (ie, serum sodium concentration $<$ 120 mEq/L) [10,11]. To avoid excessively rapid correction or normalization of serum sodium concentration during states of either hyper- or hyponatremia, the following calculations can be used.

CORRECTION OF HYPERNATREMIA

$$\text{Free water deficit} = 0.6 \times \text{kg body weight} \times \left(\left[Na^+_{current} / Na^+_{desired} \right] - 1 \right) \; [11]$$

Controversy exists as to which fluids should be used to decrease serum sodium concentration. Infusion of 5% dextrose in water actually represents administration of free water because the dextrose is metabolized to carbon dioxide and water. In cases of severe hypernatremia, however, reduction in serum sodium concentration can be achieved by first using solutions with higher concentrations of sodium such as 0.9% saline (154 mEq/L), progressing to lactated Ringer's solution (130 mEq/L) and, ultimately, to 5% dextrose in water to avoid excessively rapid correction of hypernatremia. Severe hypernatremia can occur when an animal has chronic free water or hypotonic fluid loss, such as an animal with chronic diabetes mellitus or renal insufficiency whose serum sodium concentration may approach 200 mEq/L.

A second formula determines the effect of 1 L of a solution (infusate) on the decrease in serum sodium concentration:

$$\text{Change in serum sodium (mEq/L)} = \left[Na^+_{infusate} / Na^+_{patient} \right] / [(\text{kg body weight} \times 0.6) + 1] \; [11]$$

Ideally, the change in serum sodium concentration should not exceed 0.5 mEq/kg/h or 10 to 12 mEq/kg/d. By using this calculation, one can estimate how quickly to administer 1 L of fluid. This formula predicts what the animal's serum sodium concentration should be after administration of a liter of the infusate solution.

When faced with an animal with severe chronic hyponatremia, the same approach of careful and slow correction of serum sodium concentration should be followed. Although it may seem reasonable to administer a fluid that contains large amounts of sodium (eg, 0.9% NaCl with 154 mEq/L) to an animal with a serum sodium concentration of less than 120 mEq/L, gradual administration of a fluid with a moderate amount of sodium (eg, lactated Ringer's with 130 mEq/L or Normosol-R with 140 mEq/L) is more appropriate to avoid overly rapid correction of serum sodium concentration and the risk of central pontine myelinolysis.

HYPOKALEMIA

Unless an animal has been rapidly infused with a fluid that contains added potassium chloride, hyperkalemia and resultant atrial standstill rarely are complications of intravenous fluid therapy. Severe hypokalemia can promote refractory ventricular arrhythmias, muscle cramping, muscle weakness, lethargy, ileus, and cervical ventroflexion [11]. Many isotonic crystalloids used for replacement fluid therapy contain small quantities of potassium (3–4 mEq/L). Hypokalemia, however, is a common occurrence during fluid therapy, and unless commonly used crystalloid replacement solutions are supplemented with potassium chloride, an animal can become hypokalemic as a result of intravenous fluid administration. As a rule, potassium supplementation should not exceed 0.5 mEq/kg/h. Potassium supplementation typically is performed according to the animal's serum potassium concentration (Table 1). If an animal (eg, a patient with diabetic ketoacidosis) has refractory hypokalemia despite appropriate potassium supplementation, magnesium chloride also should be administered at a rate of 0.75 mEq/kg/d by constant rate infusion. Hypomagnesemia is a common occurrence in critical illness and can lead to dysfunction of sodium-potassium-ATPase with resultant refractory hypokalemia.

INTRAVASCULAR VOLUME OVERLOAD

In normal individuals, total body water comprises approximately 60% of the animal's body weight. Most of this water (67% of total body water) is located intracellularly, whereas the rest of it is located in the intravascular and

Table 1
Serum potassium concentration and recommended amount of potassium supplementation (mEq/L)

Serum potassium (mEq/L)	KCl (mEq/L) supplementation
< 2.0	80
2.1–2.5	60
2.6–3.0	40
3.1–3.5	30
3.6–5.0	20
> 5.0	0

interstitial spaces. Of the 33% of water that is located extracellularly, 24% of total body water is located in the interstitial space and 8% to 10% of total body water is located in the intravascular space. Fluid flux between compartments is determined by the balance between hydrostatic and oncotic forces within each compartment and vascular endothelial pore size. Hydrostatic force is the pressure exerted by water on either side of a blood vessel wall. Increases in hydrostatic forces favor extravasation of fluid from one fluid compartment to the other, especially if oncotic forces are suboptimal. Conversely, oncotic forces favor retention of fluid within a fluid compartment, helping to avoid interstitial edema if a healthy vasculature is present.

Starling's Law of Diffusion largely determines the movement of fluid from one compartment to another and states that

$$\text{Fluid flux} = k[(P_c + \pi_i) - (\pi_c + P_i)]$$

where k is filtration coefficient, P_c is hydrostatic pressure in the capillary, P_i is hydrostatic pressure in the interstitium, π_c is capillary oncotic pressure, and π_i is oncotic pressure of the interstitial space.

The filtration coefficient is determined by the capillary fenestration or pore size. The oncotic pressure is the force that attracts fluid or water and is determined by the size and number of particles in solution relative to the size and number of particles in the interstitial space. Forces that favor filtration of fluid out of the vessel into the interstitial space are the interstitial oncotic pressure and the capillary hydrostatic pressure. Forces that favor retention of fluid within the intravascular space are the intravascular oncotic pressure and the interstitial hydrostatic pressure. The balance between the forces that favor filtration versus forces that favor fluid absorption determines the net direction of fluid flux.

Interstitial edema occurs when intravascular hydrostatic forces exceed intravascular oncotic forces. Infusion of crystalloid fluids alone (which do not contribute to intravascular oncotic pressure) can dilute serum albumin and other proteins and increase the risk of interstitial edema [12]. This is particularly true in the lungs when pulmonary capillary pressures exceed 25 mm Hg and the pulmonary lymphatic drainage system becomes overwhelmed. The use of direct cardiac output monitoring and measurement of pulmonary capillary occlusion pressures is not advocated in all critically ill animals. Central venous pressure measurements, however, are simple and easy to perform with minimally invasive equipment and can be used indirectly to measure trends in intravascular fluid volume, provided that right heart function, vascular compliance, and intrathoracic pressures are normal [13]. Colloid osmometry also is a useful monitoring technique to determine a patient's colloid osmotic (oncotic) pressure (COP) and response to colloid therapy [14]. Although attempts have been made to extrapolate serum oncotic pressure from total serum protein concentration in animals, results are variable and do not correlate well [15–17]. Intravascular oncotic pressure and intravascular fluid volume must be carefully titrated to meet the patient's fluid therapy needs. Consequences of edema include impaired cellular oxygen delivery and enzyme function, impaired cellular oxygen exchange, cellular swelling, and cellular lysis [13]. Clinical signs of overhydration include shivering, restlessness, serous nasal discharge, chemosis, tachypnea, cough, and pulmonary crackles. An important component of monitoring includes frequent assessment of the animal's respiratory status, because tachypnea and cough often occur before clinical signs of serous nasal discharge, chemosis (Fig. 1), peripheral edema (Fig. 2), and fulminant pulmonary edema [8].

ALBUMIN

Albumin is an important contributor to COP in the body. Unless severe hyperglobulinemia is present, albumin contributes approximately 50% of the patient's total protein concentration and contributes 80% to the serum COP. Extrapolation of COP using serum albumin concentration has been reported, but this method is largely inaccurate in animals [15–17]. Use of a colloid osmometer is considered the gold standard for assessment of COP if an animal is at risk of developing interstitial edema. When severe hypoalbuminemia (serum albumin concentration < 2.0 g/dL) is present, an animal is at risk for extravasation of fluid from the vascular space and development of interstitial edema. This degree of hypoalbuminemia has been associated with a significantly increased risk of mortality in critically ill dogs [18], enteral feeding intolerance, and delayed wound healing [19]. Consequently, increasing serum albumin concentration to 2.0 g/dL may improve clinical outcome. Increasing serum albumin concentration potentially can be accomplished by use of fresh frozen or regularly frozen plasma; administration of plasma is largely an inefficient method of increasing serum albumin concentration. Approximately

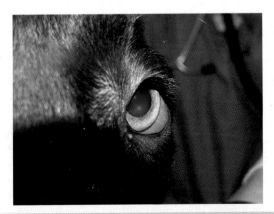

Fig. 1. Chemosis secondary to overzealous intravenous fluid administration in a dog with vasculitis. (*From* Mazzaferro EM. Fluid therapy: the critical balance between life and death. NAVC Clinician's Brief 2006;73–5; with permission.)

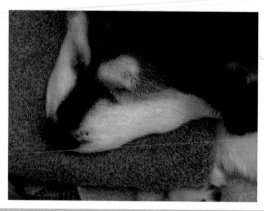

Fig. 2. Patient with severe subcutaneous edema from overhydration and renal failure.

15 to 20 mL/kg of fresh frozen plasma is necessary to increase serum albumin concentration by 0.5 g/dL, provided no ongoing losses are present [19]. Recently, concentrated human albumin has been used with success to increase serum COP and blood pressure in critically ill dogs [20]. Other research has demonstrated that concentrated human albumin and hetastarch were superior to 0.9% saline in fluid resuscitation and resulted in decreased incidence of pulmonary edema compared with saline resuscitation alone [21]. More recently, research has indicated that the use of concentrated human albumin may be detrimental in normoalbuminemic dogs [22,23]. A limitation of this study was that all experimental dogs were normoalbuminemic. The authors acknowledged that immunocompetence in normoalbuminemic dogs may have differed from that of critically ill animals and may place normoalbuminemic animals at risk for developing antihuman albumin antibodies and reactions to albumin infusion. I have used concentrated human albumin (25%) with success and minimal adverse reactions in severely hypoalbuminemic dogs in veterinary clinical practice. The potential benefits associated with the use of concentrated human albumin must be weighed against its potential risks on a case-by-case basis, however. Once serum albumin concentration has increased to 2.0 g/dL, COP can be maintained by administration of a synthetic colloid such as hydroxyethyl starch, Pentastarch, or Dextran-70.

POTENTIAL COMPLICATIONS ASSOCIATED WITH VARIOUS COLLOID FLUIDS

The various colloids available for use in veterinary patients are not without the potential for complications. In general, administration of a colloid causes any infused crystalloid fluid to be retained within the intravascular space for a longer period of time than usual. Normally, up to 80% of an infused crystalloid fluid leaves the intravascular space within 1 hour of administration. When a colloid is administered concurrently with a crystalloid, however, the crystalloid fluid volume should be decreased by 25% to 50% (ie, only 50%–75% of the crystalloid should be administered) to avoid increased intravascular hydrostatic pressure and interstitial edema, particularly within the pulmonary parenchyma. Clinically and experimentally, an increase in intravascular lung water during resuscitation from hemorrhagic shock has resulted in decreased serum COP and decreased oxygen delivery [24]. Hydroxyethyl starch or dextrans can artifactually cause small dilutional decreases in total solids as measured by refractometer, but they are known to significantly increase COP [25].

Von Willebrand factor and factor VII can be decreased to 40% of normal after an animal has received hydroxyethyl starch [26]. Activated clotting time, activated partial thromboplastin time, and platelet plug formation may be prolonged from normal in animals that have received hydroxyethyl starch [27,28]. These abnormalities likely are not clinically relevant and clinically do not cause bleeding until infusion exceeds the manufacturer's recommended dosage of 20 to 30 mL/kg/d or unless the animal has a hereditary coagulation disorder, such as a factor VII deficiency or von Willebrand's disease [29–31]. Neutrophil counts can be increased in animals that have received Dextran-70 because of neutrophil demargination [31]. Low molecular weight dextrans should be used with caution—if at all—in animals with renal impairment because of the risk of renal failure secondary to tubular obstruction [32]. Dextrans can coat red blood cells and platelets and interfere with tests of coagulation and red cell cross-match procedures. Dextran-40 has been associated with an increased risk of anaphylaxis [9] and should be avoided whenever possible because better options are available for veterinary patients.

HEMOGLOBIN-BASED OXYGEN CARRIERS

Hemoglobin-based oxygen carriers are potent colloids that have an added benefit of increasing oxygen-carrying capacity without the need for blood typing and cross-match procedures. Because hemoglobin-based oxygen carriers are potent colloids, they should be used with caution in animals with marginal cardiac function to avoid interstitial and pulmonary edema [33]. Other complications that have been reported with use of hemoglobin-based oxygen carriers include pleural effusion, discolored mucous membranes, vomiting, neurologic abnormalities, and pigmenturia. Use of hemoglobin-based oxygen carriers also artifactually alters serum and urine chemistry tests that are measured by colorimetric assays.

BLOOD PRODUCTS

Blood products, when administered correctly, can make the difference between life and death in a critically ill animal. Without care and forethought, however, administration of blood products can be associated with potentially life-threatening complications in some animals. In cats, for example, infusion of type A blood into a type B cat can result in rapid hemolysis and death [34]. In dogs, infusion of blood into an animal that has been previously sensitized can result in hemolysis, pigmenturia, and hypotension [35,36]. Other transfusion reactions that have been described include ionized hypocalcemia, fever, vomiting, urticaria, angioneurotic edema, and hypotension [37]. Ionized hypocalcemia can make the vasculature less sensitive to circulating catecholamines and potentiate vasodilatation, cardiac dysfunction, hypothermia, and hypotension. If an animal develops refractory hypotension and hypothermia after administration of blood products, citrate toxicity and ionized hypocalcemia must be considered. Treatment consists of replenishing calcium by administration of calcium gluconate (1 mL/kg of a 10% solution given slowly) [38]. Dogs that have received massive transfusions, defined as administration of blood products in an amount more than the animal's blood volume (ie, > 90 mL/kg), have been shown to develop ionized hypocalcemia, thrombocytopenia, and coagulopathy [37].

Minimally, blood typing should be performed before administration of any blood product to a dog or cat. Ideally, a cross-match procedure also should be performed to prevent adverse complications [39]. Nausea, ptyalism, and vomiting also can be caused by accumulation of nitrogenous waste products, such as urea in stored blood [40]. Unless severe hemorrhage has occurred, administration of blood products should proceed slowly, and personnel should monitor the recipient carefully for early signs of a transfusion reaction. If a reaction occurs, diphenhydramine (0.5–1 mg/kg intramuscularly) and a glucocorticoid such as dexamethasone sodium phosphate (0.25 mg/kg intravenously or subcutaneously) should be administered and the transfusion rate decreased. Severe reactions that result in collapse and hypotension should be treated by rapid discontinuation of the blood product and prompt administration of epinephrine (0.01 mg/kg intravenously). A rare complication of hemochromatosis (iron toxicity) has been reported in a Miniature Schnauzer with pure red cell aplasia that received multiple red blood cell transfusions over several years' time [41]. Transmission of infectious diseases, such as leishmaniasis, to dogs from infected blood donors also has been reported [42,43].

COMPLICATIONS ASSOCIATED WITH ADMINISTRATION OF PARENTERAL NUTRITION PRODUCTS

Nutrition is one of the most important aspects of therapy in a critically ill or injured patient. Whenever possible, enteral nutrition is preferred, but in some cases, parenteral nutrition must be administrated because of enteral feeding intolerance or a malfunctioning gastrointestinal tract. Many parenteral nutrition products are hyperosmolar and can contribute to thrombophlebitis. As a general rule, parenteral nutrition solutions with osmolalities of 600 mOsm/L or less can be administered short-term though a peripheral venous catheter, whereas solutions with osmolality of more than 600 mOsm/L should be administered through a central venous catheter. Perivascular administration of dextrose-containing fluids, including parenteral nutrition solutions, can cause erythema and pain. Catheter-related complications during the administration of parenteral nutrition include kinks in the catheter, disconnected lines, and clogged catheters [44]. Catheter-related sepsis also can occur, particularly with frequent disconnection of the fluid line for blood sampling or injection of drugs through a catheter used for parenteral nutrition. Guidelines for avoiding the potential for catheter-induced sepsis include not disconnecting the parenteral nutrition fluid line, designating the catheter and line solely for parenteral nutrition, and changing the parenteral nutrition fluid line every 24 hours (or if it becomes contaminated). Hyperglycemia has been associated with administration of parenteral nutrition and represents an increased risk for morbidity and mortality in critically ill cats [45]. Careful monitoring of the parenteral nutrition catheter and catheter site and acid-base, electrolyte, and glucose monitoring should be performed at least once a day to avoid these potential complications.

References

[1] Bliss SP, Bliss SK, Harvey KJ. Use of recombinant tissue-plasminogen activator in a dog with chylothorax secondary to catheter-associated thrombosis of the cranial vena cava. J Am Anim Hosp Assoc 2002;38:431–5.

[2] Marsh-Ng ML, Burney DP, Garcia J. Surveillance of infections associated with intravenous catheters in dogs and cats in an intensive care unit. J Am Anim Hosp Assoc 2007;43(1): 13–20.

[3] Lobetti RG, Joubert KE, Picard J, et al. Bacterial colonization of intravenous catheters in young dogs suspected to have parvoviral enteritis. J Am Vet Med Assoc 2002;220(9): 1321–4.

[4] Coolman BR, Marretta SM, Kakoma I, et al. Cutaneous antimicrobial preparation prior to intravenous catheter preparation in healthy dogs: clinical microbiological, and histopathological evaluation. Can Vet J 1998;39(12):757–63.

[5] Mathews KA, Brooks MJ, Valliant AE. A prospective study of intravenous catheter contamination. J Vet Emerg Crit Care 1996;6(1):33–42.

[6] Bregenzer T, Conen D, Sakmann P, et al. Is routine replacement of peripheral intravenous catheters necessary? Arch Intern Med 1998;158(2):151–6.

[7] Syring RS, Otto CM, Drobatz KJ. Hyperglycemia in dogs and cats with head trauma: 122 cases (1997–1999). J Am Vet Med Assoc 2001;218(7):1124–9.

[8] Mathews KA. The various types of parenteral fluids and their indications. Vet Clin North Am Small Anim Pract 1998;28(3):483–513.

[9] Griffel MI, Kaufman BS. Pharmacology of colloids and crystalloids. Crit Care Clin 1992;8(2):235–53.

[10] Brady CA, Vite CH, Drobatz KJ. Severe neurologic sequelae in a dog after treatment of hypoadrenal crisis. J Am Vet Med Assoc 1999;15(2):222–5.

[11] Macintire DK, Drobatz KJ, Haskins SC, et al. Part II: chapter 15, Endocrine and metabolic emergencies. In: Macintire DK, Drobatz KJ, Haskins S, editors. Manual of small animal emergency and critical care medicine. Philadelphia: Lippincott Williams & Williams; 2004. p. 323–6.

[12] Chan DL, Freeman LM, Rozanski EA, et al. Colloid osmotic pressure of parenteral nutrition components and intravenous fluids. J Vet Emerg Crit Care 2001;11(4):269–73.

[13] Rudloff E, Kirby R. Crystalloid and colloid resuscitation. Vet Clin North Am Small Anim Pract 2001;31(6):1207–29.

[14] Rudloff E, Kirby R. Colloid osmometry. Clin Tech Small Anim Pract 2000;15(3):119–25.

[15] Gabel JC, Scott RL, Adair TH, et al. Errors in calculated oncotic pressure in the dog. Am J Physiol 1980;239(Heart Circ Physiol 8):H810–2.

[16] Navar PD, Navar LG. Relationship between colloid osmotic pressure and plasma protein concentration in the dog. Am J Physiol 1977;233(2):H295–8.

[17] Brown SA, Dusza K, Boehmer J. Comparison of measured and calculated values for colloid osmotic pressure in hospitalized animals. Am J Vet Res 1994;55(7):910–5.

[18] Drobatz KJ, Macintire DK. Heat-induced illness in dogs: 42 cases (1976–1993). J Am Vet Med Assoc 1996;209(11):1894–9.

[19] Mazzaferro EM, Rudloff E, Kirby R. The role of albumin replacement in the critically ill veterinary patient. J Vet Emerg Crit Care 2002;12(2):113–24.

[20] Mathews KA, Barry M. The use of 25% human serum albumin: outcome and efficacy in raising serum albumin and systemic blood pressure in critically ill dogs and cats. J Vet Emerg Crit Care 2005;15(2):110–8.

[21] Rackow EC, Falk JL, Fein IA. Fluid resuscitation in circulatory shock: a comparison of the cardiorespiratory effects of albumin, hetastarch, and saline solutions in patients with hypovolemic and septic shock. Crit Care Med 1983;11(11):839–50.

[22] Francis AH, Martin LG, Haldorson GJ, et al. Adverse reactions suggestive of type III hypersensitivity in six healthy dogs given human albumin. J Am Vet Med Assoc 2007;230(6): 873–9.

[23] Cohn LA, Kerl ME, Lenox CE, et al. Response of healthy dogs to infusions of human serum albumin. Am J Vet Res 2007;68(6):657–63.

[24] Suda S. Hemodynamic and pulmonary effects of fluid resuscitation from hemorrhagic shock in the presence of mild pulmonary edema. Masui 2000;49(12):1339–48.

[25] Bumpus SE, Haskins SC, Hass PH. Effect of synthetic colloids on refractometric readings of total solids. J Vet Emerg Crit Care 1998;8(1):21–6.

[26] Thyes C, Madjdpour C, Frascarolo P, et al. Effect of high- and low-molecular weight low-substituted hydroxyethyl starch on blood coagulation during acute normovolemic hemodilution in pigs. Anesthesiology 2006;105(6):1228–37.

[27] Madjdpour C, Thyes C, Buclin T, et al. Novel starches: single dose pharmacokinetics and effects on blood coagulation. Anesthesiology 2007;106(1):132–43.

[28] Wierenga JR, Jandrey KE, Haskins SC, et al. In vitro comparison of the effects of two forms of hydroxyethyl starch solutions on platelet function in dogs. Am J Vet Res 2007;68:605–9.

[29] Cheng C, Lerner MA, Lichtewnstein S, et al. Effect of hydroxyethylstarch on hemostasis. Surgical Forum: Metabolism 1966;17:48–50.

[30] Smiley LE, Garvey MS. The use of hetastarch as adjunct therapy in 26 dogs with hypoalbuminemia: a phase two clinical trial. J Vet Intern Med 1994;8(3):195–202.

[31] Modig J. Beneficial effects of dextran 70 versus Ringer's acetate on pulmonary function, hemodynamics and survival in porcine endotoxin shock model. Resuscitation 1988;16: 1–12.

[32] Mailloux L, Swartz CD, Cappizzi R, et al. Acute renal failure after administration of low-molecular weight dextran. N Engl J Med 1967;277:1113–8.

[33] Gibson GR, Callan MB, Hoffman V, et al. Use of a hemoglobin-based oxygen carrying solution in cats: 72 cases (1998–2000). J Am Vet Med Assoc 2002;221(1):96–102.

[34] Castellanos I, Couto CG, Gray TL. Clinical use of blood products in cats: a retrospective study (1997–2000). J Vet Intern Med 2004;18(4):529–32.

[35] Callan MB, Jones LT, Giger U. Hemolytic transfusion reactions in a dog with alloantibody to a common antigen. J Vet Intern Med 1995;9(4):277–9.

[36] Giger U, Gelens CJ, Callan MB, et al. An acute hemolytic transfusion reaction caused by dog erythrocyte antigen 1.1 incompatibility in a previously sensitized dog. J Am Vet Med Assoc 1995;206(9):1358–62.

[37] Jutkowitz LA, Rozanski EA, Moreau JA, et al. Massive transfusion in dogs: 15 cases (1997–2001). J Am Vet Med Assoc 2002;220(11):1664–9.

[38] Haldane S, Roberts J, Marks SL, et al. Transfusion medicine. Comp Cont Educ Pract Vet 2004;26(7):502–17.

[39] Hoenhaus AE. CH 24 blood transfusion and blood substitutes. In: DiBartola SP, editor. Fluid, electrolyte and acid-base disorders in small animal practice. 3rd edition. St Louis (MI): Saunders Elsevier; 2006. p. 567–83.

[40] Waddell LS, Holt DE, Hughes D, et al. The effect of storage on ammonia concentration in canine packed red blood cells. J Vet Emerg Crit Care 2001;11(1):23–6.

[41] Sprague WS, Hackett TB, Johnson JS, et al. Hemochromatosis secondary to repeated blood transfusions in a dog. Vet Pathol 2003;40(3):334–7.

[42] Owens SD, Oakley DA, Marryott K, et al. Transmission of visceral leishmaniasis through blood transfusions from infected English foxhounds to anemic dogs. J Am Vet Med Assoc 2001;219(8):1076–83.

[43] Giger U, Oakley DA, Owens SD, et al. *Leishmania donovani* transmission by packed RBC transfusion to anemic dogs in the United States. Transfusion 2002;42(3):381–3.

[44] Chandler ML, Payne-James JJ. Prospective evaluation of peripheral administered three-in-one parenteral nutrition product in dogs. J Small Anim Pract 2006;47(9):518–23.

[45] Pyle SC, Marks SL, Kass PH. Evaluation of complications and prognostic factors associated with administration of total parenteral nutrition in cats: 75 cases (1994–2001). J Am Vet Med Assoc 2004;225(2):242–50.

Pediatric Fluid Therapy

Douglass K. Macintire, DVM, MS

Department of Clinical Sciences, Auburn University Critical Care Program, College of Veterinary Medicine, Auburn University, Auburn, AL 36849, USA

In dogs and cats, the term "pediatric" generally refers to the first 12 weeks of life [1]. This period can be further divided into the neonatal stage (0–2 weeks), the infant stage (2–6 weeks), and the juvenile stage (6–12 weeks) [2]. Fluid therapy often is required in sick pediatric patients, but the methods and specific conditions that require fluid support vary according to the stage of life and severity of the underlying condition. Pediatric patients differ from adult patients in many ways [3]. This article addresses specific considerations and indications for fluid therapy in each of the stages of life in pediatric patients.

FLUID THERAPY IN NEONATES

Indications for fluid therapy in neonates include postpartum resuscitation, shock, trauma, dehydration, hypoglycemia, hypothermia, separation from the dam, sepsis, malnutrition, and inability to nurse [4]. Compared with adult animals, neonates are much more prone to dehydration for several reasons [3]. They have a greater surface area-to-volume ratio and increased skin permeability, which make them susceptible to rapid fluid losses. Neonates also have higher total body water content (80% of body weight compared with 60% in adult animals) and have immature renal function. Neonates are unable to concentrate their urine until 8 weeks of age in kittens and 12 weeks of age in puppies. Because of rapid water turnover, dehydration can occur much more acutely in neonates than in older animals [3].

In addition to being prone to dehydration, neonates also are at much higher risk for hypoglycemia than adult animals. Neonates have inefficient hepatic gluconeogenesis and limited glycogen stores, and they are unable to maintain glucose homeostasis if deprived of food for more than a few hours. The need for glucose always must be taken into consideration during rehydration and resuscitation of sick neonates.

Neonates also are much more predisposed to hypothermia than adult animals because of their increased surface area and lack of shivering response (the shivering response does not develop until day 6 of life) [3]. The normal body temperature of neonates also ranges from 95° to 97°F during the first week of life, and does not reach normal "adult" body temperature until after

0195-5616/08/$ – see front matter

doi:10.1016/j.cvsm.2008.01.004

2 weeks of age [1]. It is important to always administer warmed fluids to treat or prevent hypothermia. Hypothermic neonates develop bradycardia and gastrointestinal ileus. Oral feeding is not effective until normothermia is restored.

Initial Assessment of the Sick Neonate

Typical methods for assessing hydration in adult animals may be unreliable in neonates [3]. Whereas tenting of the skin is used to detect dehydration in adult animals, skin turgor is less reliable in neonates because of increased water content and decreased fat content of the skin. The thin skin on the ventral abdomen is the best place to evaluate hydration status in neonates. In adult animals, severe dehydration causes tachycardia and concentrated urine. These variables cannot be relied on in neonates because the heart rate normally is rapid and urine is not concentrated in neonates. Mucous membranes often remain moist in neonates until dehydration is severe. Mucous membrane color and capillary refill time are good indicators of perfusion in neonates and adult animals. Neonates normally have hyperemic mucous membranes for the first week of life [4]. Pale mucous membranes and slow capillary refill time ($>$ 1.5 sec) are seen when dehydration is severe enough to cause hypovolemic shock. Puppies with poor perfusion still may have normal skin turgor even when mucous membrane color and capillary refill time indicate shock. Clinical signs of sepis, hypovolemia, or shock in neonates include pale mucous membranes, decreased urine output, cold extremities, limp body tone, constant crying, and reluctance to suckle [5]. The veterinarian should determine whether the animal has simple dehydration or actual perfusion deficits. The sicker the animal, the more aggressive the route chosen for fluid therapy. Neonates with sepsis or severe hypovolemia need rapid and aggressive fluid resuscitation by either the intravenous or intraosseous route [2]. Neonates with mild to moderate dehydration can receive fluids orally (by stomach tube), subcutaneously, or intraperitoneally.

Oral Fluids

Stomach tube feeding can be used to give fluids and nutrition to neonates that are not hypothermic, hypoglycemic, or dehydrated. It is an effective method of providing hydration and nutrition to neonates that cannot suckle from the dam. A 5- to 8-Fr feeding tube is used to measure from the tip of the nose to the last rib (Fig. 1). The tube is marked, lubricated, and passed down the left side of the mouth. It should pass easily, but it is important to remember that a gag reflex is not present until approximately 10 days of age [1]. Proper placement can be assured by instilling a small amount of sterile saline first and making sure that it does not come out of the nose. The stomach capacity of the neonate is approximately 50 mL/kg [1], although filling the stomach to capacity is not recommended because the risk of aspiration increases with a full stomach. Commercial milk replacer can be used, and the amount fed can be determined from the label on the can. Initially, puppies can be fed 10 mL every 2 to 4 hours, increasing the amount by 1 mL per feeding. Kittens can be started at 5 mL every 2 to 4 hours, increasing by 1 mL per day. Food should be warmed to approximately 100°F. If diarrhea occurs, the formula should be diluted 1:2

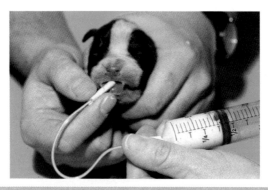

Fig. 1. Oral feeding through a stomach tube can be an effective way of maintaining nutrition and fluid requirements in neonates that are unable to nurse.

with balanced electrolyte solution until diarrhea resolves. When removing the stomach tube after feeding, it is important to kink it to prevent aspiration of liquid that otherwise could drain from the tube as it is being pulled out.

Neonates also can be fed with a syringe, eye dropper, or bottle. If using a syringe or eye dropper, care must be taken not to administer the liquid too fast because aspiration pneumonia is a common complication. If using a bottle or pet nurser, the hole in the nipple may need to be enlarged with a hot needle so that a drop of milk forms easily when the bottle is turned upside down.

Subcutaneous Fluids

Neonates with mild to moderate dehydration but normal perfusion can be treated by subcutaneous administration of fluids. Maintenance requirements are two to three times higher than for adult animals (120–180 mL/kg/d) [3]. This amount of fluid plus the dehydration deficit (% dehydration × body weight in kg = liters of crystalloid fluid) can be divided into several equal portions and administered subcutaneously at the intrascapular space. Dextrose should not be added to isotonic fluids because the resultant fluid becomes hypertonic and actually draws fluid into the subcutaneous space. The best fluid to correct mild dehydration is a balanced electrolyte solution, such as lactated Ringer's solution or Normosol-R. If dextrose supplementation is desired, 0.45% NaCl with 2.5% dextrose can be administered safely by the subcutaneous route. If hypokalemia is present, up to 30 mEq/L of KCl can be added to fluids for subcutaneous administration.

Neonates that are unable to nurse for the first 24 hours are deprived of colostrum and develop failure of passive transfer, which puts them at high risk for developing infections [6]. Subcutaneous administration of serum from the dam or some other well-vaccinated adult dog can supply protective antibodies. The recommended dose to supply adequate immunity is 16 mL for puppies and 15 mL for kittens. This volume can be divided into two to three equal portions and administered subcutaneously every 6 to 8 hours [6,7].

Intraperitoneal Fluids

Colostrum, whole blood, or crystalloid fluids can be administered intraperitoneally. Hypertonic dextrose solutions should not be given intraperitoneally, especially to dehydrated neonates, because fluid is pulled from the intravascular space and interstitium into the abdominal cavity. Blood given intraperitoneally is not absorbed for 48 to 72 hours, so it is not an effective method for treating animals with life-threatening anemia [2]. Instillation of warm fluids into the peritoneal cavity can be a useful method of treating hypothermia and increasing core body temperature.

Intravenous Fluids

Neonates with perfusion deficits do not absorb subcutaneously administered fluids well because of the peripheral vasoconstriction associated with hypovolemic shock. Aggressive resuscitation and restoration of intravascular volume can be accomplished with intravenously administered fluids. A 24-gauge catheter sometimes can be placed in a cephalic vein, but more commonly the jugular vein is the best site for intravenous catheterization. A 20- to 22-gauge cephalic catheter usually can be placed in the jugular vein (Fig. 2). If a gram scale is available, an initial bolus of 1 mL per 30 g of body weight (30–45 mL/kg) is administered by slow intravenous push over 5 to 10 minutes. Fluid loading is continued until mucous membrane color and capillary refill time have improved to a bright pink color with 1-second refill time. Warmed crystalloid fluid, such as lactated Ringer's solution or Normosol-R with 5% dextrose added, is the fluid of choice. After the initial bolus, fluid therapy is continued at a rate of 80 to 120 mL/kg/d.

Intraosseous Fluids

Sometimes it is impossible to place an intravenous catheter, but the patient has poor perfusion or shock and requires aggressive, rapid resuscitation. Any fluid

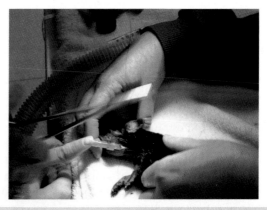

Fig. 2. A cephalic catheter can be placed in the jugular vein to provide an effective means for delivering intravenous fluids to critically ill neonates.

that can be given intravenously (eg, blood, balanced electrolyte solution, glucose) also can be given by the intraosseous route. A 1- or 2-in spinal needle (18–22 gauge) can be placed easily into the greater trochanter and threaded down the shaft of the femur. The area over the hip must be clipped and surgically prepared before inserting the needle into the femur. The cortical bone is fairly hard compared with the softer medullary cavity. Once the needle is firmly seated in the shaft of the femur, the stylet is removed from the needle and the fluid injected at the same dose and rate as with intravenous resuscitation (Fig. 3). Once the vascular volume has been restored, it is easier to place an intravenous catheter, and the intraosseous needle can be removed. In some instances, the intraosseous catheter can be bandaged in place for continued fluid therapy support. Once the animal becomes more active, however, the needle is easily dislodged and intraosseous fluid therapy must be discontinued. The intraosseous needle rarely stays in place more than 24 hours.

Neonatal Isoerythrolysis

Neonatal isoerythrolysis is a specific condition that occurs when type A or AB kittens are born to type B queens. Type B cats (usually purebred cats of British breed descent) have naturally occurring anti-A antibodies. The kittens are born normally, but when they begin to nurse, they ingest anti-A antibodies in the colostrum, which results in acute life-threatening hemolysis. Clinical signs develop within hours to days and may include sudden death, fading kittens, tail tip necrosis, hemoglobinuria, icterus, and severe anemia. If possible, neonatal isoerythrolysis should be prevented by blood-typing breeding pairs and not breeding type A males to type B females. If the condition does occur, however, the kittens should be removed from the queen for the first 24 hours as soon as a problem is suspected and managed with supportive care as outlined previously. If anemia is severe and a transfusion is required, washed red blood cells from the queen or other type B cat can be administered at a dose of 5 to 10 mL per kitten

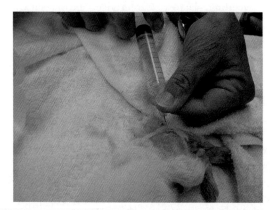

Fig. 3. Resuscitation of critically ill neonates can be accomplished by placing a spinal needle in the shaft of the femur and administering warmed fluids by the intraosseous route.

administered over several hours. This blood is not lysed by the colostral anti-bodies. The red cells should be suspended in saline rather than plasma to prevent further administration of anti-A antibodies. Subsequent transfusions adminis-tered later in life to kittens that survive should consist of type A blood.

THE INFANT PERIOD

The infant period in pediatric patients ranges from 2 to 6 weeks of age. During this time, the most life-threatening problems are internal and external parasites, juvenile hypoglycemia, dehydration from diarrhea, and trauma [1]. Because re-nal function does not mature until at least 8 weeks of age, infants remain prone to drug toxicity from decreased renal elimination and dehydration from de-creased ability to concentrate their urine.

Hookworms and fleas can cause severe anemia in infant animals and result in pale mucous membranes, tachycardia, weakness, hematocrit less than 15%, and hypoproteinemia. A blood transfusion may be required to stabilize the animal. Blood is diluted 9:1 with a citrate anticoagulant and given through a millipore blood filter at a dosage of 20 mL/kg over 2 to 4 hours. Intraosseous or intrave-nous administration is preferred in critical patients, but blood can be adminis-tered by the intraperitoneal route as a last resort. Iron supplementation should be given in addition to transfusion in animals with blood-loss anemia [2].

Juvenile hypoglycemia can occur because of immature hepatic enzyme sys-tems, lack of glycogen stores, and increased metabolic requirements for glucose [4]. Clinical signs include weakness, tremors, seizures, stupor, and coma. Treat-ment involves intravenous or intraosseous administration of glucose (0.5–1 g/kg) diluted to a 5% to 10% solution followed by supportive care.

Dehydration is always a potential problem in juvenile animals that develop diarrhea. Severe consequences can be avoided by administering subcutaneous fluids at one to two times maintenance requirements while attempting to deter-mine the cause of the diarrhea. Common reasons for diarrhea in juvenile ani-mals include overfeeding, lactose intolerance, excess saturated fatty acids, giardiasis, coccidiosis, hookworms, roundworms, coronavirus, rotavirus, par-vovirus, campylobacter, salmonella, clostridia, or improper handing of the milk replacement diet [4]. If dehydration is severe, hypovolemia and perfusion deficits should be corrected as outlined previously for neonates.

THE JUVENILE PERIOD

Juveniles are pediatric patients aged 6 to 12 weeks [1]. They are more similar to adults in terms of renal function and vital signs but still have increased main-tenance water requirements (120–200 mL/kg/d) and caloric requirements (180 kcal/kg/d). Because maternal antibody is lost during this time, juvenile patients often are susceptible to infectious diseases unless protected by vaccination. Fe-line panleukopenia and canine parvovirus are life-threatening diseases that re-quire aggressive fluid therapy support. General concerns regarding prevention of hypoglycemia, dehydration, hypoproteinemia, and anemia need to be ad-dressed during treatment as described for neonates and infants. Young animals that are not eating generally require potassium supplementation in their fluids (20 mEq KCl/L) to prevent hypokalemia [2]. Animals with severe enteritis also often develop hypoproteinemia and need colloid support. Plasma transfusions or hetastarch (20 mL/kg/d) can be administered to maintain colloid osmotic pressure in the range of 16 to 25 mm Hg.

SUMMARY
Pediatric patients have higher maintenance requirements for fluid therapy than adult animals and are more prone to dehydration and hypovolemic shock because of higher total body water content and immature renal function. Aggressive treatment with intravenous or intraosseous fluids or preventive strategies using subcutaneous fluids can be life-saving techniques in these fragile patients.

References
[1] Hoskins JD, editor. Veterinary pediatrics. 3rd edition. Philadelphia: WB Saunders Co.; 2001.
[2] Macintire DK. Pediatric intensive care. Vet Clin North Am Small Anim Pract 1999;29: 971–88.
[3] Poffenbarger EM, Ralston AL, Chandler ML, et al. Canine neonatology: part 1. Physiologic differences between puppies and adults. Compendium on Continuing Education for the Practicing Veterinarian 1990;12:601–9.
[4] Lawler DF. Care and diseases of neonatal puppies and kittens. In: Kirk RW, editor. Current veterinary therapy x: small animal practice. Philadelphia: WB Saunders Co.; 1989. p. 1325–33.
[5] Poffenbarger EM, Ralston AL, Chandler ML, et al. Canine neonatology: part 2. Disorders of the neonate. Compendium on Continuing Education for the Practicing Veterinarian 1991;13: 25–37.
[6] Poffenbarger EM, Olson PN, Chandler ML, et al. Use of adult dog serum as a substitute for colostrum in the neonatal dog. Am J Vet Res 1992;53:230–3.
[7] Levy JK, Crawford PC, Collante WR, et al. Use of adult cat serum to correct failure of passive transfer in kittens. J Am Vet Med Assoc 2001;219:1401–5.

Vet Clin Small Anim 38 (2008) 629–643

VETERINARY CLINICS
SMALL ANIMAL PRACTICE

Assessment and Treatment of Hypovolemic States

Garret E. Pachtinger, VMD*, Kenneth Drobatz, DVM, MSCE

Section of Critical Care, Department of Clinical Studies–Philadelphia,
School of Veterinary Medicine, University of Pennsylvania,
3900 Delancey Street, Philadelphia, PA 19104, USA

H ypovolemia refers to decreased intravascular circulating fluid volume relative to the total vascular space [1]. This may be a result of absolute fluid volume deficiency (eg, loss of blood, vomiting, polyuria without adequate polydipsia); relative fluid volume deficiency, as seen in distributive states in which there is expansion of the vascular space without a change in blood volume (eg, vasodilation); or a combination of the two. Physiologically, the most devastating consequence of this abnormality is an absolute or relative decrease in cardiac preload (Fig. 1) resulting in poor cardiac output (CO), inadequate tissue perfusion, and decreased tissue oxygen delivery. Decreased oxygen delivery to the tissues results in impaired cellular function. The term *shock* is used when global tissue perfusion is impaired. The most troublesome consequences of shock are cellular failure resulting in the systemic inflammatory response syndrome (SIRS) and multiple-organ dysfunction syndrome (MODS). Hence, one of the "holy grails" of assessment of the critically ill patient is adequacy of tissue perfusion.

CLINICAL ASSESSMENT OF TISSUE PERFUSION STATUS

No single variable provides an accurate and consistent estimate of the adequacy of global tissue perfusion despite advances in technology and availability of medical monitoring. Hence, we are left with "surrogate markers" for assessing tissue perfusion. Subjective physical examination variables in assessing tissue perfusion include mucous membrane color, capillary refill time, heart rate, pulse quality, and the gradient between extremity and core body temperature. More objective variables to assess perfusion status include arterial blood pressure measurement, urine output, and blood lactate concentration. Ultimately, placement of a pulmonary artery catheter and measurement or calculation of CO, peripheral vascular resistance, right atrial pressure, central venous oxygen saturation, total oxygen delivery, and total oxygen consumption can be done, but these techniques are not practical in most clinical veterinary practices [2].

*Corresponding author. E-mail address: garretp@vet.upenn.edu (G.E. Pachtinger).

0195-5616/08/$ – see front matter
doi:10.1016/j.cvsm.2008.01.009

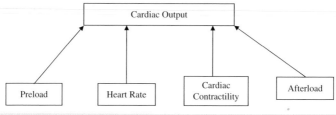

Fig. 1. Determinants of cardiac output.

BLOOD PRESSURE: INDIRECT AND DIRECT

Blood pressure, indirect and direct, is a useful surrogate marker for the assessment of global tissue perfusion. Examples of indirect blood pressure measurement include Doppler ultrasonic blood pressure and oscillometric blood pressure measurements (eg, Dinamap, GE Heathcare Systems Inc., Waukesha, Wisconsin; Cardell, CAS Medical Systems Inc., Branford, Connecticut). Although blood pressure measurement is a valuable tool, the clinician must keep in mind that normal arterial pressure does not rule out altered tissue perfusion. Using the equation, $MAP = CO \times SVR$, it is easy to see that mean arterial pressure (MAP) is not an isolated value, but depends on CO and systemic vascular resistance (SVR). States like acute blood loss can lead to a dramatic compensatory response that increases CO and SVR, resulting in adequate MAP despite an altered state of perfusion. Consequently, the clinician should use blood pressure as one of many measurements along with the subjective physical examination findings (discussed previously) when evaluating the patient.

DOWNSTREAM PARAMETERS

Aside from the methods listed previously, other variables can guide clinical treatment of the patient. Downstream variables do not contribute to perfusion but rather depend on having adequate perfusion. Although these tests do not identify a specific cause, they can alert the clinician to the likelihood of inadequate perfusion.

Lactate

Lactate is a normal metabolic end product of glycolysis and is produced in low concentrations throughout the body. Although all body tissues can produce lactate, skeletal muscle, brain, and erythrocytes are responsible for most lactate production and the liver and kidneys are responsible for most of its metabolism [3,4]. Lactic acidosis develops when production of lactate exceeds use. Lactate occurs in two isomeric forms: L-lactate and D-lactate. The D isomer has been reported in cases of short bowel syndrome in people [5] and in cats fed propylene glycol [5–7] and also is present in lactated Ringer's solution. The L isomer is thought to be clinically more important than the D isomer and can now be reliably measured by many point-of-care analyzers available to veterinarians.

When hypoperfusion develops, tissues become hypoxic and anaerobic metabolism ensues. In anaerobic metabolism, lactate is generated from pyruvate and hyperlactatemia occurs [8]. Blood lactate concentrations greater than 2 mmol/L warrant investigation. Although clinical disorders characterized by hypoperfusion can cause increased blood lactate concentrations, other states, such as acute liver failure, severe sepsis, cancer, seizures, poisoning, and drugs, also can increase blood lactate concentrations [3,4,9–17].

Urine Output and Urine Concentration
Urine output and urinary concentrating ability (as assessed by urine specific gravity) are readily accessible and useful downstream indicators of renal perfusion and indirectly assess patient response to therapy. Normal urine output is 1 to 2 mL/kg/h. Without adequate perfusion, the kidneys aggressively conserve fluid, concentrate the urine, and decrease production of urine. If the clinician is concerned that urine production is inadequate despite volume resuscitation, an indwelling urinary catheter should be considered [18]. Complicating factors to consider when using urine output and urine specific gravity to assess perfusion include impaired renal function and administration of diuretics or corticosteroids.

HYPOVOLEMIA AND SHOCK CLASSIFICATION
Although hypovolemic shock can lead to inadequate perfusion, other types of shock also can lead to hypoperfusion. Numerous classification schemes have been developed to describe shock syndromes, and clinically useful categories in small animal emergency medicine include hypovolemic shock, cardiogenic shock, obstructive shock, and distributive shock (sepsis or SIRS) (Table 1) [19,20].

Table 1
Causes of hypoperfusion in small animal patients

Hypovolemia	Cardiogenic	Obstructive	Distributive
Hemorrhage	Cardiomyopathy	Pericardial tamponade	SIRS
Trauma	Dilated	Restrictive pericarditis	Pancreatitis
Coagulation	Hypertrophic	Pulmonary	Neoplasia
Disorders	Valvular disease	thromboembolism	Burns
Neoplasia	Severe dysrhythmias	Gastric	Sepsis
Burns		dilatation-volvulus	Severe tissue
Vomiting and diarrhea			trauma
Severe polyuria			
Marked internal			
fluid Losses			
Pleural			
Peritoneal			
Intestinal			
Severe dehydration			

Hypovolemic Shock

Hypovolemic shock can be absolute or relative in nature. Hemorrhage leading to loss of intravascular volume is an absolute cause of hypovolemic shock. Common causes of hemorrhage include trauma leading to external blood loss, hemoperitoneum attributable to splenic or hepatic neoplasia, coagulopathies (anticoagulant rodenticide), gastrointestinal hemorrhage, and epistaxis [21–24]. Other causes of absolute fluid loss include vomiting, diarrhea, and severe polyuria. A relative state of hypovolemia can be caused by increased volume capacity or vasodilatation, such as may occur in anaphylaxis, with the use of vasodilatory drugs, or in severe burns, leading to SIRS and increased microvascular permeability.

Cardiogenic Shock

Cardiogenic shock is caused by decreased CO and often is associated with cardiac disease. Examples of cardiac diseases potentially associated with cardiogenic shock include severe valvular disease, dysrhythmias, and primary ventricular disease. The end result of cardiogenic shock is global hypoperfusion. Although clinical signs of cardiogenic shock are similar to those of other shock syndromes, physical examination abnormalities specific to cardiogenic shock include cardiac murmurs, cardiac arrhythmias, pulmonary edema, bilateral crackles on thoracic auscultation, jugular vein distention, and cyanotic mucous membranes [18,25].

Distributive Shock

Distributive shock is most commonly associated with SIRS, sepsis, or anaphylaxis. Distributive shock is triggered by dysfunction in the microcirculation that leads to inappropriate widespread vasodilatation and relative hypovolemia. Although clinical signs may be similar to those of other shock syndromes, unique characteristics of distributive shock and systemic vasodilatation include warm extremities, hyperemic (ie, brick red) mucous membranes, and bounding pulses in the early stage of the disease [18].

Obstructive Shock

Obstructive shock results from mechanical interference with ventricular filling. Examples include pericardial effusion leading to pericardial tamponade, caval syndrome of heartworm disease, aortic thromboembolism, intracardiac neoplasia, and gastric dilatation and volvulus (GDV) leading to decreased ventricular filling as a result of obstruction of the caudal vena cava. Clinical signs are variable and depend on the location of the obstruction [18].

TREATMENT OF HYPOVOLEMIA

Therapy for hypovolemia involves replacing the effective circulating volume deficit, ensuring return of adequate intravascular volume, and avoiding tissue damage.

Before replacement of the intravascular volume deficit is initiated, several questions must be answered:

- Does the patient require emergency therapy?
- What type of fluid should be given, and by what route?
- How much fluid should be given initially, at what fluid rate, and how much to follow-up?
- What are the goals of resuscitation?
- What ancillary therapies should be used, and when should they be considered?

DOES THE PATIENT REQUIRE EMERGENCY THERAPY?

Emergency therapy is dictated by the history, physical examination, and assessment of the "surrogate markers" of tissue perfusion described previously. When clinical signs of shock are present, the clinician must assume that the patient has lost at least 25% of its intravascular volume. Thus, if signs of hypovolemic shock are present, emergency fluid therapy is warranted. If a 10-kg dog (with an intravascular volume of 90 mL/kg) has signs of shock and at least 25% loss of fluid volume, an approximate 225-mL loss of blood volume can be anticipated (10 kg × 25% × 90 mL/kg).

WHAT KIND OF FLUID SHOULD BE GIVEN AND BY WHAT ROUTE?

There are many ways to administer fluids. The oral, subcutaneous, and intraperitoneal routes are considered inadequate for emergency therapy. Intravenous access is necessary. Although central veins (eg, jugular veins) would allow more rapid resuscitation, jugular vein catheterization is technically more demanding, is more stressful to the patient, and requires more time. Peripheral venous catheterization (eg, cephalic vein, lateral saphenous vein) should be attempted first. For immediate fluid resuscitation, the clinician should consider use of multiple, short, large-gauge catheters to administer fluid at an appropriately rapid rate. A short large-gauge catheter allows more rapid administration of fluid as compared with a longer smaller bore catheter. A classic example of when this technique should be used is in the resuscitation of a patient that has GDV. In this situation, hind limb catheters should be avoided because of inadequate venous return, and short large-gauge catheters should be placed into both cephalic veins for resuscitation. In patients weighing less than 2 kg, in which intravenous catheter placement is difficult, intraosseous placement of large-gauge needles can be considered. Common locations for intraosseous needle placement include the trochanteric fossa, tibial crest, iliac wing, and proximal humerus [18]. Once intravenous or intraosseous access is obtained, a decision must be made on the appropriate fluid therapy: crystalloids, colloids, or both.

Crystalloid fluids are low-molecular-weight solutions that initially enter the intravascular space but effectively replenish the entire extracellular space (ie, intravascular space, interstitial space). The small-molecular-weight particles in crystalloids are primarily electrolytes and buffers. The sodium concentration of the crystalloid determines its tonicity and fluid dynamics. When the osmolality of the solution is equivalent to that of the cell, the solution is called isotonic. Intravascular administration of isotonic crystalloids (eg, lactated Ringer's solution, Normosol-R [Lake Forest, Illinois], Plasmalyte-A [Deerfield, Illinois], 0.9% NaCl) results in intravascular and interstitial volume replacement and minimal intracellular fluid accumulation. Greater than 75% of the isotonic crystalloid administered intravenously is in the extravascular space (interstitial space) within 1 hour [26]. As a result of the rapid shift of isotonic crystalloid solutions from the intravascular space to the extracellular space, larger volumes must be given to replace an intravascular loss. As a general rule, the amount of isotonic crystalloid administered should be three times the estimated loss from the intravascular space [27]. Hypotonic fluids (eg, 5% dextrose in water, 0.45% NaCl) result in intracellular fluid distribution and are not effective as resuscitation fluids. Table 2 shows the composition of various crystalloid solutions [18].

Aside from electrolytes in solution, several crystalloid solutions also contain buffering anions that serve as bicarbonate precursors. Lactated Ringer's solution contains lactate as a bicarbonate precursor. It has been suggested that administration of this fluid may increase lactate concentrations in animals with severe liver disease [28]. Plasmalyte-148 (Deerfield, Illinois), Plasmalyte-A, and Normosol-R contain acetate as the alkalinizing component. Although rare and not appreciated clinically, rapid administration of acetate solutions may cause vasodilatation and hypotension in hypovolemic animals [29].

Traditionally, the shock dose for crystalloids is 90 mL/kg in the dog and 40 to 60 mL/kg in the cat. Most patients do not require the entire shock dose, and it is advisable to divide the total shock volume into two to four aliquots, giving each over 20 to 30 minutes and reassessing the patient between each increment. After the patient has been stabilized (see the section on goals of end points of resuscitation), fluid can be administered at a maintenance rate (2–4 mL/kg/h).

Table 2
Composition of several crystalloid fluids

	Na (mEq/L)	Cl (mEq/L)	K (mEq/L)	Ca (mEq/L)	Mg (mEq/L)	Buffer (mEq/L)	Osmolarity	pH
Plasma	145	105	5	5	3	24 (B)	300	7.4
0.45% NaCl	77	77	0	0	0	0	154	5
0.9% NaCl	154	154	0	0	0	0	308	5
Lactated Ringer's solution	130	109	4	3	0	28 (L)	272	6.5
Normosol-R	140	98	5	0	3	27 (A)	296	6.4
Plasma-Lyte	140	103	10	5	3	47 (A)	312	5.5
5% Dextrose	0	0	0	0	0	0	252	4.0

Buffers used are acetate (A), bicarbonate (B), and lactate (L).
Abbreviations: Ca, calcium; Cl, chloride; K, potassium; Mg, magnesium; Na, sodium.
Data from DiBartola SP. Fluid, electrolyte and acid base disorders. 3rd edition. Philadelphia: Elsevier; 2006. p. 333.

Table 3
Composition of several colloidal fluids

Solution	Na (mmol/L)	Cl (mmol/L)	K (mmol/L)	Ca (mmol/L)	Colloid	COP (mm Hg)	pH	Osmolarity
Plasma	144	107	5	5	Albumin	19.95 ± 2.1	7.5	290
Hetastarch 6% in 0.9% NaCl (HEspan)	154	154	0	0	Hydroxyethylated amylopectic, 60 g/L, MW 450 kd	31	5.5	310
Dextran 40 in 0.9% NaCl	154	154	0	0	Dextran, 100 g/L, MW 40 kd	NM	3.5–7.0	310
Dextran 70 in 0.9% NaCl	154	154	0	0	Dextran, 60 g/L, MW 70 kd	59	5.1–5.7	310
6% Albumin in 0.9% NaCl	154	154	0	0	MW 69 kd	30	5.5	310

Abbreviations: COP, colloid oncotic pressure; MW, molecular weight; NM, not measurable because of diffusion of smaller particles.
Data from DiBartola SP. Fluid, electrolyte and acid base disorders. 3rd edition. Philadelphia: Elsevier; 2006. p. 408–15.

Table 4
Ancillary therapy constant rate infusion chart

Drug	Dose
Dobutamine	2–15 µg/kg/min
Dopamine	0.5–20 µg/kg/min
Epinephrine	0.1–0.3 µg/kg/min
Phenylephrine	1–3 µg/kg/min
Norepinephrine	0.1–10 µg/kg/min
Vasopressin	0.5–5 µg/kg/min

Other calculations can be used to assess patient needs beyond maintenance, including the fluid deficit as a result of dehydration (% dehydration × body weight in kg × 1000 mL) and estimations of ongoing losses (eg, vomiting, diarrhea, polyuria).

Colloid solutions contain large-molecular-weight substances and can be divided into two categories: natural and synthetic (Table 3). Albumin is the only naturally occurring colloid. At this time, no species-specific albumin is available for dogs and cats. Although administration of plasma is the optimal choice for albumin replacement, the cost of plasma, its limited supply, and the amount necessary to increase colloid osmotic pressure make plasma an unrealistic choice for colloid fluid therapy. Canine fresh-frozen plasma contains approximately 25 to 30 g/L of albumin. If a 20-kg dog has a serum albumin value of 1.5 g/dL, the patient would require 2 L of fresh-frozen plasma to replace the albumin deficit according to the following formula: albumin deficit = 10 × (desired albumin − patient albumin) × body weight in kg × 0.3 [30–32]. Pooled human albumin formulations are commercially available as 5% and 25% solutions for states of severe hypoalbuminemia when albumin therapy is desired. Volume for volume, 5% albumin is approximately four times as effective in expanding plasma volume as is a sodium-containing crystalloid [30].

There are three types of synthetic colloids (gelatins, hydroxyethyl starches, and dextrans), and they vary in their molecular weights and duration of action. When compared with crystalloids, colloids remain in the intravascular space longer, increase oncotic pressure, and also increase vascular volume by retaining fluid within the vascular space [32,33]. Their presence in the vasculature pulls water from the interstitium, aiding in more efficient volume resuscitation. Colloid therapy often is used in conjunction with crystalloid fluid therapy, because colloids provide intravascular volume and crystalloids correct intravascular and extravascular deficits. Because of their ability to increase oncotic pressure, colloids are especially useful in patients that have disease processes causing increased microvascular permeability, such as systemic vasculitis attributable to SIRS or sepsis. If the site of the vascular leak exceeds the size of the molecule, however, the colloid also leaks from the vascular space. Initial boluses of hydroxyethyl starch (hetastarch) or dextran 70 at a dosage of 5 mL/kg in the dog or 2 mL/kg in the cat given over 15 to 20 minutes can be used. The main adverse effect of synthetic colloid administration is coagulopathy. Hydroxyethyl starch administration can lead to decreased circulating factor VIII and von Willebrand factor concentrations and also may have a dilutional effect on other coagulation factors. The risk for coagulopathy with dextrans may be related to dilutional effects on coagulation factors, coating of platelets and interference with platelet function, and decreased activity of von Willebrand factor. When dosages greater than 20 mL/kg administered every 24 hours are used, coagulopathic effects become apparent [18,33–35].

Hypertonic saline is another option for fluid resuscitation in hypovolemic states. Introduction of hypertonic saline into the vascular space increases the osmotic gradient. The osmotic gradient pulls water from the interstitial space and intracellular space into the intravascular space, expanding intravascular volume. Although evidence for use of hypertonic saline in states of hypovolemia and specific states, such as head trauma, is accumulating, no study has clearly established the clinical benefits of hypertonic saline as compared with other methods of fluid resuscitation [36,37]. Compared with crystalloids, in which three times the estimated loss from the intravascular space must be administered for replacement, a much smaller volume needs to be administered when using hypertonic saline. In a canine hemorrhagic shock model, administration of hypertonic saline at a dose equal to only 10% of the shed blood volume provided full resuscitation [38]. Based on these data, doses of 3 to 5 mL/kg of 7.5% hypertonic saline in dogs and 2 to 3 mL/kg in cats have been recommended.

Hemoglobin-based oxygen-carrying solutions (HBOCs) also can be used as a fluid therapy choice. This fluid can carry and release oxygen in a similar manner to red blood cells. Oxyglobin (Biopure Corporation, Cambridge, Massachusetts) has been used successfully in different species (eg, dogs, cats, ferrets, horses, some birds) [39–43]. Oxyglobin requires no cross-matching. It has immediate oxygen-carrying capability, because there is no requirement for 2,3-diphosphoglycerate. It contributes to osmotic pressure, offering an additional advantage in hypotensive patients. Dosages from 5 to 30 mL/kg have been reported, and titration in 5-mL/kg increments is advised. Oxyglobin is available in 125-mL bags, and the product only has a 24-hour shelf life once opened. Although this product has several advantages, it is expensive, has become increasingly difficult to stock, and has several potential drawbacks. The nitric oxide scavenging properties of Oxyglobin have been suggested to result in vasoconstriction, increased blood pressure, and an overall failure in its goal of expanding intravascular volume. At this time, Hemopure (Cambridge, Massachusetts) (a more polymerized and refined HBOC that was developed for use in people) is still not approved by the US Food and Drug Administration (FDA) [44]. Because of difficulty in gaining FDA approval, Hemopure currently is being considered for use in other countries [45,46] and by the United States Navy for trauma in emergency situations [47]. Because of the higher colloid osmotic pressure of Oxyglobin (43 mm Hg) as compared with that of hetastarch (32 mm Hg), rapid administration, especially in cats, may cause circulatory overload and pulmonary edema [48].

Blood products, such as packed red blood cells or whole blood transfusions, can also be considered in hypovolemic states caused by hemorrhage. The decision to administer red blood cells or whole blood should not be based solely on absolute measurements of hematocrit or hemoglobin. Instead, a clinical indication for use should be present. Examples of clinical indications include anemia associated with tachycardia, tachypnea, hypoxemia, active bleeding, and hyperlactatemia. Determination of the ideal laboratory test to evaluate in making the decision to transfuse blood or packed red cells has been ongoing in human and veterinary medicine. In 1942, a threshold was developed in human medicine based on clinical experience with surgical patients at the Mayo Clinic [49]. At that time, the clinical threshold for red blood cell transfusion (ie, transfusion trigger) was set at a hemoglobin concentration of 10 g/dL or a hematocrit of 30%. With recent concerns about the risks and complications of transfusion therapy, studies showed survival using lower threshold values in animals [50] and people [51]. Because there are no evidence-based transfusion triggers yet defined for dogs or cats, the clinician must consider the signalment, duration of illness, clinical signs attributed to anemia (eg, tachycardia, hypotension, hyperlactatemia, hypoxemia), and underlying disease process before recommending transfusion.

GOALS AND END POINTS OF RESUSCITATION

During resuscitation, basic monitoring should be performed, including heart rate, respiratory rate, pulse quality, capillary refill time, mucous membrane color, temperature, and overall patient mentation. Urine production should be monitored with a goal of urine production at greater than 1 to 2 mL/kg/h. Urine specific gravity also can be measured. Packed cell volume and total solids can be monitored. Arterial blood pressure should be measured whenever possible. Optimal resuscitation results include MAP of 80 to 100 mm Hg and systolic blood pressure of 100 to 120 mm Hg. Blood lactate concentrations can be used to assess perfusion and should be normalized to less than 2.0 mmol/L. If available, central venous pressure (CVP) should be monitored. Unless markedly increased and indicative of abnormal cardiac function, volume overload, or inappropriate catheter placement (ie, >15 mm Hg), a single measurement of CVP provides little useful information. Dynamic CVP measurements (ie, measurement of CVP in animals after a fluid challenge) yield important information about cardiovascular status, however. When evaluating CVP, fluid challenges are administered until the CVP increases greater than 3 cm H_2O. If the CVP increases 3 to 6 cm H_2O, wait 10 minutes and re-evaluate, but if it increases more than 6 cm H_2O, fluid infusion should be stopped. Fluid challenges of 5 to 10 mL/kg can be used.

In situations in which a more than appropriate administered fluid volume has not successfully resuscitated the patient to normal values, ancillary therapy should be considered. Evidence of poor perfusion despite resuscitation includes sustained hypotension, increased CVP, and decreased urine production (<1 mL/kg/h) [52].

ANCILLARY THERAPIES

Positive inotropes, such as dobutamine and dopamine, are pharmacologic agents that are most useful when adequate intravascular fluid resuscitation has occurred but tissue perfusion parameters still indicate hypoperfusion (Table 4). Dobutamine is a synthetic sympathomimetic agent and direct β_1-adrenergic agonist, causing an increase in the force of myocardial contractions. It also has mild β_2 effects causing vasodilatation. The combination of increased myocardial contractility and increased arterial vasodilatation results in an increase in CO with minimal change in arterial blood pressure. The dosage range of dobutamine is wide (2–15 μg/kg/min). Most clinicians begin administration at 2 to 5 μg/kg/min and titrate as needed [18,53]. Anecdotally, seizures have been reported in cats receiving dobutamine. Seizures as a result of dobutamine can be treated with diazepam and should stop once dobutamine therapy is discontinued.

Dopamine is a catecholamine and immediate precursor to norepinephrine. At extremely low intravenous dosages (0.5–2 μg/kg/min), dopamine acts predominantly on dopaminergic receptors and dilates the renal, mesenteric, coronary, and intracerebral vascular beds. At dosages from 2 to 10 μg/kg/min, dopamine also stimulates β_1-adrenergic receptors. The net effect in this dosage range is to exert positive inotropic effects and to increase organ perfusion, renal blood flow, and urine production. At these lower dosages, SVR remains largely unchanged. At higher dosages (>10–12 μg/kg/min), the dopaminergic effects are overridden by α-adrenergic effects. Systemic peripheral resistance is increased and hypotension may be corrected in animals with decreased SVR; renal and peripheral blood flow thus is decreased [18,53]. The rate of dopamine administration should be titrated to the desired clinical effect in each patient and re-evaluated frequently. End points of resuscitation (as discussed previously) should be used to evaluate the effectiveness of the dopamine infusion, and the infusion should be increased or decreased to achieve the desired effect.

Additional vasopressors, such as epinephrine (0.1–0.3 μg/kg/min), phenylephrine (1–3 μg/kg/min), or norepinephrine (0.1–10 μg/kg/min), also may be used. The use of these vasopressors should be considered a temporary solution because they cause vasoconstriction and can lead to decreased tissue and organ perfusion [18,53] (see Table 4).

Vasopressin, also known as antidiuretic hormone, is a relatively new therapeutic agent for shock. Vasopressin is a peptide synthesized in the hypothalamus and stored in the posterior pituitary gland. It is important in the maintenance of blood volume and water balance by virtue of its effects on the kidneys, and it helps to restore blood pressure in hypotensive states by its vasoconstrictor effects. Other functions of vasopressin include effects on body temperature, insulin release, corticotropin release, memory, and social behavior. In experimental studies in dogs, vasopressin has shown promising results, including the restoration of renal blood flow and oxygen delivery [54] in addition to an increase in MAP and a trend toward increased CO [55]. Although positive effects have been reported, negative effects also were documented, including worsening of underlying metabolic and hemodynamic derangements from prolonged shock [56]. For this reason, the use of vasopressin currently is being debated.

As with fluid administration, the same basic monitoring techniques (discussed previously) should be used to determine the effectiveness of therapy. The following formulas may aid in constant rate infusion (CRI) calculation and administration [57]:

$$M = DWV/(R \times 16.67) \tag{1}$$

where M is the milligrams of drug to add to the base solution, D is the dosage of drug (μg/kg/min), W is the body weight in kilograms, R is the fluid rate (mL/h), and 16.67 is the conversion factor.

To determine the appropriate R if the dosage is adjusted, the formula is R = D(adjusted)WV/M(16.67) [57]:

$$\text{Dosage } (\mu g/kg/min) \times BW \text{ (kg)} = \\ \text{mg to add to base solution (250 mL) at a rate of 15 mL/}h \tag{2}$$

$$\text{Dosage } (\mu g/kg/min) \times 0.36 = \text{mg needed for 6-hour infusion} \tag{3}$$

Hypovolemia and hypoperfusion are common life-threatening problems in animals presented to the emergency veterinarian. Physical findings are the immediate mainstay of assessment of tissue perfusion. Rapid recognition and treatment of abnormal tissue perfusion and correction of the underlying cause are the keys to optimizing outcome. Multiple factors contribute to the prognosis for patients with abnormal tissue perfusion. Ongoing hypoperfusion, persistently high blood lactate concentration, and the continued requirement for vasoactive support to maintain blood pressure despite adequate intravascular volume resuscitation all indicate a refractory shock state and poor prognosis. Overall, prognosis also depends on the underlying cause that resulted in poor tissue perfusion.

Suggested Readings

Available at: http://www.vin.com/Members/calculators/calc.plx?CalcID=7. Accessed July 1, 2007.
Available at: http://www.cvmbs.colostate.edu/clinsci/wing/fluids/cri.htm. Accessed July 1, 2007.
Available at: http://www.apg-software.com/index_files/CIC_Main.htm. Accessed July 1, 2007.
PDA Version http://vetpda.ucdavis.edu/Projects/VetPDA-Calcs.cfm. Accessed July 1, 2007.

References

[1] Cottingham C. Resuscitation of traumatic shock. AACN Adv Crit Care 2006;17(3): 317–26.
[2] Boag AK, Hughes D. Assessment and treatment of perfusion abnormalities in the emergency patient. Vet Clin North Am Small Anim Pract 2005;35(2):319–42.

[3] Cohen RD, Woods RF. Clinical and biochemical aspects of lactic acidosis. Boston (MA): Blackwell Scientific; 1976. p. 42.

[4] Kriesberg RA. Pathogenesis and management of lactic acidosis. Annu Rev Med 1984;35: 36–48.

[5] Hudson M, Pocknee R, Mowat NA. D-lactic acidosis in short bowel syndrome—an examination of possible mechanisms. Q J Med 1990;74(274):157–63.

[6] Christopher MM, Eckfeldt JH, Eaton JW. Propylene glycol ingestion causes D-lactic acidosis. Lab Invest 1990;62:114–8.

[7] Christopher MM, Perman V, White JG, et al. Propylene glycol-induced Heinz Body formation and D-lactic acidosis in cats. Prog Clin Biol Res 1989;319:88–92.

[8] Cilley R, Scharenberg A, Bongiourno P, et al. Low oxygen delivery produced by anemia, hypoxia and low cardiac output. J Surg Res 1991;51:425–33.

[9] Berry MN, Scheuer J. Splanchnic lactic acid metabolism in hyperventilation, metabolic alkalosis and shock. Metabolism 1967;16:537–47.

[10] Cain S. Appearance of excess lactate in anesthetized dogs during anemia and hypoxic hypoxia. Am J Physiol 1965;209:604–10.

[11] Cucinell SA, O'Brien JC, Bryant GH, et al. Lactate generation by liver in hemorrhagic shock. Proc Soc Exp Biol Med 1981;168(2):222–7.

[12] dePapp E, Drobatz KJ, Hughes D. Plasma lactate concentration as a predictor of gastric necrosis and survival among dogs with gastric dilatation-volvulus: 102 cases (1995–1998). J Am Vet Med Assoc 1999;215(1):49–52.

[13] Lagutchik MS, Ogilvie GK, Hacket TB, et al. Increased lactate concentrations in ill and injured dogs. J Vet Emerg Crit Care 1998;8:117–26.

[14] Lagutchik MS, Ogilvie GK, Wingfield WE, et al. Lactate kinetics in veterinary critical care; a review. J Vet Emerg Crit Care 1996;6(2):81–95.

[15] Orringer CE, Eustace JC, Wunsch CD, et al. Natural history of lactic acidosis after grand mal seizures. A model for the study of an anion-gap acidosis not associated with hyperkalemia. N Engl J Med 1977;297(15):796–9.

[16] Rose RJ, Bloomberg MS. Responses to sprint exercises in the greyhound: effects on hematology, serum biochemistry and muscle metabolites. Res Vet Sci 1989;47:212–8.

[17] Weil MH, Afifi AA. Experimental and clinical studies in lactate and pyruvate as indicators of the severity of acute circulatory failure. Circulation 1970;41(6):989–1001.

[18] DiBartola SP. Fluid, electrolyte and acid base disorders. 3rd edition. Philadelphia: Elsevier; 2006.

[19] Kumar A, Parillo JE. Shock classification, pathophysiology, and approach to management. In: Parillo JE, Dellinger RP, editors. Critical care medicine: principles of diagnosis and management in the adult. 2nd edition. Philadelphia: Mosby; 2001. p. 371–420.

[20] Muir WW. Overview of shock. In: Proceedings of the 14th Annual Kal Kan Symposium Emergency/Critical Care. Columbus (OH); 1990. p. 7–13.

[21] Crystal MA, Cotter SM. Acute hemorrhage: a hematologic emergency in dogs. Compend Contin Educ Pract Vet 1992;14:60–7.

[22] Moore KE, Murtaugh RJ. Pathophysiologic characteristics of hypovolemic shock. Vet Clin North Am Small Anim Pract 2001;31:1115–28.

[23] Gutierrez G, Reines HD, Wulf-Gutierrez ME. Clinical review: hemorrhagic shock. Crit Care. 2004;8(5):373–81 [Epub Apr 2, 2004].

[24] Rixen D, Siegel JH. Bench-to-bedside review: oxygen debt and its metabolic correlates as quantifiers of the severity of hemorrhagic and post-traumatic shock. Crit Care 2005;9(5): 441–53 [Epub Apr 20, 2005].

[25] Cote E. Cardiogenic shock and cardiac arrest. Vet Clin North Am Small Anim Pract 2001;31:1129–45.

[26] Griffel MI, Kaufman BS. Pharmacology of colloids and crystalloids. Crit Care Clin 1992;8: 235–53.

[27] Elgart HN. Assessment of fluids and electrolytes. AACN Clin Issues 2004;15(4):607–21.

[28] Deb S, Martin B, Sun L, et al. Resuscitation with lactated Ringer's solution in rats with hemorrhagic shock in wounds induces immediate apoptosis. J Trauma 1999;46: 582–8.

[29] Pascoe PJ. Perioperative management of fluid therapy. In: DiBartola S, editor. Fluid therapy in small animal practice. 2nd edition. Philadelphia: WB Saunders; 2000. p. 307.

[30] Mendez CM, McClain CJ, Marsano LS. Albumin in clinical practice. Nutr Clin Pract 2005;20(3):314–20.

[31] Rahilly L. Hypoalbuminemia: pathophysiology and treatment. In: Conference Proceedings, International Veterinary Emergency and Critical Care Symposium 2006.

[32] Rizoli SB. Crystalloids and colloids in trauma resuscitation; a brief overview of the current debate. J Trauma 2003;54(Suppl 5):S82–8.

[33] Concannon KT, Haskins SC, Feldman BF. Hemostatic defects associated with two infusion rates of dextran 70 in dogs. Am J Vet Res 1992;53(8):1369–75.

[34] Glowaski MM, Moon-Massat PF, Erb HN, et al. Effects of oxypolygelatin and dextran 70 on hemostatic variables in dogs. Vet Anaesth Analg 2003;30(4):202–10.

[35] Vercueil A, Grocott MP, Mythen MG. Physiology, pharmacology, and rationale for colloid administration for the maintenance of effective hemodynamic stability in critically ill patients. Transfus Med Rev 2005;19(2):93–109.

[36] Bunn F, Roberts I, Tasker R, et al. Hypertonic versus near isotonic crystalloid for fluid resuscitation in critically ill patients. Cochrane Database Syst Rev 2004;(3):CD002045.

[37] Johnson AL, Criddle LM. Pass the salt: indications for and implications of using hypertonic saline. Crit Care Nurse 2004;24(5):36–8, 40–4, 46 passim.

[38] Velasco IT, Pontieri V, Rocha e Silva M. Hypertonic NaCl and severe hemorrhagic shock. Am J Physiol 1980;239:H664–73.

[39] Abou-Madi N, Garner M, Kollias GV, et al. The use of Oxyglobin in birds: preliminary pharmacokinetics and effects on selected blood parameters and tissues. In: Proceedings AAZV, AAWV, ARAV, NAZWV Joint Conference; 2001. p. 77–9.

[40] Vin R, Bedenice D, Rentko V, et al. The use of ultrapurified bovine hemoglobin solution in the treatment of two cases of presumed red maple toxicosis in a miniature horse and a pony. Journal of Veterinary Emergency and Critical Care 2002;12(3):169–75.

[41] Gibson GR, Callan MB, Hoffman V, et al. Use of a hemoglobin-based oxygen-carrying solution in cats: 72 cases (1998–2002). Journal of the American Veterinary Medical Association 2002;221(1):96–102.

[42] Kelly N, Rentko VT. Comparative cardiovascular response by Oxyglobin versus packed red blood cells in acute anemia. Journal of Veterinary Emergency and Critical Care 1998;8(3): 252.

[43] Day TK. Current development and use of hemoglobin-based oxygen-carrying (HBOC) solutions. J Vet Emerg Crit Care 2003;13(2):77–93, (2).

[44] Krasner J. FDA may seek more Biopure tests. The Boston Globe. January 9, 2004. Vol 265, No. 9. p. C3.

[45] Krasner J. Biopure switches direction on blood product in bid to right itself. The Boston Globe. Vol 266, No. 16. p. D1.

[46] Associated Press. Biopure: British agency to review Biopure drug. The Boston Globe September 12, 2006. Available at: http://www.boston.com/business/healthcare/articles/2006/09/12/british_agency_to_review_biopure_drug/.

[47] Kerber R. Biopure, navy seek blood-substitute study. The Boston Globe. July 4, 2005. Vol. 268, No. 4. p. B5.

[48] Walton RS. Polymerized hemoglobin versus hydroxyethyl starch in an experimental model of feline hemorrhagic shock. In: Proceedings IVECCS. San Antonio (TX): 1996. p. 5–10.

[49] Adams RC, Lundy JS. Anesthesia in cases of poor surgical risk. Some suggestions for decreasing the risk. Surg Gynecol Obstet 1942;74:1011–9.

[50] Wilkerson DK, Rosen AL, Lakshman RS, et al. Limits of cardiac compensation in anemic baboons. Surgery 1998;103:665–70.

[51] Weiskopf RB, Viele MK, Feiner J, et al. Human cardiovascular and metabolic response to acute, severe isovolemic anemia. JAMA 1998;279:217–21.

[52] Vincent JL, Weil MH. Fluid challenge revisited. Crit Care Med 2006;34(5):1333–7.

[53] Plumb DC, editor. Veterinary drug handbook. 5th edition. Wiley, John & Sons Incorporated; 2005.

[54] Guzman JA, Rosado AE, Kruse JA. Vasopressin vs norepinephrine in endotoxic shock: systemic, renal, and splanchnic hemodynamic and oxygen transport effects. J Appl Physiol 2003;95(2):803–9.

[55] Morales D, Madigan J, Cullinane S, et al. Reversal by vasopressin of intractable hypotension in the late phase of hemorrhagic shock. Circulation 1999;100:226–9.

[56] Johnson KB, Pearce FJ, Jeffreys N, et al. Impact of vasopressin on hemodynamic and metabolic function in the decompensatory phase of hemorrhagic shock. J Cardiothorac Vasc Anesth 2006;20(2):167–72 [Epub Mar 9, 2006].

[57] Macintire D, Drobatz K, Haskins S, et al. Manual of small animal emergency and critical care medicine. Baltimore (MD): Lippincott Williams & Wilkins; 2005. p. 422–3.

Fluid Resuscitation and the Trauma Patient

Elke Rudloff, DVM*, Rebecca Kirby, DVM

Animal Emergency Center and Specialty Services, 2100 West Silver Spring Drive, Glendale, WI 53209, USA

Traumatic events, such as motor vehicle accidents, penetrating injuries, animal bites, and surgical procedures, are common in small animal emergency medicine and surgery. The incidence of trauma in dogs and cats (13% of hospital accessions) is similar to that seen in human emergency rooms [1]. The degree of physiologic compensation should be proportional to the extent of trauma experienced. Although, superficially, an animal may seem to have incurred only mild injury, life-threatening trauma may have occurred.

Traumatic injuries, such as pneumothorax, pericardial tamponade, ongoing hemorrhage, burns, and brain injury, complicate therapy and increase the possibility of treatment failure. All animals that have experienced trauma are at greater risk for complications related to fluid therapy. A sudden increase in intravascular hydrostatic pressure can lead to tissue edema as a result of increased capillary permeability, hemorrhage from disruption of a clot, and heart failure attributable to increased preload in an injured heart. When developing a fluid therapy plan, it is important to recognize the systemic changes that can occur as a consequence of the traumatic event.

PATHOPHYSIOLOGY OF TRAUMA

Trauma stimulates the hypothalamic-pituitary-adrenal axis, immune system, and metabolic systems in an effort to restore homeostasis (Fig. 1). These compensatory mechanisms can be called "stress responses" and are modulated by the extent of tissue injury, volume of blood loss, pain experienced, fear, shock, hypoxia, hypotension, and hypothermia [2,3]. The metabolic responses to trauma occur within the first few hours of injury and are characterized by hypovolemia, decreased blood flow, and the initial compensatory physiologic reactions to shock and trauma [4,5]. A catabolic phase is initiated after reperfusion of hypoxic tissues and lasts days to weeks. It is characterized by a hyperdynamic response, fluid retention and edema, catabolism, and hypermetabolism. An anabolic phase is initiated once volume deficits have been restored, wounds have been closed, and infection has been controlled. The anabolic phase is

*Corresponding author. E-mail address: aecerdvm@aol.com (E. Rudloff).

0195-5616/08/$ – see front matter
doi:10.1016/j.cvsm.2008.01.018

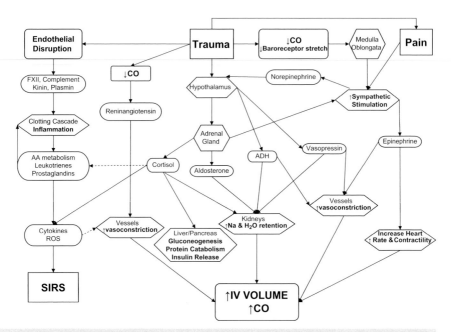

Fig. 1. Hormonal, immune, and metabolic responses to a traumatic event. Trauma results in tissue injury, pain, hemorrhage, and hypovolemia, which decrease cardiac output (CO) or trigger the sympathetic nervous system through afferent stimulation. Subsequent epinephrine and norepinephrine release increases heart rate, cardiac contractility, minute ventilation, and vasoconstriction. Trauma and sympathetic stimulation trigger the hypothalamic-pituitary-adrenal axis, resulting in the release of hormones that promote energy production, vasoconstriction, and renal retention of water. These actions are meant to increase intravascular volume (IV) and CO. Local mediators are produced in response to endothelial disruption in injured and ischemic tissue. Circulating factor XII (FXII), kinin, plasmin, and complement are activated, initiating the clotting cascade and inflammation. Arachidonic acid (AA) metabolism results in the production of leukotrienes and prostaglandins, which are potent mediators of vascular tone, inflammation, and coagulation. Cortisol tempers these reactions (*dashed line*). Activation of local mediators during trauma is designed to restore vascular integrity and promote wound healing, but excessive stress can result in microthrombi formation that inhibits blood flow and exacerbates ischemia in tissues other than those injured. Local production of cytokines (tumor necrosis factor and interleukins-1, -6, and -8) by neutrophil activation and production of radical oxygen species (ROS) after reperfusion can culminate in a systemic inflammatory response syndrome (SIRS), counteract vasoconstriction (*dashed line*), cause vasodilatation, and increase capillary permeability. ADH, antidiuretic hormone; Na, sodium.

characterized by diuresis, resumption of normal cardiovascular dynamics, and restoration of body protein and fat stores. This final stage can last for weeks.

The initial responses to trauma are designed to preserve body water and decrease blood loss. Local and systemic inflammation from tissue injury and hypoxia can lead to a systemic inflammatory response syndrome (SIRS) characterized by loss of capillary integrity, loss of protein (primarily albumin) into the extravascular space, and postcapillary venoconstriction with an increase in capillary hydrostatic pressure. Tissue edema, in conjunction with intravascular hypovolemia, alters oxygen delivery to the cells.

Careful patient evaluation is required to determine the initial responses to trauma and create a fluid therapy plan specific for the individual patient. As the patient's condition changes, the types and volumes of fluids may require adjustment.

ASSESSMENT AND THERAPY

Initial Assessment

On arrival, triage parameters (eg, airway, breathing, circulation, level of pain, level of consciousness) are immediately assessed. Life-threatening complications of trauma include airway obstruction, tension pneumothorax, fulminant hemorrhage, brain injury, and bradyarrhythmia or tachyarrhythmia. The patient's history, vital signs, and physical examination findings and the emergency laboratory database provide clues that can be used to guide therapy of the trauma patient. Pale, gray, or blue mucous membrane color; capillary refill time shorter than 1 second or longer than 2 seconds; weak pulse quality; and tachycardia are clinical signs associated with perfusion abnormalities. Rapid intervention is based on assessment of perfusion and correction of the causes of perfusion abnormalities [6].

Internal (less obvious) hemorrhage is assumed when there is evidence of a hemothorax on thoracocentesis, increased or moist lung sounds or hemoptysis caused by pulmonary contusions, an abdominal fluid wave, or decreased total protein concentration with or without anemia. Gross evidence of hemorrhage, traumatized tissue, and decreased packed cell volume (PCV) and total protein concentration are indicators of hypovolemia attributable to blood loss. An initial total protein concentration less than 6.5 g/dL in the trauma patient, with or without anemia, suggests hemorrhage. Splenic contraction after catecholamine release during shock and pain can release sequestered red blood cells into the circulation in the dog and mask laboratory signs of hemorrhage. Increased lactate concentration indicates inadequate tissue perfusion, and failure to respond to corrective measures may indicate a poor prognosis [7–10].

Resuscitation

The resuscitative approach to the trauma patient is outlined in Fig. 2. Consequences of trauma that can affect perfusion include airway compromise, pneumothorax, pulmonary contusions, myocardial contusions, hemorrhage, massive tissue damage, pain, and head injury. Major bleeding vessels are clamped or ligated, and bleeding wounds are covered with a compression wrap. Abdominal hemorrhage may be slowed using hind limb abdominal counterpressure [11].

Virtually every animal that has experienced a traumatic event benefits from analgesia. Pain stimulates the sympathetic nervous system, magnifying the shock response. The level of pain is evaluated by examining posture, response to palpation, heart rate, and respiratory rate. Intravenous administration of

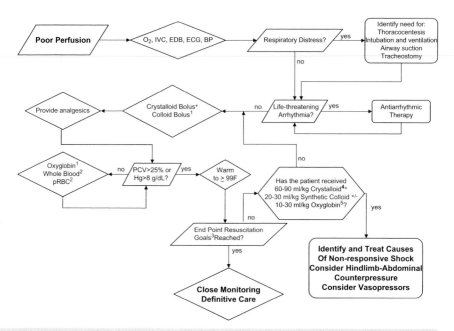

Fig. 2. Resuscitation algorithm for the trauma patient. This resuscitation algorithm is a guide for immediate stabilization and fluid resuscitation of the trauma patient with poor perfusion variables. O₂, oxygen; IVC, intravenous catheter; EDB, emergency database (PCV, total protein, blood glucose, venous blood gas, electrolyte panel, lactate, and blood urea nitrogen); ECG, electrocardiogram; BP, blood pressure; Hg, hemoglobin; HES, hetastarch; pRBC, packed red blood cell transfusion. [1]Buffered isotonic replacement crystalloid (eg, Plasmalyte-7.4 or Normosol-R at a rate of 10–15 mL/kg) and HES (3–5 mL/kg) or Oxyglobin (dog: 3–5-mL/kg boluses up to 30 mL/kg; cat: 1–3-mL/kg boluses up to 10 mL/kg). [2]Calculation of volume of blood transfusion to administer [dog: weight (lb) × 40 × (desired PCV − patient PCV)/donor PCV = milliliters to administer; cat: weight (lb) × 30 × (desired PCV − patient PCV)/donor PCV = milliliters to administer]. [3]See Table 1. [4]60 mL/kg for the cat and 90 mL/kg for the dog. [5]10 mL/kg for the cat and 30 mL/kg for the dog.

pure opioids (eg, morphine, hydromorphone, fentanyl) provides a high level of analgesia and can be titrated to effect. Adverse effects are rare, but titration of the reversal agent (naloxone, 0.02 mg/kg, administered intravenously) can be used to decrease unwanted effects of the opioid. Combining opioids with midazolam or diazepam (0.2 mg/kg administered intravenously) benzodiazepines, which also are reversible (flumazenil, 0.01 mg/kg, administered intravenously), provides a combined effect that can decrease the overall requirement for opioids.

Hypothermia can reduce vasoreactivity and platelet adhesion, especially in cats. Rapid passive external rewarming of the patient to at least 99°F should occur after administration of the initial fluid dose (see Fig. 2) [12].

Hypovolemia can result from maldistribution of blood flow, increased vascular permeability, hemorrhage, or some combination of these problems.

A combination of crystalloids, colloids, and blood products is the cornerstone of resuscitation of perfusion deficits. Many types of fluids are available. Therapy must be individualized, and monitoring must be continuous. The type and dose of fluid depend on the condition of the patient, severity of trauma, volume of blood lost, and anticipated complications. Selecting the appropriate fluids to administer is the first step in creating the fluid therapy plan. Catastrophic hemorrhage requires rapid infusion of whole blood, packed red blood cells, or Oxyglobin (Biopure, Cambridge, Massachusetts) while hemostasis is achieved (see Fig. 2).

In the absence of catastrophic hemorrhage, balanced isotonic crystalloids (eg, Plasmalyte 148 (Baxter Healthcare, Deerfield, Illinois) or Normosol-R (Hospira, Lake Forest, Illinois)) are infused to provide water and electrolytes to the intravascular compartment and interstitium. Although lactated Ringer's solution contains a buffer, there is some evidence that it can exacerbate neutrophil superoxide burst activity and increase neutrophil adherence, potentially promoting the inflammatory phase of trauma [13]. The extent of vascular damage may not be recognized during the initial assessment. With doses necessary to restore and maintain intravascular volume, using crystalloids alone may result in additional edema as fluid exudes into the interstitial space through leaking capillaries. Using colloids in conjunction with crystalloids preserves intravascular colloid osmotic pressure (COP) and decreases the total fluid volume needed [14].

Natural colloids include whole blood, plasma products, concentrated human albumin solutions, and Oxyglobin, whereas synthetic colloids include dextran 70 and hydroxyethyl starch (HES), such as Hespan (Braun, Irvine, California), Hextend (Hospira, Lake Forest, Illinois), or 10% pentastarch. The authors prefer to use HES products (Hespan or Hextend) or Oxyglobin during fluid resuscitation of the trauma patient. Experience has shown that the amount of Oxyglobin required for resuscitation is approximately one third of the volume required when using HES because of the vasoconstrictive properties of Oxyglobin. Bleeding times may increase in animals given colloids and should be monitored in patients requiring surgery or with possible hemorrhage. Plasma transfusion can restore clotting times when necessary.

In general, when the PCV acutely decreases to less than 25% (ie, hemoglobin <8 g/dL) in the trauma patient, a blood transfusion is needed. Ideally, crossmatching and blood typing are performed to decrease the risk for a transfusion reaction; however, time may not permit testing during catastrophic hemorrhage. When blood typing is not possible, administration of dog erythrocyte antigen 1.1-negative blood is ideal because this blood type invokes the least antigenic response in the untyped dog that requires several transfusions. Oxyglobin can be administered when blood products are not immediately available.

Hypertonic (7%) saline (4–7 mL/kg) can be used as an adjunct for rapid volume resuscitation. The concentrated salt solution provides an instant osmotic pull, transferring interstitial and intracellular fluid into the intravascular compartment. This osmotic effect may decrease intracranial pressure in the head-injured patient with intracranial signs. It also may blunt immunologic and inflammatory effects when used in conjunction with dextran in people experiencing traumatic hemorrhagic shock [15]. The rapid increase in intravascular volume is analogous to large-volume isotonic crystalloid infusion, however, and may increase bleeding from injured vessels. Hypertonic fluids may be most useful combined with colloids for immediate resuscitation after catastrophic trauma.

Aggressive or excessive rate and volume of fluids have been reported to result in clinically relevant consequences for the patient, including a rapid increase in hydrostatic pressure, displacement of tenuous clots, dilution of coagulation and oxygen-carrying factors, decreased blood viscosity, and increased mortality [16–23]. Fluid infusion volumes are titrated to prevent rapid increases in hydrostatic pressure (see Fig. 2). End-point resuscitation variables (Table 1) are used to gauge adequate blood flow to vital organs without exacerbation of hemorrhage [24]. Low normal arterial blood pressure is targeted. This approach may decrease the need for surgical intervention to control internal hemorrhage. Once end point resuscitation variables have been achieved, rigorous monitoring is instituted for early detection of potential relapse.

MONITORING

The trend of change in physical, measured, and laboratory variables of perfusion must be evaluated and a clinical judgment made. Focusing on a single variable leads to under- or overresuscitation and can contribute to morbidity and mortality. For example, it is easy to misinterpret normal arterial blood pressure as an indicator of adequate perfusion. When associated with increased

Table 1
Targeted end point resuscitation parameters in the trauma patient

Variable	Resuscitation end point
Mentation	Alert
Heart rate (beats per minute)	Dog: 80–140
	Cat: 180–220
Mucous membrane color	Pink
Capillary refill time (seconds)	1–2
Rectal temperature (°F)	99–101
Mean arterial blood pressure (mm Hg)	60–80
Systolic arterial blood pressure (mm Hg)	90–100
Central venous pressure (cm H_2O)	5–10
Urine output (mL/kg/h)	>1
SpO_2 (%)	>97
$ScvO_2$ (%)	<65
PCV (%)	>25
Hemoglobin (g/dL)	>8
Lactate (mmol/L)	<2
pH	>7.32
Base deficit (mEq/L)	−2 to +2
COP (mm Hg)	14–20

Abbreviations: SpO_2, arterial oxygen saturation; $ScvO_2$, central venous oxygen saturation.

heart rate, however, blood pressure is being maintained at the expense of tachycardia.

Physical examination variables (eg, heart rate, pulse palpation, mucous membrane color, capillary refill time, rectal temperature) are the most reliable indicators of change in perfusion status. Evaluation of respiratory and neurologic status may identify noncirculatory influences on perfusion. Measured variables that can provide information regarding intravascular perfusion status include arterial blood pressure, central venous pressure, oximetry (pulse and central venous), and urine output.

Despite normalization of physical and measured variables, up to 85% of severely injured human victims of trauma can have inadequate tissue oxygenation [25]. Metabolic acidosis, lactatemia, base deficit, and abnormal central venous hemoglobin oxygen saturation variables indicate local tissue ischemia, and the need for additional resuscitative measures, such as blood transfusion, should be considered. Frequent and repeated monitoring of the PCV can indicate ongoing hemorrhage if a decrease seems to exceed that expected as a result of dilution from fluid administration.

Ongoing fluid loss is the most common cause of shock relapse or failure to reach resuscitation end points. Hemorrhage, compartment syndrome, and third space fluid loss all are potential causes of circulating volume depletion in the trauma patient. Control of ongoing hemorrhage may require emergency surgical intervention [11].

When large volumes of fluid have been administered or central venous pressure is 8 to 10 cm H_2O, causes other than inadequate fluid resuscitation must be investigated. Hypoxia (attributable to pulmonary contusions or anemia), hypothermia, myocardial dysfunction (eg, dysrhythmias, cardiac tamponade, contusions), and brain trauma may occur in the trauma patient and can contribute to inadequate perfusion. Vasopressors, such as Oxyglobin (3–5 mL/kg administered intravenously), arginine vasopressin (0.5-µg/kg/min continuous rate infusion) or dopamine (5–10-µg/kg/min continuous rate infusion administered intravenously), and, occasionally, positive inotropes, such as dobutamine (2.5–5-µg/kg/min continuous rate infusion administered intravenously), may be necessary once there is adequate intravascular volume.

After perfusion is restored, fluid infusion is continued using a continuous infusion of an isotonic replacement crystalloid solution and a synthetic colloid. Postresuscitation fluid therapy now is focused on meeting the metabolic needs of healing tissue, replacing ongoing losses, maintaining COP, and limiting loss of fluid. In general, replacement crystalloids are infused at rates necessary to maintain hydration and replace ongoing losses. HES (0.8–1.0 mL/kg/h) can maintain COP during the catabolic phase. Nutritional support should be provided as soon as possible.

References

[1] Kolata RJ, Johnston DE. Motor vehicle accidents in urban dogs: a study of 600 cases. J Am Vet Med Assoc 1975;167(10):938–41.

[2] Hume DM, Egdahl RH. The importance of the brain in the endocrine response to injury. Ann Surg 1959;150:697–712.

[3] Gann DS, Lilly MP. The neuroendocrine response to multiple trauma. World J Surg 1983;7(1):101–18.

[4] Cuthbertson DP. Post-shock metabolic responses. Lancet 1942;1:433–6.

[5] Wilmore DW. Homeostasis: bodily changes in trauma and surgery. In: Sabiston DC Jr, editor. Textbook of surgery. 13th edition. Philadelphia: WB Saunders; 1986. p. 23–37.

[6] Boag AK, Hughes D. Assessment and treatment of perfusion abnormalities in the emergency patient. Vet Clin North Am Small Anim Pract 2005;35(2):319–42.

[7] Davis JW, Kaups KL, Parks SN. Base deficit is superior to pH in evaluating clearance of acidosis after traumatic shock. J Trauma 1998;44(1):114–8.

[8] Eberhard LW, Morabito DJ, Matthay MA, et al. Initial severity of metabolic acidosis predicts the development of acute lung injury in severely traumatized patients. Crit Care Med 2000;28(1):125–31.

[9] Abramson D, Scalea TM, Hitchcock R, et al. Lactate clearance and survival following injury. J Trauma 1993;35(4):584–9.

[10] McNelis J, Marini CP, Jurkiewick A, et al. Prolonged lactate clearance is associated with increased mortality in the surgical intensive care unit. Am J Surg 2001;182(5):481–5.

[11] Herold L, Devey J, Kirby R, et al. Clinical evaluation and management of hemoperitoneum in dogs. Journal of Veterinary Emergency and Critical Care 2008;18(1):40–53.

[12] Kirby R, Rudloff E. Crystalloid and colloid fluid therapy. In: Ettinger S, Feldman E, editors. Textbook of veterinary internal medicine. 6th edition. St. Louis (MO): Saunders-Elsevier; 2005. p. 412–23.

[13] Rhee PD, Burris C, Kaufman M, et al. Lactated Ringer's solution causes neutrophil activation after hemorrhagic shock. J Trauma 1998;44(2):313–9.

[14] Silverstein D, Aldrich J, Haskins SC, et al. Assessment of changes in blood volume in response to resuscitative fluid administration in dogs. Journal of Veterinary Emergency and Critical Care 2005;15(3):185–92.

[15] Rizoli SB, Rhind SG, Shek PN, et al. The immunomodulatory effects of hypertonic saline resuscitation in patients sustaining traumatic hemorrhagic shock. Ann Surg 2006;243(1): 47–57.

[16] Heckbert SR, Vedder NB, Hoffman W, et al. Outcome after hemorrhagic shock in trauma patients. J Trauma 1998;45(3):545–9.

[17] Mapstone J, Roberts I, Evans P. Fluid resuscitation strategies: a systemic review of animal trials. J Trauma 2003;55(3):571–89.

[18] Bickell WH, Bruttig SP, O'Benar J, et al. The detrimental effects of intravenous crystalloid after aortotomy in swine. Surgery 1991;110(3):529–36.

[19] Kowalenko T, Stern SA, Dronen SC. Improved outcome with hypotensive resuscitation of uncontrolled hemorrhagic shock. J Trauma 1992;33(3):349–53.

[20] Stern SA, Wang X, Mertz M, et al. Under-resuscitation of near lethal uncontrolled hemorrhage: effects on mortality and end-organ function at 72 hours. Shock 2001;15(1):16–23.

[21] Krausz MM, Bashenko Y, Hirsh M. Crystalloid or colloid resuscitation of uncontrolled hemorrhagic shock after moderate splenic injury. Shock 2000;13(3):230–5.

[22] Riddez L, Johnson L, Hahn RG. Central and regional hemodynamics during crystalloid fluid therapy after uncontrolled intraabdominal bleeding. J Trauma 1998;44(3):433–9.

[23] Solomonov E, Hirsh M, Krausz MM. The effect of vigorous fluid resuscitation in uncontrolled hemorrhagic shock after massive splenic injury. Crit Care Med 2000;28(3):749–54.

[24] Pritte J. Optimal endpoints of resuscitation and early goal directed therapy. Journal of Veterinary Emergency and Critical Care 2006;16(4):329–39.

[25] Abou-Khalil B, Scalea TM, Trooskin SZ, et al. Hemodynamic responses to shock in young trauma patients: need for invasive monitoring. Crit Care Med 1994;22(4):633–9.

Fluid Therapy in Vomiting and Diarrhea

Andrew J. Brown, MA, VetMB, MRCVS[a],*,
Cynthia M. Otto, DVM, PhD[b]

[a]Department of Small Animal Clinical Sciences, College of Veterinary Medicine, Michigan State University, East Lansing, MI 48824, USA
[b]University of Pennsylvania School of Veterinary Medicine, Philadelphia, PA, USA

V omiting and diarrhea are two of the most common reasons for an animal to be presented to a veterinarian. A wide variety of disease processes and conditions can cause these signs, and the underlying condition may be mild and self-limiting or severe and life threatening. Vomiting and diarrhea may be caused by a primary gastrointestinal (GI) condition (eg, canine parvoviral enteritis [CPVE]) or may be secondary to an underlying systemic disease process (eg, renal failure, septic peritonitis). The fluid and electrolyte losses from vomiting and diarrhea can contribute to morbidity and mortality associated with the underlying condition. Additionally, septic complications can result from aspiration pneumonia associated with vomiting and bacterial translocation associated with some types of diarrhea. This article focuses on the pathophysiology and treatment of hypovolemia, dehydration, electrolyte disturbances, and acid-base derangements resulting from and associated with vomiting and diarrhea.

MECHANISMS OF VOMITING AND DIARRHEA

Vomiting

Vomiting is a physical response characterized by contraction of the abdominal muscles, descent of the diaphragm, and opening of the gastric cardia, resulting in expulsion of stomach contents from the mouth. It is a coordinated process involving multiple afferent and efferent neurologic pathways.

Coordination of vomiting occurs at the level of the medulla oblongata of the hindbrain [1]. The nucleus tractus solitarius (NTS) receives central and peripheral afferent fibers (Fig. 1).

Sensory vagal

Peripheral sensory fibers are predominantly vagal, with glossopharyngeal (oropharynx) and sympathetic (urogenital) fibers also contributing. Sensory vagal fibers are directly stimulated by GI distention or compression and by release of serotonin (5-HT) secondary to inflammation (GI or peritoneal) and drugs

*Corresponding author. E-mail address: andrewjb@msu.edu (A.J. Brown).

0195-5616/08/$ – see front matter
doi:10.1016/j.cvsm.2008.01.008

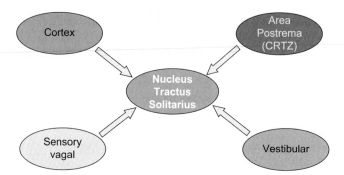

Fig. 1. The nucleus tractus solitarius receives central and peripheral afferent fibers.

or toxins. Local irritants (inflammatory cells or toxins) stimulate the release of serotonin from enterochromaffin cells, which then exerts its effects by means of 5-HT3 receptors on the sensory vagal fibers. Activation of gastric vagal afferents stimulates neurons in the NTS and the area postrema [2,3].

Chemoreceptor trigger zone
The chemoreceptor trigger zone (CRTZ) is located in the area postrema near the floor of the fourth ventricle. Chemoreceptors in the area postrema are functionally outside of the blood-brain barrier and are sensitive to circulating emetic agents [4]. Detection of circulating toxins causes a reflex action to expel these ingested toxins, and this reflex represents a long-preserved evolutionary survival technique for many species.

Vestibular
The NTS receives sensory input from the vestibular apparatus. Animals with vestibular disorders can have persistent vomiting that may lead to clinical consequences of hypovolemia, dehydration, and electrolyte disturbances. If balance, mentation, or other cranial nerves also are compromised in these animals, they may be unable to protect their airway, and thus be at increased risk for aspiration during vomiting.

Efferent pathways
The NTS receives and modulates sensory input by means of many receptors (dopaminergic, 5-HT3, neurokinin, muscarinic, and histaminergic). The coordinated contraction of abdominal muscles and relaxation of the gastric cardia then occur by means of the dorsal vagal complex (Fig. 2).

Diarrhea
Diarrhea is an increase in fecal volume caused by an increase in fecal water [5]. Pathophysiologic mechanisms include increased intestinal secretion; decreased intestinal absorption; decreased transit time; and mesenteric, vascular, or lymphatic disease [6].

Damage to the intestinal epithelial barrier may lead to decreased absorptive capacity. Infectious agents (eg, parvovirus), cellular infiltration, or surgery may

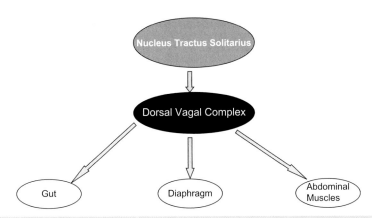

Fig. 2. Coordination of vomiting occurs by means of the dorsal vagal complex.

lead to a decrease in intestinal surface area and absorption [7]. When the absorptive capacity of the intestines is overwhelmed, osmotically active molecules retain water in the intestinal lumen, resulting in excessive fecal water loss (ie, osmotic diarrhea). An increase in intestinal osmolality and resultant osmotic diarrhea also may occur after dietary indiscretion or lactulose administration.

Bacterial enterotoxins, unconjugated bile acids, and hydroxylated fatty acids all stimulate intestinal secretion. Diarrhea ensues when absorptive capacity is overwhelmed by hypersecretion.

Diagnostically, diarrhea is commonly characterized as small- or large-bowel diarrhea. Fluid and electrolyte loss can be extensive in patients with acute or peracute small-bowel diarrhea.

CONSEQUENCES OF VOMITING AND DIARRHEA
Dehydration
Fluid loss from animals with vomiting and diarrhea can be severe, because large volumes of fluid are secreted and reabsorbed by the GI tract. Approximately 2.5 L of fluid enters the duodenal lumen of a 20-kg dog each day from diet and normal secretions, and more than 98% of this fluid is reabsorbed [8]. Fluid loss from GI disease thus can be extensive, and together with decreased intake leads to progressive dehydration. Severe complications, such as hypovolemia, may result. Clinical signs of dehydration can be subtle, and the ability to detect dehydration based on physical examination depends on the age and nutritional status of the animal, acuteness of onset of the vomiting or diarrhea, and any prior treatment. Table 1 provides guidelines for clinical assessment of dehydration. Typical clinical signs result from a loss of interstitial fluid, leading to a loss of tissue pliability and lubrication. Dehydration often can be detected first on examination of the mucous membranes. Assessment may be confounded by nausea-induced hypersalivation, however. Physical examination findings may include depression, dry or tacky mucous

Table 1
Clinical assessment of estimated dehydration in the dog

Clinical signs	Estimate of dehydration
Dry mucous membranes	5%
Reduced skin turgor	6%–8%
Mild hypoperfusion (tachycardia)	8%–10%
Moderate hypoperfusion (hypotension)	10%–12%
Severe hypoperfusion (collapse)	>12%

membranes, and a prolonged skin tent. Clinicians must consider body condition score and age when assessing skin tent; subcutaneous fat provides greater lubrication than lean tissue. Consequently, the top of the head and axillary region rather than the more commonly evaluated dorsal cervical region may provide more information about hydration status. When the eye of a normal cat is retropulsed, the nictitans should immediately slip back into place after release of the eye. With a dehydrated cat, however, the nictitans "sticks" to the globe and slides back more slowly. The most objective assessment of hydration status is body weight. Evaluation of this variable is most valuable when normal body weight can be documented on the same scale before the onset of fluid loss.

Dehydration in dogs with vomiting and diarrhea results from isotonic or hypertonic fluid loss and may be evident in changes to blood constituents. Loss of fluid from the blood results in hemoconcentration, manifested by a simultaneous increase in packed cell volume (PCV) and plasma total protein concentration or total solids (TS) by refractometry. The normal values for PCV and TS are lower in neonates than in adults. This difference is important to remember when assessing dehydration in puppies and kittens.

Animals with incessant vomiting and diarrhea become progressively more dehydrated and eventually lose sufficient volumes of fluid so as to develop a clinically relevant decrease in circulating blood volume.

Hypovolemia

Fluid loss with vomiting and diarrhea may lead to hypovolemia and compromised perfusion of organs and tissues. Hypovolemic shock is one of the most life-threatening consequences of vomiting and diarrhea. Activation of normal physiologic responses protects against impaired tissue perfusion associated with hypovolemia. First, dietary sodium intake and water intake normally are greater than basal needs, and, second, the kidney is able to enhance sodium and water reabsorption to expand circulating volume [9]. Hypovolemia is the result of such severe volume loss that fluid shifts and renal compensatory responses are unable to maintain circulating blood volume. Relatively large volumes of fluid must be lost, or the rate of loss must exceed the potential for compensatory responses, before a patient becomes hypovolemic.

When vomiting and diarrhea occur secondary to a systemic disease (eg, septic peritonitis), the volume of fluid loss that results in clinical signs of hypovolemia may be much smaller than in otherwise healthy animals. Tissue perfusion depends on vascular volume, which, in turn, is influenced by plasma volume, red blood cell volume, colloid osmotic (oncotic) pressure (COP), and vascular tone. A decrease in plasma volume can result from decreased fluid intake, fluid losses from vomiting or diarrhea, third space accumulation of fluid (eg, pooling in the GI tract), or inadequate renal compensation. Red blood cell volume may be decreased in some animals with vomiting or diarrhea associated with gastric ulcers or a bleeding disorder. Surprisingly, hemorrhagic diarrhea associated with parvovirus infection rarely causes severe anemia, and, conversely, the syndrome of hemorrhagic gastroenteritis (HGE) results in profound polycythemia that interferes with perfusion as a result of hyperviscosity. Diseases that lead to systemic vasodilatation result in signs of shock with limited fluid loss.

Clinically, hypovolemia may be demonstrated by a decrease in central venous pressure (CVP). This decreased venous pressure translates to a reduction in preload (end-diastolic volume) and inability of the heart to eject a normal stroke volume. The reflex response to a decrease in stroke volume is to increase heart rate, and therefore restore cardiac output. Thus, tachycardia is a frequent clinical finding in animals with hypovolemia. Another compensatory response is peripheral vasoconstriction that manifests clinically as pale mucous membranes with prolonged capillary refill time, depressed mentation, cold extremities, and, frequently, low rectal temperature.

Decreased delivery of oxygen to tissues secondary to hypovolemia results in anaerobic metabolism. Lactate is the metabolic end product of anaerobic metabolism, allowing the regeneration of cytosolic nicotinamide adenine dinucleotide (NAD^+) [10]. The production of lactate by hypoperfused tissues results in a high anion gap metabolic acidosis. Lactate concentration can be measured by point-of-care analyzers, and therefore may be used as a marker of decreased tissue perfusion caused by vomiting or diarrhea.

Electrolyte Disorders

Electrolyte disorders are common in patients with vomiting, diarrhea, or both. A large volume of fluid containing electrolytes is secreted and reabsorbed by the normal GI tract. Loss of these electrolytes by vomiting or malabsorption can thus lead to severe electrolyte abnormalities.

Gastric contents contain high concentrations of sodium and chloride, and hyponatremia and hypochloremia commonly result from loss of these fluids. The typical findings of hyponatremia and hypochloremia are most common when only gastric contents are lost. If biliary secretions also are present in the vomitus, electrolyte changes are less predictable. Most episodes of diarrhea result in isonatremic dehydration. Hypotonic fluid loss may occur with osmotic diarrhea (eg, secondary to lactulose administration), however, resulting in hypernatremic dehydration [11].

Hypokalemia may occur as a result of decreased intake and increased GI tract losses. The concentration of potassium in canine gastric secretions ranges from 10 to 20 mEq/L, increasing with increased rates of secretion [12]. Loss of potassium through vomiting thus results in hypokalemia. Normal feces contain a high concentration of potassium, and protracted diarrhea may lead to severe fecal potassium loss [13].

Specific diseases may result in atypical electrolyte patterns. For example, patients with vomiting and diarrhea attributable to hypoadrenocorticism typically are hyperkalemic as a consequence of mineralocorticoid deficiency. Electrolyte abnormalities depend on the underlying disease process causing the vomiting and are covered in more detail in the specific conditions discussed next.

Acid-Base Disturbances

Acid-base disturbances frequently occur with GI losses [9]. A variety of disturbances may exist and depend on the solutes lost from the GI tract and the patient's volume status. Mixed acid-base disturbances are relatively common. Although lactic acidosis may be assumed in the hypoperfused dog with vomiting and diarrhea, acid-base status cannot be predicted from history and physical examination only. Blood gas analysis therefore is recommended.

Acid secretion in dogs has been estimated at 30 mL/kg/d [14], with a peak of hydrogen chloride (HCl) at 4.1 $mEq/kg^{0.75}/h$ [7]. Patients with vomiting of gastric origin typically have metabolic alkalosis because of loss of chloride and proton-rich fluid and retention of bicarbonate by the kidneys. Intestinal, pancreatic, and biliary secretions have high concentrations of HCO^{3-}, and therefore are alkaline. Bicarbonate secretion increases and chloride secretion decreases with an increased rate of pancreatic secretion [15]. Loss of HCO^{3-} in these secretions may balance the loss of hydrogen ions from the stomach, making it difficult to predict the acid-base disturbance in the vomiting patient.

Animals with severe fluid loss from diarrhea likely have metabolic acidosis [9]. Patients with both vomiting and diarrhea may have gastric loss of chloride and hydrogen ions with intestinal loss of HCO^{3-} in the diarrhea. Accurate prediction of acid-base status in these patients is thus not possible.

Patients with vomiting, diarrhea, or both may have an increase in blood lactate concentration as a consequence of hypoperfusion. Lactic acidosis may be suspected based on clinical signs consistent with hypoperfusion or may be detected in whole blood using a point-of-care analyzer.

FLUID CHOICES

Fluid therapy in the patient with vomiting, diarrhea, or both can be complex. Animals may be presented with mild dehydration or may be profoundly hypovolemic. Patients may have a normal electrolyte and acid-base status or have life-threatening abnormalities. Each animal must therefore be considered individually, with careful attention paid to physical examination in addition to electrolyte and acid-base status.

Crystalloids

Crystalloid solutions may be hypotonic, isotonic, or hypertonic. Animals with vomiting and diarrhea typically have isotonic or hypertonic fluid loss. Replacement isotonic fluids provide sodium and water; as such, they correct volume and hydration deficits. Maintenance solutions contain a lower concentration of sodium, and therefore do not correct the volume and hydration deficits in animals with vomiting and diarrhea. Hypertonic saline (7.2% sodium chloride [NaCl]) draws fluid from the interstitium into the intravascular space, and therefore should not be used in dehydrated patients. Hypertonic saline has limited use in animals with vomiting and diarrhea.

Different crystalloid solutions have different concentrations of electrolytes and different buffers (Table 2).

Colloids

Oncotic support can be achieved using natural or synthetic colloids. Synthetic colloids include gelatins, starches, and dextrans. Natural colloids include whole blood, fresh-frozen plasma (FFP), and human albumin (HA) solutions. Table 3 illustrates the properties of colloidal solutions.

Blood products

Blood products, including packed red blood cells (PRBCs) and FFP, are rarely used in the treatment of vomiting and diarrhea.

Route of Administration

Oral

Oral rehydration therapy (ORT) can be used to correct mild to moderate dehydration. Orally administered fluids should not be used to correct hypovolemia. Oral administration has the advantage of being the most physiologic route in addition to being economic and safe. Large volumes of nonsterile fluids, electrolytes, drugs, and nutrition can be administered orally. The animal may voluntarily drink the fluids, or an enteral feeding tube can be placed. ORT

Table 2
Properties of isotonic crystalloid solutions commonly administered to dogs and cats with vomiting and diarrhea

Fluid	pH	Na^+ (mEq/L)	Cl^- (mEq/L)	K^+ (mEq/L)	Ca^{2+} (mEq/L)	Mg^{2+} (mEq/L)	Buffer
0.9% NaCl	5.0–5.5	154	154	0	0	0	None
Lactated Ringer's solution	6.5	130	109	4	3	0	Lactate
Normosol R	5.5–7.0	140	98	5	0	3	Acetate, gluconate
Plasmalyte-A	7.0–7.4	140	98	5	0	3	Acetate, gluconate

Adapted from Driessen B, Brainard B. Fluid therapy for the traumatized patient. Journal of Veterinary Emergency and Critical Care 2006;16:283; with permission.

Table 3
Properties of colloidal solutions

Fluid	pH	Na$^+$ (mEq/L)	Cl$^-$ (mEq/L)	K$^+$ (mEq/L)	Molecular weight (kd)	COP (mm Hg)	Buffer
Dextran 70	5.1–7.0	154	154	0	15–160	61	None
6% Hetastarch in 0.9% NaCl	5.5	154	154	0	10–3400	29–32	None
10% Pentastarch	7.4	154	100	0	5.6–100	45–47	None
Oxypolygelatin	5.0	154	154	0	10–1000	25	None
25% HA	6.4–7.4	130–160	130–160	<1	66–69	23.2	HCO$_3^-$, NaOH, or acetic acid
5% HA	6.4–7.4	130–160	130–160	<1	66–69	>200	HCO$_3^-$, NaOH, or acetic acid
Whole blood	Variable	140	100	4		20	HCO$_3^-$, protein
FFP	Variable	140	100	4		17–20	HCO$_3^-$, protein

Adapted from Driessen B, Brainard B. Fluid therapy for the traumatized patient. Journal of Veterinary Emergency and Critical Care 2006;16:284; with permission.

is recommended by the American Academy of Pediatrics as first-line therapy for pediatric patients with mild to moderate dehydration secondary to viral gastroenteritis [16].

The rationale for use of ORT is retention of water secondary to coupled transport of sodium with glucose in the small intestine. This reabsorption occurs even in the face of acute infectious causes of diarrhea. Controversy exists in the human literature as to the benefit of ORT compared with rapid intravenous rehydration. One recent trial in children presented to the emergency department for gastroenteritis demonstrated that ORT was as effective as intravenous fluid therapy for the correction of mild to moderate dehydration [17]. Reports on the use of ORT in veterinary patients are limited, with no randomized blind trials available.

Subcutaneous

Isotonic crystalloid solutions can be administered subcutaneously to treat mild dehydration in animals with vomiting and diarrhea. Patient selection includes patients that cannot be hospitalized and animals with self-limiting conditions that are likely to benefit from rehydration. Large volumes of fluid can be administered easily at various sites. Solutions must be isotonic, sterile, and nonirritating. Hypertonic and hypotonic crystalloids, colloids, and dextrose-containing solutions should not be given subcutaneously. Skin necrosis may occur if fluids are given subcutaneously to a vasoconstricted, hypovolemic, or immunocompromised patient. Septic necrosis of the skin and abscessation may occur if dextrose-containing fluids are administered.

Intravenous

Intravenous fluid administration should be used to correct hypovolemia and moderate to severe dehydration because it allows precise titration of fluids to meet fluid requirements. Caloric requirements also can be met with parenteral nutrition. Crystalloids (isotonic, hypertonic, and hypotonic), colloids, and blood products all can be administered intravenously. Hyperosmolar solutions should be administered into a central vein.

Intraosseous

Intraosseous access is useful in patients that require rapid fluid and drug administration when intravenous access is not possible. Intravenous catheterization in the hypovolemic puppy or kitten with vomiting and diarrhea may be technically challenging, and provision of isotonic crystalloids and dextrose by means of the intraosseous route may be life-saving.

INDICATIONS FOR FLUID THERAPY IN THE TREATMENT OF VOMITING AND DIARRHEA
Dehydration

Dehydration from vomiting and diarrhea can be corrected with oral, subcutaneous, or intravenous administration of fluids. Moderate to severe dehydration, electrolyte or acid-base derangements, and hypovolemia should be corrected by intravenous fluid therapy.

Correction of interstitial fluid deficits should begin during fluid resuscitation for hypovolemia. Crystalloid fluid in the intravascular space rapidly equilibrates with the interstitial space, with only 20% to 25% of the infused volume remaining within the intravascular space after 1 hour [18].

After restoration of normovolemia, the remaining interstitial fluid deficits should be corrected over 12 to 24 hours. Maintenance needs and ongoing losses over that period should be estimated and added to the volume to be infused. Animals should be resuscitated with an isotonic replacement crystalloid and not a hypotonic maintenance fluid. The specific choice of fluid depends on the acid-base and electrolyte status of the animal.

Assessment of the patient, including physical examination and objective assessments of volume status (eg, CVP, arterial blood pressure, urine output), should be performed frequently. Hemoconcentration should resolve (ie, PCV and TS should decrease with fluid administration) and body weight should increase as hydration is restored.

Treatment of Hypovolemia

The primary focus of fluid therapy in the patient with vomiting or diarrhea is restoration of normovolemia. In the case of a patient with clinical signs consistent with shock, a short large-gauge intravenous catheter should be placed and fluid therapy instituted without delay.

The selection of resuscitation fluid is based on the goals of therapy. The fluid of choice in most patients is an isotonic crystalloid, because fluid loss is a major component of the disease process. The next decision is to determine whether a buffered crystalloid would be beneficial. In animals with acidosis, a buffered solution provides the potential benefit of correcting the acidosis. If the acidosis is a result of hypoperfusion, the primary goal of treatment is volume replacement, and, ideally, a buffered electrolyte solution should be used. If the patient is hypochloremic and has metabolic alkalosis with a chloride deficit, 0.9% NaCl represents a more physiologic resuscitation fluid.

Resuscitation should be accomplished by administering multiple small volumes of fluid with frequent physical examination and close monitoring of end points of resuscitation. Dogs that have signs consistent with mild hypoperfusion may only require isotonic crystalloids at a dose of 20 to 30 mL/kg, whereas those with evidence of severe hypoperfusion may require 70 to 90 mL/kg and the addition of colloids. Hypovolemic cats may respond to a single 10- to 20-mL/kg bolus of an isotonic crystalloid solution or may require repeated boluses of isotonic crystalloids and addition of a colloid. Resuscitation should be more conservative if the animal has concurrent heart disease. Physical examination findings consistent with an improvement in perfusion status include a decrease in heart rate, restoration of normal mucous membrane color and capillary refill time, stronger pulses, improvement in mentation, and increase in urine production. More objective variables, including CVP, arterial blood pressure, and quantification of urine output, provide further evidence that normovolemia has been restored. Lactate concentration should decrease after cessation of anaerobic metabolism.

Colloidal therapy may be an important component of treating the hypovolemic patient. Some patients already may be hypoalbuminemic because of GI loss from diarrhea and are not tolerant of large volumes of isotonic crystalloids. Other patients become hypoproteinemic after administration of large volumes of crystalloid fluids and require colloids as part of fluid resuscitation. The authors typically consider a colloid bolus in the hypovolemic patient when total protein concentration is less than 4.5 g/dL. Caution must be exercised to avoid rapid changes in serum electrolyte concentrations.

Correction of Acid-Base and Electrolyte Abnormalities

Treatment of acid-base and electrolyte disturbances is often necessary in the patient with vomiting or diarrhea. Treatment depends on the nature and severity of the abnormality, the underlying disease process, and the chronicity of the condition. Volume status, acid-base imbalance, and severe electrolyte disturbances should be corrected before induction of anesthesia for any necessary procedures.

Hyponatremia should be corrected slowly so as to avoid delayed central pontine myelinolysis. Serum sodium concentration, fluid rate, and chronicity of the hyponatremia determine the optimal concentration of sodium in administered fluids.

Correction of hypokalemia should be achieved with supplemental potassium added to intravenous fluids. A sliding scale has been developed to determine the amount of potassium to be added to fluids (Table 4). The rate of intravenous infusion of potassium-containing fluids should not exceed 0.5 mEq/kg/h, and fluids with supplemental potassium should not be given as boluses.

Oncotic Support

Animals with vomiting and diarrhea may have decreased COP and require colloidal support. Loss of protein into a compromised GI tract, increased vascular permeability with the systemic inflammatory response syndrome (SIRS), decreased albumin production, and aggressive crystalloid therapy all contribute to decreased COP. Hypotensive dogs that are being aggressively resuscitated

Table 4
Amount of potassium to be added to intravenous fluids to correct hypokalemia

Serum potassium (mmol/L)	Potassium (mEq)m to add to 0.9% NaCl, 250 mL
<2.0	20
2.0–2.5	15
2.5–3.0	10
3.0–3.5	7

Rate of potassium administration should not exceed 0.5 mEq/kg/h.

with isotonic crystalloids commonly require colloidal support. Colloidal support is required in the adult hypotensive dog when total plasma protein concentration is less than approximately 4.5 g/dL.

Administration of crystalloids and colloids can result in dilutional coagulopathy, and colloids can decrease concentrations of factor VIII and von Willebrand factor more than would be expected from dilution alone [18]. Use of colloids at higher rates (>20 mL/kg/d) may result in prolongation of clotting times.

FFP is a natural colloid commonly recommended in the veterinary literature to treat hypoalbuminemia. It is a poor source of albumin, however, and evidence supporting its recommendation is lacking. Two liters of FFP would be required to increase the serum albumin concentration in a 20-kg dog from 1.5 to 2.5 g/dL. With ongoing loss of albumin, this dose still would be inadequate. As is the case with all fluids, blood products, and drugs, FFP is not without potential complications. Because of concern about transfusion-related immunomodulation and transfusion reactions, lack of efficacy, and ready availability of synthetic colloids, FFP is not recommended as a treatment to increase a patient's COP or serum albumin concentration.

HA solutions are increasingly being used for treatment of hypoalbuminemia. Solutions have a higher COP (25% HA = 200 mm Hg) than synthetic colloids and provide a carrier protein for the transport, thereby limiting the toxicity of bilirubin, some drugs, and long-chain fatty acids [19]. Patients with vomiting and diarrhea attributable to SIRS (eg, septic peritonitis, pancreatitis) may have endothelial or alveolar epithelial cell injury or dysfunction [20]. These animals may have severe hypoalbuminemia and could benefit from HA. Although critically ill patients have been given HA safely, its use is associated with some risk [21,22].

Nutritional Support

Nothing per os (NPO) has commonly been recommended for all people and animals with vomiting and diarrhea. Growing evidence, however, supports the use of early enteral nutrition. Cited advantages include decreased intestinal mucosal permeability [23], decreased incidence of multiple organ failure [24], and improved clinical outcome [25]. In one study of dogs with CPVE, animals fed by means of a nasoesophageal tube experienced shorter hospital stays, decreased morbidity, and increased weight gain as compared with dogs in which feeding was delayed [26]. Some advocate instituting enteral nutrition as early as possible during the course of illness and using it in preference to parenteral nutrition whenever possible [27].

Enteral nutrition can be provided by esophageal, gastric, or jejunal feeding tubes. Nasoesophageal or nasogastric tubes can be easily placed with minimal or no sedation. Two techniques for minimally invasive placement of nasojejunal tubes also have been described recently [28,29]. A benefit of jejunal feeding tubes over esophageal or gastric feeding tubes is the ability to provide enteral nutrition to animals with protracted vomiting. Jejunal feeding does require use of an elemental diet, however.

SPECIFIC CONDITIONS

Case Example 1: Gastrointestinal Obstruction

A 3-year-old Jack Russell terrier is referred with a 7-day history of vomiting. Initial physical examination findings are listed in Table 5.

The findings of abdominal radiographs are consistent with an intestinal obstruction. Assessment of physical examination findings is consistent with dehydration and hypovolemia secondary to protracted vomiting and reduced fluid intake. After just 24 hours of intestinal obstruction, abnormal secretion and absorption of fluid occur oral and aboral to the obstruction [30]. Instead of absorption, net secretion of electrolytes and water occurs. After 60 minutes of complete obstruction, secretion of fluid can reach 13 mL/min [30]. The presence of a foreign body, intestinal dilatation, and local inflammation all activate sensory pathways that induce vomiting, and fluid and electrolyte losses rapidly occur. In this case example, increased losses secondary to vomiting and luminal fluid sequestration and decreased intake of fluid have resulted in dehydration and hypovolemia.

The first priority is to correct hypovolemia and restore normal tissue perfusion. The dog is given a 30-mL/kg intravenous bolus of a buffered isotonic crystalloid solution over 20 minutes. The results of an emergency database are listed in Table 6.

Dehydration results in increased PCV and total plasma protein concentration (hemoconcentration). In one study, 30% of dogs with GI obstruction had evidence of hemoconcentration [31]. Severity depends on the nature (partial or complete obstruction) and chronicity of the obstruction in addition to time to presentation.

Acid-base and electrolyte abnormalities are common in animals with GI disease [32]. Hypochloremia is the most common electrolyte abnormality in dogs with GI foreign bodies because of the high chloride load lost through GI sequestration and vomiting [31]. Hyponatremia is seen in approximately 20% of dogs and may occur in the presence of hemoconcentration [31]. The decrease in serum sodium concentration suggests a hypertonic loss of fluid or, more likely, a gain in free water. Two mechanisms may contribute to hyponatremia. First, bowel distention causes an increase in the secretion of sodium into the lumen [33]. Affected dogs are still able to drink water, and

Table 5	
Initial physical examination of case example 1	
Heart rate (beats per minute)	180
Respiratory rate (breaths per minute)	32
Temperature (°C)	38.0
Mucous membrane color	Pale
Capillary refill time (seconds)	3
Pulse quality	Weak
Abdominal palpation	Midabdominal pain

Table 6
Initial emergency database of case example 1

	Patient	Laboratory reference range
Na$^+$ (mEq/L)	124	144–150
K$^+$ (mEq/L)	2.5	3.1–4.7
Cl$^-$ (mEq/L)	84	113–125
pH (at 38°C)	7.54	7.35–7.45
Base excess	17.3	±4
Glucose (mg/dL)	248	57–108
Lactate (mmol/L)	3.1	0.3–3.2
PCV (%)	54	37–55
TS (g/dL)	8.2	5.5–7.0

therefore reabsorb free water despite sodium-rich losses into the GI tract. Second, release of vasopressin (antidiuretic hormone) in response to decreased effective circulating volume causes increased reabsorption of water in the collecting tubules of the kidney [34]. Patients with linear foreign bodies are more likely to develop hyponatremia, possibly as a result of development of a partial obstruction [31].

Hypokalemia is common in dogs with intestinal obstruction attributable to the high potassium load lost from vomiting and fluid sequestration. Hypovolemia and secondary aldosterone-induced sodium reabsorption and potassium excretion in the principal cells of the collecting duct further worsen the hypokalemia.

Metabolic alkalosis is the most common acid-base disturbance in patients with intestinal obstruction [31]. Metabolic alkalosis is thought to occur secondary to the loss of chloride and proton-rich fluid in the vomitus and concurrent hypovolemia. Under normal conditions, the secretion of HCl in the stomach is balanced by secretion of an equal amount of HCO_3^- by the pancreas. Loss of the chloride and proton-rich fluid by vomiting leads to metabolic alkalosis. Metabolic alkalosis persists as a result of limited renal excretion of bicarbonate secondary to decreased effective circulating volume and decreased chloride delivery to the collecting tubules. In an attempt to prevent sodium loss and further depletion of effective circulating volume, sodium is reabsorbed with bicarbonate in the cortical collecting tubule. Chloride depletion also increases net distal bicarbonate reabsorption by means of increased hydrogen ion secretion and decreased bicarbonate secretion [35]. The result is persistent hypochloremic metabolic alkalosis. High (proximal) GI obstruction is often said to result in hypochloremic hypokalemic metabolic alkalosis, whereas more distal obstruction is said to be more likely to result in metabolic acidosis [36]. Boag and colleagues [31] found no significant association between electrolyte or acid-base abnormalities and the site of the foreign body in dogs with GI obstruction, however.

Hyperlactatemia has been reported to occur in 40% of patients with GI foreign bodies [31]. Hyperlactatemia may cause primary metabolic acidosis or contribute to mixed metabolic acidosis and alkalosis. Hypovolemia secondary to increased GI losses leads to a decrease in organ perfusion with resultant tissue hypoxia and an increase in lactate production. Lactic acidosis occurs when production of lactate in the muscle and the gut exceeds its use by the liver and kidneys [10].

The dog responds well to the fluid bolus, with an improvement in mentation and normalization of heart rate, pulse strength, and mucous membrane color. The mean arterial blood pressure is 70 mm Hg. The dog is started on 0.9% NaCl at a dosage of 5 mL/kg/h.

Further patient stabilization is essential before anesthetizing the patient for exploratory laparotomy. Intravenous isotonic crystalloid therapy is necessary to continue restoration of normovolemia and to correct dehydration. Provision of chloride is essential when correcting hypochloremic metabolic alkalosis. The initial treatment of choice is thus 0.9% NaCl. With volume expansion, more bicarbonate and chloride ions are delivered to the distal nephron, which possesses a greater capacity to reabsorb chloride than bicarbonate [37]. Chloride is retained, bicarbonate is excreted, and the metabolic alkalosis is corrected [38]. Correction of hypochloremic metabolic alkalosis typically is rapid (see Table 6; Table 7), and patients then can be switched to a solution with a lower concentration of sodium.

A venous blood gas measurement repeated after 4 hours of fluid therapy is provided in Table 7. After further stabilization, the dog is anesthetized for an exploratory laparotomy. Pieces of cloth are removed by means of a jejunal enterotomy, and the dog recovers uneventfully.

Case Example 2: Hypoadrenocorticism

A 5-year-old, male, castrated American Eskimo dog is presented to the veterinary hospital with a 1-week history of lethargy, anorexia, vomiting, bloody diarrhea, and weakness. The findings of the initial physical examination and emergency database are listed in Tables 8 and 9.

The clinical picture of decreased perfusion with an inappropriately low heart rate is the classic presentation of a dog with hypoadrenocorticism. Immune-

Table 7		
Emergency database of case example 1 after fluid therapy		
	Patient	Laboratory reference range
Na$^+$ (mEq/L)	128	144–150
K$^+$ (mEq/L)	2.9	3.1–4.7
Cl$^-$ (mEq/L)	100	113–125
pH (at 38.8°C)	7.47	7.35–7.45
Base excess	1.4	±4
Glucose (mg/dL)	130	57–108
Lactate (mmol/L)	1.3	0.3–3.2
PCV (%)	38	37–55
TS (g/dL)	5.7	5.5–7.0

Table 8
Initial physical examination of case example 2

Heart rate (beats per minute)	68
Respiratory rate (breaths per minute)	24
Temperature (°C)	36.5
Mucous membrane color	Pale pink
Capillary refill time (seconds)	2
Pulse quality	Weak

mediated destruction of the adrenal cortex, resulting in deficiencies in glucocorticoids and mineralocorticoids, is the most common cause of hypoadrenocorticism [39]. Hypoperfusion results from hypovolemia, decreased systemic vascular resistance (glucocorticoids aid in maintenance of vascular tone), and bradycardia. There are two main mechanisms responsible for the severe hypovolemia observed in patients that have hypoadrenocorticism. First, increased losses from the GI tract and decreased intake lead to progressive dehydration and hypovolemia. Second, the absence of adrenal production of the mineralocorticoid aldosterone results in failure of the normal mechanisms of sodium and water retention in addition to potassium and hydrogen ion secretion in the connecting segment and principal cells of the cortical collecting tubule [34]. Sodium and water are lost in the urine, whereas potassium and hydrogen ions are retained, resulting in progressive dehydration, hyponatremia, hypovolemia, hyperkalemia, and metabolic acidosis. The hyperlactatemia is consistent with anaerobic metabolism resulting from decreased tissue perfusion. Patients commonly are azotemic and also may be hypoglycemic and hypercalcemic [39].

An electrocardiogram is performed and reveals prolongation of the PR interval, widened QRS complexes, and tented T waves. The dog is infused with a buffered isotonic crystalloid solution (30 mL/kg) containing sodium (140 mEq/L) over 20 minutes.

Table 9
Initial emergency blood screen of case example 2

	Patient	Laboratory reference range
Na^+ (mEq/L)	130	144–50
K^+ (mEq/L)	7.46	3.1–4.7
Cl^- (mEq/L)	104	113–125
pH (at 38°C)	7.35	7.35–7.45
Base excess	−5.4	±4
Glucose (mg/dL)	121	57–108
Lactate (mmol/L)	4.1	0.3–3.2
Blood urea nitrogen (mg/dL)	109	10–31
Creatinine (mg/dL)	7.1	0.7–1.8
PCV (%)	45	37–55
TS (g/dL)	5.4	5.5–7.0

The primary goals of fluid therapy in the patient that has vomiting and diarrhea secondary to hypoadrenocorticism are to restore normovolemia, correct hyperkalemia, and resolve metabolic acidosis.

Correction of hypovolemia should be achieved with repeated boluses of an isotonic crystalloid solution. Because the patient is hyponatremic and hyperkalemic, 0.9% NaCl often is cited as the most appropriate fluid. Improvement of metabolic acidosis may not be as rapid as may occur with administration of a balanced isotonic crystalloid solution, however, and the serum sodium concentration may increase too rapidly, resulting in delayed central pontine myelinolysis [40]. The sodium concentration should not be corrected at a rate greater than 0.5 mEq/h [41]. Other cited benefits of 0.9% NaCl include the absence of potassium in the fluid. However, severe hyperkalemia should immediately be treated with calcium (for its cardioprotective effects), with or without insulin and dextrose (to decrease extracellular potassium concentration). Additionally, the low concentration of potassium delivered in balanced solutions (4 mEq/L in lactated Ringer's solution) still dilutes the serum potassium concentration, and the buffering effects also may help to drive potassium into cells. A buffered isotonic crystalloid solution with a sodium concentration of 140 mEq/L or less is appropriate for resuscitation of the hypovolemic patient that has hypoadrenocorticism.

Hyperkalemia can be a life-threatening emergency. Hypoadrenocorticism should be suspected in any dog that has clinical signs consistent with hypoperfusion and an inappropriately low heart rate. Hyperkalemia may be confirmed with venous blood analysis or observation of typical electrocardiographic (ECG) changes. The earliest ECG change is a symmetric increase in T wave amplitude (tenting). As serum potassium concentration increases further, conduction slows and is manifest by prolongation of the PR interval and widening of the QRS complex. Eventually, P waves flatten and disappear, and T waves merge with the preceding QRS complex, resulting in a sine wave pattern [42]. Fluid therapy decreases the serum potassium concentration sufficiently in most patients that have hypoadrenocorticism. Occasionally, more aggressive therapy to protect the heart or decrease serum potassium concentration rapidly is necessary. Treatment with 10% calcium gluconate (0.5 mL/kg) does not decrease serum potassium concentration but restores the difference between resting and threshold potentials and allows normal cardiac conduction to occur. This therapy is rapid but short-lived. Intravenously administered dextrose (0.5 g/kg) and regular insulin (0.2 IU/kg) decrease the serum potassium concentration by promoting intracellular translocation of potassium. Fluid therapy, as described previously, further decreases the serum potassium concentration by means of dilution. Sodium bicarbonate therapy often is recommended for correction of hyperkalemia and metabolic acidosis. Because of the efficacy of appropriate fluid therapy (calcium gluconate and dextrose with insulin), however, the authors rarely use sodium bicarbonate in the treatment of hyperkalemia. Adverse effects of sodium bicarbonate, such as metabolic alkalosis, paradoxical central nervous system acidosis, and ionized hypocalcemia, must be considered before its use [10].

After two 30-mL/kg boluses (each over 20 minutes) of an isotonic crystalloid solution, the dog's heart rate is 120 beats per minute and pulses are improved. Indirect blood pressure (Doppler) is 90 mm Hg. After jugular catheter placement, the CVP is 3 mm Hg, PCV is 38%, and total plasma protein concentration is 3.8 g/dL. The dog is given a 5-mL/kg intravenous bolus of a synthetic colloid in 0.9% NaCl over 30 minutes. An indwelling urinary catheter is placed.

Multiple small-volume boluses with frequent reassessment of physical examination, objective hemodynamic monitoring, and collection of emergency laboratory data provide the clinician with the information necessary to provide optimal therapy. Blood volume commonly is assessed indirectly by arterial pressure, CVP, PCV, TS, and determination of urine output. Monitoring CVP is important when multiple boluses of fluids have not corrected perfusion and a more objective assessment of preload is necessary. Resuscitation to normovolemia is reflected by a CVP of 8 to 10 mm Hg, although trends may be more important than an absolute number [43].

Repeated measurement of TS permits resuscitation with the most appropriate fluid. A decrease in TS secondary to aggressive crystalloid therapy necessitates the provision of colloidal support. Colloidal support to the hypotensive patient is warranted when the TS value is less than 4.5 g/dL.

After administration of the colloid bolus, the heart rate is 100 beats per minute, CVP is 7 mm Hg, mean arterial pressure is 86 mm Hg, and urine output is greater than 2 mL/kg/h. Repeated venous blood gas results are listed in Table 10.

Variables indicative of perfusion (eg, physical examination, lactate concentration) have normalized after restoration of normovolemia. The sodium concentration has not increased by more than 0.5 mEq/h, the maximum recommended. The potassium concentration has been decreased with fluid therapy alone.

Case Example 3: Canine Parvoviral Enteritis

A 6-month old, 25-kg, unvaccinated, male American pit bull terrier is presented with a 4-day history of lethargy, anorexia, vomiting, and diarrhea. Initial

Table 10		
Emergency blood screen of case example 2 after fluid therapy		
	Patient	Laboratory reference range
Na^+ (mEq/L)	131	144–150
K^+ (mEq/L)	5.64	3.1–4.7
Cl^- (mEq/L)	104	113–125
pH (at 38°C)	7.37	7.35–7.45
Lactate (mmol/L)	2.6	0.3–2.5
Blood urea nitrogen (mg/dL)	78	10–31
Creatinine (mg/dL)	5.2	0.7–1.8
PCV (%)	34	37–55
TS (g/dL)	4.0	5.5–7.0

physical examination findings and an emergency database are provided in Tables 11 and 12. A fecal antigen test for parvovirus is positive. A 20-mL/kg intravenous bolus of a buffered isotonic crystalloid solution is administered over 30 minutes.

CPVE is a common cause of severe vomiting and diarrhea. Fluid therapy is crucial to patient survival, and without treatment, mortality is as high as 90% [44]. In contrast, with appropriate and aggressive treatment, survival can exceed 90% [45]. Fluid therapy is the mainstay of this treatment.

As a result of the increased losses (ie, vomiting, diarrhea) and decreased intake, affected dogs typically are dehydrated and hypovolemic. Hypoglycemia is commonly observed in patients that have CPVE and is considered to be secondary to profound malnutrition, hypermetabolism, inadequate liver function, and sepsis [46]. Restoration of normovolemia and correction of hypoglycemia should be the immediate treatment priorities. Resuscitation with multiple boluses of a balanced isotonic crystalloid solution at a rate of 20 to 30 mL/kg and frequent reassessment of the patient as outlined previously are recommended. The dog in this case example was presented with signs consistent with 8% to 10% dehydration and mild hypovolemia (eg, prolonged skin tent, increased heart rate, pale pink mucous membranes, mildly prolonged capillary refill time, good pulse quality).

After the initial fluid bolus, the heart rate is 120 beats per minute and the capillary refill time is approximately 1 second. A fluid rate is calculated to restore deficits, provide maintenance needs, and replace ongoing losses (vomiting and diarrhea) over a 24-hour period.

> Replacement (restore deficits)
>   Fluid deficit = [body weight (kg)] × [% dehydration] (25 kg × 10% = 2.5 L)
> Maintenance
>   Maintenance requirements = 60 mL/kg/d (60 × 25 kg/d = 1500 mL/d or
>   1.5 L/d)
> Ongoing losses (vomiting and diarrhea)
>   Vomiting: 10 times a day with estimated volume of 50 mL = 500 mL/d
>   Diarrhea: five times per day with an estimated volume of 125 mL = 625 mL/d
>   Total = 1125 mL/d or 1.125 L/d
> Total fluid requirement
>   Replacement + maintenance + ongoing losses (2.5 L + 1.5 L + 1.125 L)
>   = 5.125 L or 213 mL/h

The dog is placed on a buffered isotonic crystalloid solution at a rate of 213 mL/h. K^+ (28 mEq) and 50% dextrose (25 g) are added to fluids (1 L) to create a 2.5% dextrose solution. Heart rate, respiratory rate, mucous membrane color, capillary refill time, pulse quality, auscultation, and temperature are recorded every 6 hours. PCV, TS, blood glucose, and body weight are measured every 6 hours, and venous blood gas and serum electrolyte concentrations are repeated after 12 hours. Frequency of urination, defecation, and vomiting is noted. The fluid rate is reassessed after 6 hours. Other medications indicated in the treatment of CPVE are not discussed in this article.

Table 11
Initial physical examination of case example 3

Heart rate (beats per minute)	170
Respiratory rate (breaths per minute)	32
Temperature (°C)	39.5
Mucous membrane color	Pale pink
Capillary refill time (seconds)	3
Pulse quality	Good

Despite marked GI losses, dogs with CPVE usually have a normal or mildly decreased serum sodium concentration (Cynthia M. Otto, unpublished data, 2006). Potassium is typically within normal limits at presentation, although supplementation often is required after fluid resuscitation. Table 2 illustrates the amount of potassium chloride that should be added to fluids. The clinician should be aware of the high rates of fluids that dogs with CPVE require, however, and alter potassium supplementation accordingly to avoid excessively rapid administration of potassium and development of hyperkalemia.

After 6 hours of fluid therapy, indicators of perfusion are within normal limits. Urine output has been adequate, but the dog has continued to vomit and have diarrhea. Repeated PCV and TS values are 30% and 4.4 g/dL, respectively. The blood glucose concentration is 112 mg/dL. The dog is maintained on a balanced electrolyte solution with 2.5% dextrose and started on a synthetic colloid in 0.9% NaCl at a rate of 25 mL/h. The rate of isotonic crystalloids is reduced to 150 mL/h.

TS may be low, normal, or occasionally high at presentation in dogs with CPVE. The normal range of albumin and TS for puppies and kittens is lower than that of adult dogs. TS values rapidly decrease after fluid resuscitation, however. The serum albumin concentration may be decreased as a result of sepsis-induced SIRS and increased loss of protein through the GI tract [19].

Table 12
Initial emergency blood screen of case example 3

	Patient	Laboratory reference range
Na⁺ (mEq/L)	133	144–150
K⁺ (mEq/L)	3.5	3.1–4.7
Cl⁻ (mEq/L)	112	113–125
pH (at 38°C)	7.30	7.35–7.45
Base excess	–7.5	±4
Glucose (mg/dL)	56	70–110
Lactate (mmol/L)	4.4	0.3–2.0
Blood urea nitrogen (mg/dL)	33	10–31
Creatinine (mg/dL)	1.7	0.7–1.8
PCV (%)	40	37–55
TS (g/dL)	6.7	5.5–7.0

With critical illness, the body is in a catabolic state and generation of acute-phase proteins occurs at the expense of albumin. Increased extravasation from abnormal vascular endothelium further depletes the serum albumin concentration and TS as measured by refractometry.

Serum albumin contributes approximately 75% to 80% of COP [21]. Low COP is associated with increased fluid flux from the vasculature into the interstitium and the development of edema. Dogs with CPVE and hypoalbuminemia therefore may require colloidal support. Options include synthetic colloids or natural colloids. Synthetic colloids include hydroxyethyl starch, gelatin, and dextran, and they have the advantage of being widely available and relatively inexpensive. Synthetic colloids may prolong coagulation times; however, because dogs with CPVE have been shown to be hypercoagulable [47], this effect is rarely of clinical relevance when used at administration rates less than 1 mL/kg/h. Natural colloids include HA, FFP, and whole blood. Hypoalbuminemia in dogs with CPVE typically is mild to moderate, and given the risks associated with its use, HA is rarely indicated in this patient population. Despite the widespread recommendation that FFP be used in the treatment of hypoalbuminemia, it is a poor source of albumin and evidence supporting this recommendation is lacking. Current "Surviving Sepsis Guidelines (2004)" in human beings state that the use of FFP in septic patients should be limited to those in whom there is active bleeding or planned invasive procedures [48].

SUMMARY

Fluid therapy in the patient with vomiting and diarrhea is essential to correct hypovolemia, dehydration, acid-base imbalance, and serum electrolyte abnormalities. It is often difficult to predict acid-base or electrolyte disturbances; blood gas analysis therefore is useful. Fluid therapy should be tailored to the individual patient, with restoration of normovolemia and correction of life-threatening acid-base, electrolyte, and metabolic disturbances the primary therapeutic aim.

References

[1] Hornby PJ. Central neurocircuitry associated with emesis. Am J Med 2001;111:106S–12S.
[2] Yuan CS, Barber WD. Area postrema: gastric vagal input from proximal stomach and interactions with nucleus tractus solitarius in the cat. Brain Res Bull 1993;30:119–25.
[3] Boissonade FM, Sharkey KA, Davison JS. Fos expression in ferret dorsal vagal complex after peripheral emetic stimuli. Am J Physiol 1994;266:R1118–26.
[4] Borison HL. Area postrema: chemoreceptor circumventricular organ of the medulla oblongata. Prog Neurobiol 1989;32:351–90.
[5] Hall EJ, German AJ. Diseases of the small intestine. In: Ettinger SJ, Feldman EC, editors. Textbook of internal medicine. 6th edition. St. Louis (MO): Elsevier Saunders; 2005. p. 1332–78.
[6] Ooms L, Degryse A. Pathogenesis and pharmacology of diarrhea. Vet Res 1986;10: 355–97.
[7] Simpson KW, Birnbaum N. Fluid and electrolytes disturbances in gastrointestinal and pancreatic disease. In: DiBartola SP, editor. Fluid, electrolytes, and acid-base disorders in small animal practice. 3rd edition. St. Louis (MO): Elsevier Saunders; 2006. p. 420–36.

[8] Strombeck DR, Guilford WG. Classification, pathophysiology, and symptomatic treatment of diarrheal diseases. In: Strombeck DR, Guilford WG, editors. Small animal gastroenterology. 2nd edition. Davis (CA): Stonegate Publishing Company; 1990. p. 277–95.

[9] Rose BD, Post TW. Hypovolemic states. In: Rose BD, Post TW, editors. Clinical physiology of acid-base and electrolyte disorders. 5th edition. New York: McGraw-Hill; 2001. p. 415–46.

[10] DiBartola SP. Metabolic acid-base disorders. In: DiBartola SP, editor. Fluid, electrolytes, and acid-base disorders in small animal practice. 3rd edition. St. Louis (MO): Elsevier Saunders; 2006. p. 251–83.

[11] Nelson DC, McGrew WRG, Hoyumpa AM. Hypernatremia and lactulose therapy. JAMA 1983;249:1295–8.

[12] Strombeck DR, Guilford WG. Gastric structure and function. In: Strombeck DR, Guilford WG, editors. Small animal gastroenterology. 2nd edition. Davis (CA): Stonegate Publishing Company; 1990. p. 167–86.

[13] Fordtran JS. Speculations on the pathogenesis of diarrhea. Fed Proc 1967;26:1405–14.

[14] Burrows CF. Chronic diarrhea in the dog. Vet Clin North Am 1983;13:521–40.

[15] Strombeck DR, Guilford WG. Small and large intestine, normal structure and function. In: Strombeck DR, Guilford WG, editors. Small animal gastroenterology. 2nd edition. Davis (CA): Stonegate Publishing Company; 1990. p. 244–78.

[16] Practice parameter: the management of acute gastroenteritis in young children. American Academy of Pediatrics, Provisional Committee on Quality Improvement, Subcommittee on Acute Gastroenteritis. Pediatrics 1996;97:424–35.

[17] Spandorfer PR, Alessandrini EA, Joffe MD, et al. Oral versus intravenous rehydration of moderately dehydrated children: a randomised, controlled trial. Pediatrics 2005;115: 295–301.

[18] Hughes D, Boag AK. Fluid therapy with macromolecular plasma volume expanders. In: DiBartola SP, editor. Fluid, electrolytes, and acid-base disorders in small animal practice. 3rd edition. St. Louis (MO): Elsevier Saunders; 2006. p. 621–34.

[19] Mazzaferro EM, Rudloff E, Kirby R. The role of albumin replacement in the critically ill veterinary patient. J Vet Emerg Crit Care 2002;12:113–24.

[20] Wheeler AP, Bernard GR. Treating patients with sepsis. N Engl J Med 1999;340:207–14.

[21] Matthews KA, Barry M. The use of 25% human serum albumin: outcome and efficacy in raising serum albumin and systemic blood pressure in critically ill dogs and cats. J Vet Emerg Crit Care 2005;15:110–8.

[22] Cohn LA, Kerl ME, Lennox CE, et al. Response of healthy dogs to infusions of human serum albumin. Am J Vet Res 2007;68:657–63.

[23] Hadfield RJ, Sinclair DG, Houldsworth PE, et al. Effects of enteral and parenteral nutrition on gut mucosal permeability in the critically ill. Am J Respir Crit Care Med 1995;152:1545–8.

[24] Kompan L, Kremzar B, Gadzijev E, et al. Effects of early enteral nutrition on intestinal permeability and the development of multiple organ failure after multiple injury. Intensive Care Med 1999;25:157–61.

[25] Austrums E, Pupelis G, Snippe K. Postoperative enteral stimulation by gut feeding improves outcomes in severe acute pancreatitis. Nutrition 2003;19:487–91.

[26] Mohr AJ, Leisewitz AL, Jacobson LS, et al. Effect of early enteral nutrition on intestinal permeability, intestinal protein loss, and outcome in dogs with severe parvoviral enteritis. J Vet Intern Med 2003;19:791–8.

[27] Heyland DK, Cook DJ, Guyatt GH. Enteral nutrition in the critically ill patient: a critical review of the evidence. Intensive Care Med 1993;19:435–42.

[28] Beal MW, Jutkowitz LA, Brown AJ. Development of a novel method for fluoroscopically-guided nasojejunal feeding tube placement in dogs [abstract]. J Vet Emer Crit Care 2007;17:S1–22.

[29] Wohl JS. Nasojejunal feeding tube placement using fluoroscopic guidance: technique and clinical experience in dogs. J Vet Emer Crit Care 2006;16:S27–33.

[30] Shields R. The absorption and secretion of fluid and electrolytes by the obstructed bowel. Br J Surg 1965;52:774–9.

[31] Boag AK, Coe RJ, Martinez TA, et al. Acid-base and electrolyte abnormalities in dogs with gastrointestinal foreign bodies. J Vet Intern Med 2005;19:816–21.

[32] Cornelius LM, Rawlings CA. Arterial blood gas and acid-base values in dogs with various diseases and signs of dehydration. J Am Vet Med Assoc 1981;178:992–5.

[33] Lantz GC. The pathophysiology of acute mechanical small bowel obstruction. Compend Contin Edu Pract Vet 1981;3:910–7.

[34] Rose BD, Post TW. Effects of hormones on renal function. In: Rose BD, Post TW, editors. Clinical physiology of acid-base and electrolyte disorders. 5th edition. New York: McGraw-Hill; 2001. p. 163–238.

[35] Rose BD, Rennke HG. Acid-base physiology and metabolic alkalosis. In: Rose BD, Rennke HG, editors. Renal pathophysiology—the essentials. 1st edition. Philadelphia: Lippincott Williams & Wilkins; 1994. p. 123–51.

[36] Twedt DC, Grauer GF. Fluid therapy for gastrointestinal, pancreatic and hepatic disorders. Vet Clinic North Am Small Anim Pract 1982;12:463–85.

[37] de Morais HAS, Biondo AW. Disorders of chloride: hyperchloremia and hypochloremia. In: DiBartola SP, editor. Fluid, electrolytes, and acid-base disorders in small animal practice. 3rd edition. St. Louis (MO). Elsevier Saunders; 2006. p. 80–90.

[38] Galla JH, Luke RG. Chloride transport and disorders of acid-base balance. Annu Rev Physiol 1988;50:141–58.

[39] Hertage ME. Hypoadrenocorticism. In: Ettinger SJ, Feldman EC, editors. Textbook of internal medicine. 6th edition. St. Louis (MO). Elsevier Saunders; 2005. p. 1612–22.

[40] Brady CA, Vite CH, et al. Severe neurological sequelae in a dog after treatment of hypoadrenal crisis. J Am Vet Med Assoc 1999;215:222–5.

[41] DiBartola SP. Disorders of sodium and water: hypernatremia and hyponatremia. In: DiBartola SP, editor. Fluid, electrolytes, and acid-base disorders in small animal practice. 3rd edition. St. Louis (MO). Elsevier Saunders; 2006. p. 47–79.

[42] Arieff AI. Acid-base, electrolyte, and metabolic abnormalities. In: Parillo JE, Dellinger RP, editors. Critical care medicine—principles of diagnosis and management in the adult. 2nd edition. St. Louis (MO). Mosby; 2002. p. 1169–203.

[43] Hughes D, Beal MW. Emergency vascular access. Vet Clin North Am 2000;30:491–507.

[44] Kariuki NM, Nyaga, et al. Effectiveness of fluids and antibiotics as supportive therapy of canine parvovirus-2 enteritis in puppies. Bull Anim Health Prod Afr 1990;38:379–89.

[45] Otto CM, Jackson CB, et al. Recombinant bactericidal/permeability-increasing protein for treatment of parvovirus enteritis: a randomised double-blinded, placebo-controlled trial. J Vet Intern Med 2001;15:355–60.

[46] Prittie J. Canine parvoviral enteritis: a review of diagnosis, management, and prevention. J Vet Emer Crit Care 2004;14:167–76.

[47] Otto CM, Rieser TM, et al. Evidence of hypercoagulability in dogs with parvoviral enteritis. J Am Vet Med Assoc 2000;217:1500–4.

[48] Zimmerman JL. Use of blood products in sepsis: an evidence-based review. Crit Care Med 2004;32:S542–7.

Managing Fluid and Electrolyte Disorders in Renal Failure

Cathy Langston, DVM

Nephrology, Urology, and Hemodialysis Unit, Animal Medical Center,
510 E. 62nd Street, New York, NY 10065, USA

The kidneys are responsible for maintaining homeostasis in the body; kidney failure typically leads to derangements of fluid, electrolyte, and acid-base balance. The goal of treatment is to correct these derangements. Kidney disease is classified into acute and chronic disease, which is a convenient way to view what frequently are markedly different manifestation syndromes. Acute and chronic kidney disease (CKD) may vary from mild to severe. Many patients with acute kidney injury (AKI) require hospitalization for optimal management. Patients with CKD may present in a decompensated state and need hospitalization, or their fluid and electrolyte disturbances may be managed on an outpatient basis. Despite the different types of kidney disease, many of the principles of fluid and electrolyte management are the same regardless of the underlying cause.

Intrinsic renal failure occurs when damage to the renal parenchyma occurs. The damage may be reversible or irreversible and can include damage to the glomeruli, tubules, interstitium, or renal vasculature. Prerenal azotemia occurs when blood flow to the kidney is decreased, as may occur with hypovolemia, hypotension, or increased renal vascular resistance. Prerenal azotemia is rapidly reversible once the underlying disorder has been controlled. Postrenal azotemia occurs when there is an obstruction to urine flow, from the level of the renal pelvis to the urethra, or when urine leaks into surrounding tissue and is reabsorbed (eg, ruptured bladder, ureter, or urethra). Postrenal azotemia also can be reversed rapidly by diverting the urine with a urinary catheter or peritoneal catheter (in cases of an intra-abdominal urinary tract rupture). With prerenal and postrenal causes of azotemia, longstanding problems may progress to intrinsic renal failure. Although substantial renal disease can be present without azotemia, fluid therapy generally is not necessary in those situations. In fact, fluid therapy may not be necessary in cases of compensated chronic renal failure with mild to moderate azotemia.

E-mail address: cathy.langston@amcny.org

0195-5616/08/$ – see front matter
doi:10.1016/j.cvsm.2008.01.007

FLUID TREATMENT

Normal fluid losses consist of insensible and sensible losses. Insensible losses are those that are not easily measured, such as water lost via respiration, normal stool, or sweating. Sweating is negligible in dogs and cats. Respiratory losses vary, and dogs can lose considerable amounts of fluid by excessive panting, but 22 mL/kg/d is the average. The main sensible fluid loss in the normal patient is urine output. Additional sensible losses include the volume lost from vomiting, diarrhea, body cavity drainage, and burns. In healthy animals, these losses are replaced by drinking water and the fluid contained in food. In sick animals that may not be voluntarily consuming food or water or may be restricted from consumption because of vomiting, fluid therapy is necessary to replace these losses. With renal disease, urine volume frequently is abnormally high or low or inappropriate for the situation, and fluid therapy is tailored for the individual patient to maintain fluid balance.

FLUID THERAPY FOR HOSPITALIZED PATIENTS

Although oliguria and anuria are the classic manifestations of AKI, it may present with polyuria, which frequently portends less severe renal injury [1,2]. AKI also may be indicated by a subtle increase in serum creatinine concentration (> 50% of baseline) or urine volume inappropriate for the volume of fluid administered. In this early stage of injury, attempts to limit further renal damage are warranted. Patients with CKD may present in a decompensated uremic crisis, which may represent AKI superimposed on chronic disease.

Many drugs have been evaluated for their benefit in treating AKI, and some are helpful in certain settings. The most effective therapy of AKI is careful management of fluid balance, however, which involves thoughtful assessment of hydration, a fluid treatment plan personalized for the specific patient, repeated and frequent reassessment of fluid and electrolyte balance, and appropriate changes in the treatment plan in response to the rapidly changing clinical situation of the patient.

ASSESSING HYDRATION

The key feature to an appropriate fluid plan is accurate determination of hydration status. Blood volume can be measured using indicator dilution techniques, radioactive tracers, bioimpedance spectroscopy, or other methods. Unfortunately, readily available accurate measurement of blood volume is not feasible in general practice settings.

Despite a lack of precise objective data, there are many ways to estimate hydration. A deficit of the extravascular fluid compartment (interstitial and intracellular) causes dehydration. A severe deficit may decrease the intravascular compartment and lead to poor perfusion. Dehydration of less than approximately 5% is difficult to detect clinically. A 5% to 6% deficit leads to tacky mucous membranes. Six percent to 8% dehydration causes dry mucous membranes and decreased skin elasticity. By 8% to 10% dehydration, the eyes may be sunken; with more than 12% dehydration, the corneas are dry, mentation is dull, and perfusion is impaired [3]. Overhydration may be manifested by wet mucous membranes, increased skin elasticity (heavy or gelatinous), shivering, nausea, vomiting, restlessness, serous nasal discharge, chemosis, tachypnea, cough, dyspnea, pulmonary crackles, pulmonary edema, pleural effusion, ascites, diarrhea, or subcutaneous (SC) edema (especially in the hocks and intermandibular space) [4,5].

Interpretation of these physical findings can be difficult. Patients with uremia frequently have xerostomia, which causes dry mucous membranes independent of hydration status. Hypoalbuminemia or vasculitis may cause interstitial fluid accumulation despite an intravascular volume deficit. Emaciation or advanced age decreases elasticity of the skin.

Central venous pressure (CVP) measurement using a centrally placed intravenous (IV) catheter may provide information about intravascular filling. A volume-depleted animal has a CVP less than 0 cm H_2O. A CVP of more than 10 cm H_2O is consistent with volume overload or right-sided congestive heart failure [6]. Pleural effusion falsely increases CVP, however [7]. An accurate body weight recorded before illness is an invaluable aid to assessing hydration. Body weight should be measured at least twice a day on the same scale to monitor fluid balance. A sick animal may lose up to 0.5% to 1% body weight per day because of anorexia; changes in excess of this amount are caused by changes in fluid status [8]. An increase in blood pressure may indicate a gain of fluid. Conversely, a decrease in blood pressure may indicate a net loss of fluid. Because of the high percentage of patients with hypertension (80% of dogs with severe acute uremia and 20%–30% of dogs and cats with CKD), the trend rather than the absolute value is of more use in assessing changes in hydration status [4,9,10]. Similarly, changes in trends for packed cell volume and total solids may reflect changes in volume in the absence of bleeding or blood transfusion. Because each variable is impacted by factors other than hydration status, these factors must be viewed in aggregate.

ROUTE OF FLUID ADMINISTRATION

In most hospitalized patients, the IV route is the most appropriate route of fluid administration. In some situations, such as with extremely small patients, including neonates or young puppies or kittens, IV catheterization may be difficult. Intraosseous fluid administration can be used in that setting. In dehydrated patients, fluids administered into the peritoneal cavity are readily absorbed, but this method is not reliable for promoting diuresis or in patients with oliguria. Fluid administered SC may not be absorbed rapidly or completely, and it is not possible to administer a large volume by this route, which makes SC fluid administration inappropriate for the hospital setting. It may, however, play a role in outpatient therapy (see later discussion).

TYPE OF FLUID

A balanced polyionic solution (eg, lactated Ringer's solution, Plasmalyte-148, Normosol-R) is an appropriate choice for initial volume resuscitation and replacement of the dehydration deficit. Physiologic (0.9%) NaCl contains no potassium and is a suitable initial choice for patients with hyperkalemia. After rehydration, maintenance fluids with a lower sodium concentration are more appropriate (eg, 0.45% NaCl with 2.5% dextrose, half-strength lactated Ringer's solution with 2.5% dextrose). Dextrose 5% in water is rarely appropriate as the sole fluid choice, but it may be combined with lactated Ringer's solution or 0.9% saline to make half- or three-quarter-strength sodium solutions (25 mL lactated Ringer's solution + 25 mL dextrose 5% in water = 50 mL half-strength lactated Ringer's solution + 2.5% dextrose).

Colloidal solutions (eg, hydroxyethyl starch, 6% dextran) may be appropriate if hypoalbuminemia is present. Hypoalbuminemia may be present with protein-losing nephropathy, diseases associated with vasculitis, or severe gastrointestinal losses or bleeding. The recommended dosage is 20 mL/kg/d, and it may be used to replace the insensible portion when using the "ins-and-outs" method (see later discussion). Higher dosages may be associated with coagulopathy. An alternative to synthetic colloids is human albumin, but use of this product carries a risk of anaphylaxis [11,12].

Treatment of the patient with acute uremic crisis caused by protein-losing nephropathy with severe hypoalbuminemia presents additional considerations. The increased intravascular volume and hydrostatic pressure from crystalloid infusion are not balanced by adequate colloid osmotic (oncotic) pressure in the plasma, which enhances interstitial edema in the periphery. Even with concurrent administration of a colloid, aggressive diuresis with a crystalloid may not be possible without creating peripheral edema. Loss of antithrombin III in the urine causes a hypercoagulable state, which may cause complications associated with IV catheterization.

Anemia may be present in acute and chronic renal failure. Red cell survival is shorter in the uremic environment, blood sampling may create substantial losses, and erythropoietin production generally is suppressed. Gastrointestinal bleeding can acutely cause anemia, and if bleeding is brisk, hypotension and hypovolemia may occur and require rapid infusion of crystalloid or synthetic colloid solutions. Red blood cell transfusion may be indicated if symptomatic anemia is present. Intensive diuresis may exacerbate high output heart failure in cats with anemia. Conversely, rapid blood transfusion may cause congestive heart failure. In patients with compromised cardiovascular function or incipient volume overload, red blood cell transfusion may need to be given more slowly than usual.

A sometimes overlooked fluid choice is water given enterally. Because vomiting is a common problem with uremia, enteral food or water frequently is contraindicated, and many patients with uremia do not voluntarily consume water. Water administered through a feeding tube should be included in water calculations, however.

Ultimately, the fluid choice must be guided by monitoring the patient's fluid and electrolyte balance. A major determining factor in the appropriate fluid choice is the serum sodium concentration, because the degree of free water loss relative to sodium loss varies greatly in patients with AKI. The guiding principle in treating a sodium disorder is to reverse it at the same rate at which it developed, because rapid increases or decreases in serum sodium concentration may cause central nervous system dysfunction (see later discussion).

VOLUME AND RATE

Some patients may present in hypovolemic shock, which is manifest as dull mentation, hypotension (systolic blood pressure < 80 mm Hg), poor perfusion of the periphery (eg, cold extremities, pale or gray mucous membranes with slow capillary refill time), hypothermia, and tachycardia [6]. Immediate correction of shock is necessary to prevent irreversible organ damage. The standard dosage of crystalloids is 60 to 90 mL/kg for dogs and 45 to 60 mL/kg for cats, of which 25% is given over 5 to 15 minutes [13]. If hemodynamic parameters do not improve sufficiently with the first 25% dose, a second dose should be given. Resuscitation efforts are continued until the patient is hemodynamically stable. If the patient remains hypotensive and there are concerns about volume overload, CVP monitoring may be helpful. A CVP less than 0 cm H_2O indicates hypovolemia, whereas a CVP more than 10 cm H_2O is a contraindication to further fluid therapy. A 10- to 15-mL/kg bolus of crystalloid or 3- to 5-mL/kg bolus of colloid does not change CVP in patients with hypovolemia but transiently increases CVP by 2 to 4 cm H_2O in patients with euvolemia and causes an increase of more than 4 cm H_2O in patients with hypervolemia [6]. Adequate resuscitation (as assessed by achievement of identifiable goals) decreases renal morbidity in people as compared to standard resuscitation doses [14].

For patients that present with dehydration, the dehydration deficit is calculated as body weight (in kilograms) × estimated % dehydration = fluid deficit in liters. Because dehydration less than 5% cannot be detected by clinical examination, a 5% dehydration deficit is assumed in patients with AKI that appear normally hydrated. If a fluid bolus was used for initial resuscitation, that volume is subtracted from the dehydration deficit.

The rate at which to replace the dehydration deficit depends on the clinical situation. In patients with AKI that presumably have become dehydrated over a short period of time, rapid replacement is indicated. This approach restores renal perfusion to normal and may prevent further damage to the kidneys. In situations in which urine output may be decreased, rapid replacement of the dehydration deficit to normalize fluid status allows the clinician to quickly determine if oliguria is an appropriate response to volume depletion or is a pathologic change arising from renal damage. In this setting, replacing the deficit in 2 to 4 hours is recommended. If diastolic cardiac function is impaired, a rapid fluid bolus may precipitate congestive heart failure, and a more gradual rehydration rate (ie, over 12–24 hours) may be prudent. In patients with chronic dehydration, a more gradual replacement of the fluid deficit is acceptable to minimize the risk of cardiac problems or excessively rapid changes in serum electrolyte concentrations; 24 hours is a commonly selected time frame. In severely dehydrated, chronically debilitated patients, it may take up to 48 hours to achieve rehydration.

The concept of the maintenance fluid rate is based on average fluid losses from insensible (eg, respiration) and sensible (eg, urine output) sources. There are various published values for maintenance fluid therapy, the most commonly quoted of which is 66 mL/kg/d. Ignoring normal individual variation, the assumption with this value is that urine output is normal and there are no other sources of fluid loss, which is rarely the case in patients with renal failure. This figure provides a reasonable starting point for calculating fluid administration volumes, however. If accurate measurement of urine output and ongoing losses can be documented, fluid therapy can be adjusted precisely (see "ins-and-outs" method later). If these variables cannot be measured accurately, an estimate of the loss should be included in the fluid administration rate. In practical terms, after initial fluid resuscitation for shock, the volume of fluid to administer is calculated by adding average maintenance fluid needs (66 mL/kg/d) plus replacement of dehydration (over a selected time frame) plus ongoing losses (eg, estimated volume of polyuria, vomiting).

Because uremic toxins are retained in renal failure, administration of a volume of fluid that exceeds "maintenance" can improve excretion of some uremic toxins in animals with the ability to increase urine output in response to a fluid challenge. The volume is varied based on the clinical situation and clinician preferences, but generally ranges from 2.5% to 6% of body weight per day in addition to the maintenance fluid administration rate. In practical terms, twice the maintenance fluid rate is equivalent to a maintenance rate plus a 6% "push" for diuresis (60 mL/kg/d = 6% of body weight).

If the urine output deviates substantially from normal–whether oliguria (< 0.5 mL/kg/h) or polyuria (> 2 mL/kg/h)–a fluid plan based on these assumptions may be inadequate. Animals with renal failure may have urine output in the normal range (0.5–2.0 mL/kg/h), but if their kidneys are unable to alter urine volume to excrete a fluid load, the patient has "relative oliguria." The "ins-and-outs" method of fluid administration is appropriate in these situations. It should be used only after rehydration is complete and is not appropriate if the patient is still dehydrated. The three components of volume calculations in the "ins-and-outs" method consist of (1) insensible loss (fluid lost via respiration and normal stool = 22 mL/kg/d), (2) urine volume replacement calculated by actual measurement (see later discussion for measuring techniques), and (3) ongoing losses (eg, vomiting, diarrhea, body cavity drainage) that are usually estimated.

To write treatment orders for "ins-and-outs" using two IV catheters, divide the daily insensible loss by 4 to determine the every-6-hour dose of IV fluid for one catheter (Box 1). One may then use this fluid dose to deliver any drugs that need to be given by constant rate infusion (CRI) (eg, metoclopramide, furosemide, mannitol), being cognizant of drug incompatibilities. For the starting fluid dose, select a volume based on an estimate of the patient's needs. The fluid rate is then recalculated every 6 hours. Use the previous 6-hour urine output volume plus an estimate of losses during that time period (eg, vomiting, diarrhea) as the volume to deliver over the next every-6-hours treatment in the second

Box 1: Sample calculations for "ins-and-outs" method of intravenous fluid administration

Without fluid pump

Insensible loss: 4.5 kg cat x 22 mL/kg/d = 100 mL/d

100 mL/day ÷ 4 treatment periods per day = 25 mL per 6 hours

Urine output: 30 mL urine over previous 6 hours

Ongoing loss: vomiting approximately 3 times a day (approximately 8 mL each time) = 6 mL over 6 hours

Total: 25 + 30 + 6 mL = 61 mL to administer over next 6 hours

Readjust volume every 6 hours based on urine output and ongoing losses

With fluid pump

Insensible loss: 4.5 kg cat x 22 mL/kg/d = 100 mL/d

100 mL/day ÷ 24 h per day = 4 mL/h

Urine output: 30 mL urine over previous 6 hours ÷ 6 h = 5 mL/h

Ongoing loss: vomiting approximately 3 times a day (approximately 8 mL each time) = 1 mL/h

Total: 4 + 5 + 1 mL = 10 mL/h

Readjust volume every 6 hours based on urine output and ongoing losses

catheter. This method avoids the need to recalculate the dosage for the CRI drugs every 6 hours. If only one IV catheter is available, calculate the amount of medication to be administered by CRI over 6 hours. Add this amount to the fluid volume required over the next 6 hours (6 hours of insensible losses + previous 6-hour urine output). Divide the total volume by 6 to get the hourly rate for the CRI. If a fluid pump is available, calculate daily insensible fluid needs and divide by 24 to get the hourly rate. Add to this number the hourly volume of urine output over the previous monitoring interval plus an estimate of ongoing losses.

A patient with anuria should receive fluid administration to replace insensible loss only. If the patient is overhydrated, withhold the insensible loss. Overhydration in a patient with anuria or inability to induce diuresis in a patient with oliguria or anuria is an indication for dialysis, which is the only other effective therapeutic option.

CONVERTING OLIGURIA TO NONOLIGURIA

A decrease in urine production may be caused by prerenal, intrinsic renal, or postrenal factors. An appropriate renal response to inadequate renal perfusion from hypovolemia or hypotension includes fluid retention with a concomitant decrease in urine volume. Renal perfusion should be optimized by ensuring adequate hydration before determining whether oliguria is pathologic or physiologic. A volume of fluid equal to 3% to 5% of body weight should be administered to patients that seem normally hydrated because dehydration less than

5% cannot be detected clinically. In patients that are clearly volume overexpanded, this fluid administration is not necessary. Healthy kidneys can autoregulate renal blood flow at perfusion pressures between 80 and 180 mm Hg, but renal perfusion may be more linear in damaged kidneys [8,15]. The mean arterial pressure should be maintained above 60 to 80 mm Hg or the systolic pressure above 80 to 100 mm Hg when measured by Doppler technology. Apparent anuria caused by obstruction of the urinary tract or leakage into the peritoneal, retroperitoneal, or SC tissues should be excluded before determining that a lack of urine is caused by intrinsic renal damage.

Various values have been used to define oliguria, including less than 0.25 mL/kg/h, less than 0.5 mL/kg/h, and less than 1 to 2 mL/kg/h [4]. In a hydrated, well-perfused patient, less than 1.0 mL/kg/h can be considered absolute oliguria, and urine production between 1 and 2 mL/kg/h in a patient on fluid therapy is considered relative oliguria [4,8]. Anuria is defined as essentially no urine production [4]. Urine volume more than 2 mL/kg/h is generally considered polyuria.

If pathologic oliguria or anuria persists despite correcting prerenal factors, most clinicians attempt to convert oliguria to nonoliguria using diuretics. There is no evidence that diuretics improve outcome in acute renal failure (ARF), and some believe that the ability to respond to diuretics indicates less severe renal injury, which is associated with a better prognosis. In people, an increase in urine output with diuretic use delays referral for dialysis, perhaps inappropriately [16]. In veterinary medicine, however, in which dialysis is not as readily available to control fluid status, an increase in urine output from diuretic use may allow other medications or nutrition to be administered in larger volumes, and treatment with diuretics may be justified even without improvement in renal function.

Mannitol is an osmotic diuretic that causes extracellular volume expansion, which can increase glomerular filtration rate (GFR) and inhibit sodium reabsorption in the kidney by inhibiting renin. Mannitol also increases tubular flow, which may relieve intratubular obstruction from casts and debris. Mannitol decreases vascular resistance and cellular swelling, increases renal blood flow, GFR, and solute excretion, protects from vascular congestion and red blood cell aggregation, scavenges free radicals, induces intrarenal prostaglandin production and vasodilatation, and induces atrial natrurietic peptide release [4,8,17,18]. Mannitol may blunt the influx of calcium into mitochondria in sublethally injured renal cells, thus decreasing the risk of sublethal injury progressing to lethal damage. Despite theoretical advantages, no randomized studies have shown a better clinical response with the use of mannitol and volume expansion than with volume expansion alone in people or healthy cats [17,19].

Mannitol is administered as a slow IV bolus of 0.25 to 1.0 g/kg. If urine production increases, mannitol may be administered as a CRI of 1 to 2 mg/kg/min IV or 0.25 to 0.5 g/kg every 4 to 6 hours [4]. Doses in excess of 2 to 4 g/kg/d may cause ARF. Mannitol should not be given to patients that are dehydrated because it further exacerbates intracellular dehydration. Conversely, it is also contraindicated if overhydration is present, and it may worsen pulmonary edema. Hypertonic dextrose can be used as an osmotic diuretic if mannitol is not available. A total daily dose of 22 to 66 mL/kg of a 20% dextrose solution should cause hyperglycemia and glucosuria [20].

Loop diuretics, such as furosemide, can increase urine flow without increasing GFR [17,19,21–23]. Despite the increase in urine output, loop diuretics do not improve outcome, which suggests that patients that respond have less severe renal failure, resulting in a better outcome for recovery independent of drug therapy [17,21–24]. In one study, for example, human patients who could be converted from oliguric to nonoliguric renal failure had better Acute Physiology And Chronic Health Evaluation (APACHE) scores and higher creatinine clearance before treatment, which suggested that they had less severe renal injury [24]. Because of a perception that there is a low complication rate associated with loop diuretic administration, they often are used despite lack of proven benefit. Loop diuretics inhibit the Na^+-$2Cl^-$-K^+ pump in the luminal cell membrane of the loop of Henle, decreasing transcellular sodium transport. Basal Na^+-K^+-ATPase activity becomes less crucial and renal medullary oxygen consumption decreases, which is hypothesized to protect the kidney from further injury [24,25]. The amount of structural damage to the thick ascending limb of the loop of Henle consequently is decreased in isolated perfused kidneys [25]. Loop diuretics also have renal vasodilatory effects [26]. Despite the theoretical reasons to use loop diuretics, one retrospective study in people showed an increased risk of death or failure of renal recovery in the furosemide treatment group. Potential reasons for this finding include a detrimental effect of the drug, delay in recognizing the severity of renal failure with subsequent delay in starting dialysis, or preferential use of loop diuretics in patients with a more severe course of disease [16,21]. Loop diuretics may make fluid management easier in people without changing the outcome [24]. In animals, loop diuretics may play a larger role in management because dialysis is not universally available. Established indications for the use of furosemide in veterinary medicine include treatment of overhydration or hyperkalemia [4]. Furosemide should not be given to patients with aminoglycoside-induced ARF [8].

An increase in urine output should be apparent 20 to 60 minutes after an IV dose of furosemide of 2 to 6 mg/kg. Ototoxicity has been reported at high doses in people, and doses of 10 to 50 mg/kg may cause adverse effects in animals (eg, apathy and anorexia in cats; hypotension, apathy, and staggering in dogs) [8]. If there is no response to high doses of furosemide, therapy should be discontinued. If a response does occur, the effective dose can be administered every 6 to 8 hours. A CRI provides a more sustained diuresis with a lower cumulative dose compared to bolus administration [21]. In people, the time to maximal effect using a CRI without a loading dose is 3 hours and 1 hour with a loading dose. The dosage used in people is usually 1 to 9 mg/h (approximately 0.01–0.15 mg/kg/h), with some reports using dosages as high as 0.75 mg/kg/h [27]. In normal dogs, 0.66 mg/kg/h resulted in diuresis [28,29], and dosages of 0.25 to 1.0 mg/kg/h have been used in dogs and cats with naturally occurring renal failure [4]. Because electrolyte and fluid balance disorders can develop rapidly if a brisk diuresis ensues, frequent monitoring is necessary.

Dopamine has been shown to convert some human patients from oliguria to nonoliguria, but it does not increase GFR or improve outcome in people [17,23,30,31]. Because of lack of efficacy and adverse effects associated with dopamine, it is no longer recommended for treatment of oliguric renal failure, except for pressor control [4,32]. Selective dopamine agonists may have better efficacy and fewer adverse effects compared to dopamine. There are two dopaminergic receptors, DA-1 and DA-2. Fenoldopam is a selective DA-1 receptor agonist, and as such, it selectively increases renal cortical and medullary blood flow, sodium excretion, and urine output while maintaining GFR in people. It does not have DA-2 or alpha or beta adrenergic activity, so it does not cause vasoconstriction, tachycardia, or arrhythmias as seen with dopamine [17,26]. Although no clear benefit has been observed, studies with fenoldopam in people are encouraging, and larger clinical trials are needed [26]. Although some studies in dogs treated with fenoldopam have demonstrated an improvement in GFR, GFR may decrease within the first few hours after administration [33–35].

Calcium channel antagonists have been used to decrease damage after renal transplantation [36]. Calcium channel antagonists presumptively reverse renal vasoconstriction by causing predominantly preglomerular vasodilatation, inhibiting vasoconstriction induced by tubuloglomerular feedback mechanisms, and causing natriuresis independent of GFR [36]. Although the results of one study using diltiazem in addition to standard care in dogs with AKI caused by leptospirosis were not statistically significant, there was a trend toward increased urine output and more complete resolution of azotemia [36]. Whether calcium channel antagonists will prove beneficial is still to be determined.

Atrial natriuretic peptide increases tubular excretion of salt and water and stimulates afferent arteriolar dilatation and efferent arteriolar constriction, which increases GFR. Although atrial natriuretic peptide decreases the severity of experimental ARF from ischemic but not nephrotoxic causes, it has not been effective in clinical trials thus far [17].

MONITORING FLUID THERAPY

Monitoring fluid status is an ongoing process that must be repeated throughout the day. Physical examination and body weight should be assessed at least twice daily and the fluid plan adjusted accordingly. Blood pressure also should be monitored. Urine output and other fluid losses should be monitored and correlated with other findings of volume status.

Determining urine volume can be performed by various methods, including placing an indwelling urinary catheter with a closed collection system, collecting naturally voided urine, using a metabolic cage, and weighing cage bedding or litter pans (1 mL of urine = 1 g). An indwelling catheter is usually the most precise method, but technical issues such as urine leakage around the catheter and inadvertent disconnection may artifactually decrease measured volumes. The risk of iatrogenic urinary tract infection from the catheter can be decreased by careful attention to catheter and patient hygiene, including cleaning the external portions of the catheter with an antiseptic solution several times daily and changing the collection bag and tubing daily [37]. Complete collection of voided urine may be difficult in many patients because of lack of patient cooperation or urinary incontinence in obtunded or recumbent patients. An accurate scale is necessary to measure small volumes of urine in cats and small dogs, but weighing cage bedding or litter pans before and after use may provide adequate and noninvasive assessment of urine volume in some patients. Fluid losses from vomiting and diarrhea usually are estimated, and other losses such as body cavity drainage (eg, ascites, pleural effusion) or nasogastric tube suctioning can be measured.

DISCONTINUING FLUID THERAPY

With AKI, once a diuresis has been established, polyuria can be marked. Monitoring urine production to prevent inadequate fluid administration is necessary in this phase just as monitoring was necessary during oliguria or anuria to prevent overhydration. Weaning these patients from IV fluids is a crucial step. When azotemia has resolved or reached a plateau, the fluid dose can be decreased by 25% per day. If urine output decreases by a corresponding amount and azotemia does not return, tapering of fluid administration over 2 to 3 days should continue. If urine output does not decrease, the kidneys are not yet able to regulate fluid balance and further reduction in fluid administered will lead to dehydration. Attempts to taper fluid administration can be made again after several days, but generally at a slower rate (10%–20% per day). It can take weeks for the kidneys to regain the ability to control fluid volume in rare cases.

With CKD, once the prerenal component of the azotemia has resolved, serum creatinine concentration (generally monitored every 48 hours) usually decreases by at least 1 mg/dL/d. When serum creatinine concentration reaches a baseline value (ie, when it no longer decreases despite IV fluid therapy), fluids should be tapered in preparation for patient discharge. After a period of intensive diuresis, fluid administration should be tapered gradually over approximately 2 to 3 days.

OUTPATIENT FLUID THERAPY

Despite widespread use of SC fluid therapy, its role in managing kidney disease has never been evaluated rigorously. Empirically, chronic dehydration and persistent signs of uremia are rational indications for chronic SC fluid administration. The dosage is empirical, based on subjective assessment of the patient's well-being and hydration status. A typical starting dose for cats is 100 to 150 mL daily or every other day. Cats subjectively seem to respond more favorably to SC fluid therapy compared to dogs. Lactated Ringer's solution and 0.9% saline are appropriate fluids choices. Dextrose-containing fluids increase the risk of abscess formation, and Plasmalyte is reported to sting when administered SC. Many owners can be taught to administer fluids at home, using a new needle for each administration. An administration tube can be implanted in the SC space for fluid administration without a needle, but this method increases the risk of infection at the site where the tube exits the skin, and SC fibrosis with subsequent pain during fluid administration and decreased capacity to accommodate fluid has been observed.

NUTRITIONAL SUPPORT

Renal failure is highly catabolic. Although it is hard to identify clearly the contribution of nutritional management to outcome, poor nutritional status is a major factor that increases patient morbidity and mortality [38]. Early enteral feeding can help preserve gastrointestinal mucosal integrity [39]. Although renal diets, characterized by restricted phosphorus and restricted quantities of high-quality protein, are indicated for treating CKD, the ideal diet for ARF has not been identified [40,41]. In the absence of information, enteral diets for critically ill animals or people have been used [8].

Anorexia is a common problem in hospitalized patients that have renal failure. If appetite does not return within a few days of therapy, feeding tube placement may allow administration of an appropriate quantity of the desired diet and easy administration of oral medications. It is strongly recommended in animals not voluntarily consuming adequate calories. If vomiting cannot be controlled, partial or total parenteral nutrition may be necessary.

Whether supplementation is enteral or parenteral, the volume that can be administered may be limited in patients that are anuric or oliguric. Most liquid diets suitable for administration via a nasoesophageal or nasogastric tube have a caloric density of approximately 1 kcal/mL [42]. Provision of 100% of the basal energy requirements general requires a volume of approximately twice the insensible fluid requirement. Common formulas for calculation of total parenteral nutrition also encompass almost twice the insensible fluid requirements [43]. Dialysis can remove fluid from the patient by ultrafiltration, which may be necessary to prevent volume overload in an oliguric or anuric patient receiving nutritional support.

ELECTROLYTE ABNORMALITIES

Sodium and Chloride

The serum sodium concentration may be normal, increased, or decreased with renal failure. Hypernatremia before fluid therapy indicates excessive free water loss. Administration of sodium bicarbonate or hypertonic saline may contribute to hypernatremia. Hyponatremia may indicate excessive sodium loss associated with vomiting or may represent transient dilutional hyponatremia after administration of mannitol, hypertonic dextrose, or colloid solutions. Sodium-poor solutions (eg, 5% dextrose, total parenteral nutrition, enteral formulations) may contribute to hyponatremia. In many situations, dehydration initially is caused by isonatremic fluid loss, and the patient's serum sodium concentration is normal [4,8].

The initial fluid deficit should be replaced by an isonatremic solution such as lactated Ringer's solution, 0.9% saline, or Plasmalyte-148. Continued administration of these solutions over several days may lead to hypernatremia. A sodium-poor fluid, such as half-strength lactated Ringer's solution or 0.45%

saline with 2.5% dextrose, may be a more appropriate fluid choice after the initial rehydration phase. The serum sodium concentration should be monitored regularly and the fluid choice adjusted as needed.

Clinical signs of sodium disorders are unlikely unless rapid changes in serum sodium concentration occur, and signs generally are related to neurologic dysfunction. The rate of change in serum sodium concentration should not exceed 1 mEq/L/h [44]. Changes in serum chloride concentration tend to parallel changes in serum sodium concentration.

Potassium

Hypokalemia

Hypokalemia is more likely to be present in CKD compared to AKI and is more likely in cats compared to dogs. Between 20% and 30% of cats with CKD have hypokalemia [45–47]. Multiple mechanisms may contribute to the development of hypokalemia, including excessive renal wasting associated with polyuria. Alkalemia worsens hypokalemia because potassium shifts intracellularly in response to translocation of hydrogen ions out of the cells. Vomiting and loop diuretics can cause additional potassium loss. Decreased oral intake alone generally does not cause hypokalemia, but prolonged anorexia exacerbates hypokalemia. Hypokalemia may be present at admission, particularly with polyuric CKD, or it may develop during hospitalization, particularly in the diuretic phase of recovery from AKI or with effective diuretic therapy. Hypokalemia is a cause and effect of renal dysfunction; hypokalemia interferes with urinary concentrating ability, but the renal dysfunction generally is reversible with normalization of serum potassium concentration [48].

Signs of hypokalemia include muscle weakness (eg, stiff, stilted gait in hind limbs, cervical ventroflexion, respiratory muscle paralysis). Cardiac abnormalities occur inconsistently but may include ventricular and supraventricular arrhythmias. Rarely, U waves are noted on the electrocardiogram. Other signs include fatigue, vomiting, anorexia, and gastrointestinal ileus [4,49]. Clinical signs of hypokalemia are likely when serum potassium concentration is less than 2.5 mEq/L; a concentration of less than 2.0 mEq/L may be life threatening [4,8]. By definition, hypokalemia is diagnosed by detecting a low serum potassium concentration. Evaluation of the fractional excretion of potassium may help distinguish renal potassium loss (fractional excretion > 4%) from nonrenal loss (fractional excretion < 4%) [50,51].

Because excretion of potassium may be impaired with renal failure, treatment in this setting requires judicious supplementation with careful monitoring. Because normalization of hypokalemia can improve renal function and decrease clinical signs, treatment of hypokalemia should not be overlooked [48]. In hospitalized patients unable to tolerate orally administered medications, potassium chloride may be added to the IV fluids. The rate of supplementation is based on a patient's serum potassium concentration using an empirically derived scale (Table 1). The rate of potassium supplementation should not exceed 0.5 mEq/kg/h. Serum potassium concentration may decrease during initial fluid

Table 1	
Sliding scale of potassium supplementation	
Serum potassium concentration (mEq/L)	Potassium concentration in fluids (mEq/L)
3.5–4.5	20
3–3.5	30
2.5–3	40
2–2.5	60
< 2	80

therapy despite supplementation because of extracellular fluid volume expansion, increased distal renal tubular flow, and cellular uptake, especially if potassium is administered with dextrose-containing fluids.

In a life-threatening hypokalemic emergency (eg, respiratory muscle weakness with hypoventilation, cardiac arrhythmias), some clinicians recommend administering an IV bolus of KCl. This approach should be undertaken only with constant electrocardiographic monitoring because a rapid potassium bolus potentially could cause a fatal arrhythmia. To calculate the amount of potassium to administer, subtract the patient's serum potassium concentration from a desired serum potassium concentration of 3 mEq/L. Calculate the blood volume (8% of body weight in kg in dogs or 6% of body weight in kg in cats) and multiply the blood volume by 60% to estimate the plasma volume. Multiply the plasma volume by the difference between the measured and desired potassium concentrations to determine the number of milliequivalents of KCl to administer as an IV bolus over 1 to 5 minutes through a central vein. Check the patient's serum potassium concentration 5 minutes later. A second bolus—calculated from the new serum potassium concentration—can be administered, but caution must be used and it should be administered more slowly as the patient's serum potassium concentration approaches 3 mEq/L [49].

Once oral intake is possible, potassium gluconate can be administered. A dose of 5 to 10 mEq/d divided into two to three doses is used to replenish potassium, followed by 2 to 4 mEq/d for maintenance [50]. Potassium citrate (40–60 mg/kg/d divided into two to three doses) is an alternative to potassium gluconate that also helps to correct acidosis. Potassium chloride can be added to SC fluids at concentrations up to 35 mEq/L.

Frequent monitoring (once to several times daily) is recommended for patients on IV potassium supplementation. During potassium repletion on an outpatient basis, monitoring every 7 to 14 days is recommended until a stable maintenance dose is determined [48]. If hypokalemia persists after standard supplementation, hypomagnesemia may be present and magnesium supplementation may be necessary.

Hyperkalemia
Renal excretion is the major mechanism for removing potassium from the body, and chronic hyperkalemia is unlikely to occur with normal renal function. Hyperkalemia is more likely to develop in cases of oliguric or anuric ARF and

usually does not occur in cases of CKD unless oliguria or severe metabolic acidosis is present [8]. Metabolic acidosis from mineral acids (eg, NH_4Cl, HCl) but not organic acids (eg, lactic acid, ketoacids) causes translocation of potassium out of cells as hydrogen ions enter the cells. Patients that have CKD may have decreased ability to tolerate an acute potassium load and may take 1 to 3 days to re-establish external potassium balance after a potassium load [51]. Mild hyperkalemia is relatively common in stable patients being treated with angiotensin-converting enzyme inhibitors. My experience is that most patients on angiotensin-converting enzyme inhibitors do not develop serum potassium concentrations in excess of 6.5 mEq/L, and the clinical relevance of mild hyperkalemia in these patients is uncertain. Hyperkalemia and azotemia are common with hypoadrenocorticism and acute tumor lysis syndrome [50].

Hyperkalemia is a potentially life-threatening electrolyte disorder. The increase in extracellular potassium changes the electrical potential of excitable cells. The myocardium is relatively resistant compared to the conducting system of the heart. Typical electrocardiographic changes include bradycardia, tall spiked T waves, shortened QT interval, wide QRS complex, and small, wide, or absent P waves. Severe hyperkalemia can lead to a sinoventricular rhythm, ventricular fibrillation, or ventricular standstill. Muscle weakness may be present in patients with serum potassium concentrations more than 8 mEq/L [50]. Characteristic electrocardiographic changes may require emergency therapy before serum potassium concentration results are available from the laboratory. Pseudohyperkalemia may occur ex vivo if red cell potassium content is high, as may occur in Akita dogs.

Calcium gluconate 10% (0.5–1.0 mL/kg IV to effect, given slowly) can be used in critical situations to restore cardiac membrane excitability, but it does not decrease serum potassium concentration. During infusion, the electrocardiogram must be monitored and administration slowed or stopped if the arrhythmia worsens. The cardiac effects should be apparent within minutes. Despite a rapid onset of action, the duration of effect after administration of calcium gluconate is less than 1 hour [51]. Calcium administration increases the risk of soft tissue mineralization if hyperphosphatemia is present.

Several methods can be used to translocate potassium intracellularly. Regular insulin (0.5 U/kg IV) has an effect within 20 to 30 minutes. Dextrose (1–2 g/U insulin as an IV bolus, then 1–2 g/U insulin in IV fluids administered over the next 4–6 hours) is necessary to prevent hypoglycemia when insulin is used. Dextrose induces endogenous insulin release in patients that do not have diabetes and can be used at a dosage of 0.25 to 0.5 g/kg IV to control mild to moderate hyperkalemia without concurrent insulin administration.

Metabolic acidosis from mineral acids causes an extracellular shift of K^+ as H^+ increases intracellularly. Correction of metabolic acidosis with bicarbonate allows an intracellular shift of K^+ as the H^+ is combined with HCO_3^- and removed. The dose of sodium bicarbonate used to treat hyperkalemia is based on the base deficit, or an empirical dosage of 1 to 2 mEq/kg IV over 10 to 20 minutes can be used. Sodium bicarbonate is contraindicated if the partial pressure of carbon dioxide (PCO_2) is increased or metabolic alkalosis is present, and it may contribute to hypernatremia or paradoxical central nervous system acidosis. If serum ionized calcium concentration is low, dextrose is preferred to bicarbonate because alkalemia exacerbates hypocalcemia [8].

The beta-agonist albuterol has been used to treat hyperkalemia in people because it causes an intracellular shift of potassium [8]. The cation exchange resin sodium polystyrene sulfonate (Kayexalate) can be administered orally or by enema at a dosage of 2 g/kg in three to four divided doses as a suspension in 20% sorbitol [4]. This substance binds potassium in the gastrointestinal tract and releases sodium. It takes several hours to work, and adverse effects include hypernatremia and constipation.

The potassium-lowering effects of these drugs, with the exception of polystyrene sulfonate, are temporary. Serum potassium concentrations gradually increase again within several hours after administration unless urine production increases. Once even minimal urine production resumes, serum potassium concentrations usually decrease. Peritoneal dialysis or hemodialysis may be necessary to ultimately control serum potassium concentration if oliguria or anuria persists.

Drugs and other treatments that contribute to hyperkalemia should be avoided, including nonspecific beta-blockers, digoxin, angiotensin-converting enzyme inhibitors, angiotensin receptor antagonists, nonsteroidal anti-inflammatory drugs, potassium-sparing diuretics (eg, spironolactone, amiloride, triamterene), high doses of trimethoprim, cyclosporine, and total parenteral nutrition [50].

Calcium

Most of the body's calcium is found in the skeleton as hydroxyapatite. Serum calcium concentration consists of three fractions: (1) ionized calcium (55%), which is the biologically active form, (2) protein-bound (35%), a storage form generally bound to albumin, and (3) complexed calcium (10%), which is bound to citrate, lactate, bicarbonate, or phosphate in serum. Serum total calcium concentration (including all three fractions) is most commonly measured, but measurement of serum ionized calcium concentration is becoming more readily available in practice settings.

Disturbances of serum calcium concentration may occur in renal failure for several reasons. An acute decrease in GFR may lead to an abrupt increase in serum phosphorus concentration, causing a decrease in serum calcium concentration by the law of mass action. The decrease in serum ionized calcium concentration stimulates parathyroid hormone synthesis and release, which act to increase the calcium concentration back to normal. On the other hand, chronic renal failure may cause parathyroid hyperplasia which rarely leads to hypercalcemia. Metabolic acidosis increases the ionized calcium fraction, but more than 50% of dogs with CKD and metabolic acidosis were hypocalcemic [52].

Based on serum ionized calcium concentration, 36% to 56% of dogs with CKD are hypocalcemic, 20% to 55% are normocalcemic, and 9% to 24% are hypercalcemic [52,53]. Based on serum total calcium concentration, 8% to 19% are hypocalcemic, 60% to 76% are normocalcemic, and 16% to 22% are hypercalcemic. The concordance between serum ionized calcium and serum total calcium concentrations is poor, especially in dogs with CKD [52,53].

Symptomatic hypocalcemia (tetany) occurs infrequently in renal disease. Hypocalcemia may be more severe with ethylene glycol-induced ARF, because antifreeze contains phosphate that can cause severe hyperphosphatemia, and ethylene glycol is converted to oxalate, which complexes with calcium. Treatment with calcium increases the risk of soft tissue mineralization in patients with hyperphosphatemia. The minimal dose of calcium gluconate that controls clinical signs should be used when therapy is needed. A 10% solution of calcium gluconate can be used at a dosage of 0.5 to 1.5 mL/kg IV over 20 to 30 minutes. As when treating hyperkalemia, the electrocardiogram should be monitored during infusion.

In patients with renal failure, hypercalcemia based on total serum calcium concentration usually is mild and associated with normal serum ionized calcium concentration. No specific treatment is necessary. If serum ionized calcium concentration is increased, treatment is warranted. Hypercalcemia may respond to fluid therapy, although calcium-containing fluids (eg, lactated Ringer's solution) should be avoided. Normal saline (0.9% NaCl) is an ideal fluid choice because its high sodium content facilitates calciuresis. Furosemide also promotes urinary calcium loss. Sodium bicarbonate therapy decreases serum ionized calcium concentration as more calcium ions bind to serum proteins. Hypercalcemia associated with renal failure is not likely to be glucocorticoid responsive [54]. Calcitonin or bisphosphonates could be considered if hypercalcemia is severe, although bisphosphonates also can induce renal failure [54].

MAGNESIUM

Serum magnesium concentrations may be increased in severe renal failure because the kidneys are the major route of excretion of magnesium, but specific therapy generally is not necessary. Supplemental magnesium, such as that found in some phosphate binders, should be avoided in these situations. Hypomagnesemia may occur with polyuric renal failure. Hypokalemia may be refractory to therapy if concurrent hypomagnesemia is present. In this situation, correction of the magnesium deficit may be necessary before correction of the hypokalemia can occur. Magnesium sulfate or magnesium chloride can be used for IV supplementation, and various formulations of magnesium are available for oral supplementation [55].

PHOSPHORUS

Dietary phosphorus is readily absorbed from the gastrointestinal tract and excreted by the kidneys. Decreased excretion commonly leads to hyperphosphatemia in patients with ARF and chronic renal failure. Intravenous fluid therapy may partially control serum phosphorus concentration by improving renal blood flow and correcting prerenal azotemia. No other specific treatments are available to decrease serum phosphorus concentration in the early stages of ARF. A phosphate-restricted diet is recommended for long-term control of hyperphosphatemia. Because protein is phosphate-rich, adequate phosphorus restriction necessitates a protein-restricted diet. Although diet may be sufficient to control serum phosphorus concentration in mild to moderate renal failure, diet alone generally is not sufficient as renal disease progresses.

Phosphate binders prevent absorption of dietary phosphorus in the gastrointestinal tract. Aluminum-containing phosphate binders are commonly used in veterinary medicine. They are rarely used in people because of the potential for complications from long-term exposure to aluminum, including anemia and neurologic disorders. These effects are rarely noted in animals unless they are receiving chronic hemodialysis. Aluminum hydroxide or aluminum carbonate can be administered at a dosage of 30 to 90 mg/kg/d divided and given with meals. Calcium acetate and calcium carbonate are alternatives to aluminum-containing phosphorus binders. They may cause hypercalcemia and should be avoided in patients with increased serum calcium concentrations. Calcium carbonate combined with chitosan is a veterinary product for binding phosphorus. Several newer phosphate binders, such as sevelamer hydrochloride and lanthanum carbonate, are available for people, but there is limited veterinary experience with them. With all phosphate binders, the dosage is adjusted by serial determination of serum phosphorus concentration. Because of their binding properties, they can interfere with absorption of orally administered medications, especially antibiotics.

METABOLIC ACIDOSIS

Metabolic acidosis is a common acid-base disturbance in renal failure. The daily H^+ load is excreted in the urine with NH_3 as NH_4^+ or with phosphate as $H_2PO_4^-$. With renal failure, the kidneys are less able to excrete H^+ and cannot reabsorb adequate amounts of HCO_3^-. Lactic acidosis from dehydration and poor tissue perfusion also may contribute to acidosis in some patients with renal failure. If acidosis persists after correcting dehydration and perfusion, IV sodium bicarbonate therapy can be considered. Sodium bicarbonate therapy usually is reserved for patients with pH less than 7.2 or HCO_3 less than 12 mEq/L. Treatment with sodium bicarbonate causes H^+ to combine with HCO_3^- to form H_2CO_3, which dissociates into H_2O and CO_2. If the lungs are unable to adequately eliminate the CO_2, treatment is not effective. Bicarbonate administration in this situation can increase PCO_2 and lead to paradoxical central nervous system acidosis because of the ability of CO_2 to more easily diffuse into the central nervous system and lower pH. Sodium bicarbonate treatment also is contraindicated in patients with hypernatremia. The bicarbonate dose can be calculated from the formula: $0.3 \times$ body weight (kg) $\times$ base deficit, where the base deficit $= 24 -$ the patient's serum bicarbonate concentration. Give 25% to 50% of the dose IV and an additional 25% to 50% of the dose in the IV fluids over the next 2 to 6 hours. Adjust any subsequent doses based on serial evaluation of blood gas determinations.

Oral alkalinizing agents can be used for treatment of chronic acidosis. Potassium citrate (40–75 mg/kg orally every 12 hours) simultaneously addresses metabolic acidosis and hypokalemia. Oral sodium bicarbonate (8–12 mg/kg orally every 12 hours) is more palatable in tablet form compared to powder. Doses should be adjusted based on the individual patient response.

SUMMARY

Careful fluid therapy is the most important aspect of treating a uremic crisis and involves careful assessment of hydration status with frequent reassessment, use of the appropriate fluid type and rate, and flexibility to respond to changes in the patient's clinical status. Electrolyte and acid-base disturbances are common with renal failure and frequently require specific therapy.

References

[1] Worwag S, Langston CE. Feline acute intrinsic renal failure: 32 cats (1997–2004). J Am Vet Med Assoc, in press.

[2] Behrend E, Grauer GF, Mani I, et al. Hospital-acquired acute renal failure in dogs: 29 cases (1983–1992). J Am Vet Med Assoc 1996;208(4):537–41.

[3] Kirby R, Rudloff E. Crystalloid and colloid fluid therapy. In: Ettinger SJ, Feldman EC, editors. 6th edition, Textbook of veterinary internal medicine, vol 1. St. Louis (MO): Elsevier Saunders; 2005. p. 412–24.

[4] Cowgill LD, Francey T. Acute uremia. In: Ettinger SJ, Feldman EC, editors. 6th edition, Textbook of veterinary internal medicine, vol 2. Philadelphia: Elsevier Saunders; 2005. p. 1731–51.

[5] Mathews KA. Monitoring fluid therapy and complications of fluid therapy. In: DiBartola SP, editor. Fluid, electrolyte, and acid-base disorders in small animal practice. 3rd edition. St. Louis (MO): Saunders Elsevier; 2006. p. 377–91.

[6] Waddell LS. Hypotension. In: Ettinger SJ, Feldman EC, editors. 6th edition, Textbook of veterinary internal medicine, vol 1. St. Louis (MO): Elsevier Saunders; 2005. p. 480–3.

[7] Gookin JL, Atkins CE. Evaluation of the effect of pleural effusion on central venous pressure in cats. J Vet Intern Med 1999;13(6):561–3.

[8] Chew DJ, Gieg JA. Fluid therapy during intrinsic renal failure. In: DiBartola SP, editor. Fluid, electrolyte, and acid-base disorders in small animal practice. 3rd edition. St. Louis (MO): Saunders Elsevier; 2006. p. 518–40.

[9] Syme HM, Barber PJ, Markwell PJ, et al. Prevalence of systolic hypertension in cats with chronic renal failure at initial evaluation. J Am Vet Med Assoc 2002;220(12): 1799–804.

[10] Jacob F, Polzin DJ, Osborne CA, et al. Association between initial systolic blood pressure and risk of developing a uremic crisis or of dying in dogs with chronic renal failure. J Am Vet Med Assoc 2003;222(3):322–9.

[11] Cohn LA, Kerl ME, Lenox CE, et al. Response of healthy dogs to infusions of human serum albumin. Am J Vet Res 2007;68(6):657–63.

[12] Francis AH, Martin LG, Haldorson GJ, et al. Adverse reactions suggestive of type III hypersensitivity in six healthy dogs given human albumin. J Am Vet Med Assoc 2007;230(6):873–9.

[13] Otto CM. Shock. In: Ettinger SJ, Feldman EC, editors. 6th edition, Textbook of veterinary internal medicine, vol 1. St. Louis (MO): Elsevier Saunders; 2005. p. 455–7.

[14] Lin SM, Huang CD, Lin HC, et al. A modified goal-directed protocol improves clinical outcomes in intensive care unit patients with septic shock: a randomized controlled trial. Shock 2006;26(6):551–7.

[15] Conger JD. Vascular alterations in acute renal failure: roles in initiation and maintenance. In: Molitoris BA, Finn WF, editors. Acute renal failure: a companion to Brenner & Rector's the kidney. Philadelphia: W.B. Saunders; 2001. p. 13–29.

[16] Mehta RL, Pascual MT, Soroko S, et al. Diuretics, mortality, and nonrecovery of renal function in acute renal failure. JAMA 2002;288(20):2547–53.

[17] Finn WF. Recovery from acute renal failure. In: Molitoris BA, Finn WF, editors. Acute renal failure: a companion to Brenner & Rector's the kidney. Philadelphia: W.B. Saunders; 2001. p. 425–50.

[18] Better OS, Rubinstein I, Winaver JM, et al. Mannitol therapy revisited (1940–1997). Kidney Int 1997;51:866–94.

[19] McClellan JM, Goldstein RE, Erb HN, et al. Effects of administration of fluids and diuretics on glomerular filtration rate, renal blood flow, and urine output in healthy awake cats. Am J Vet Res 2006;67:715–22.

[20] Ross LR. Fluid therapy for acute and chronic renal failure. Vet Clin North Am Small Anim Pract 1989;19:343–59.

[21] De Vriese AS. Prevention and treatment of acute renal failure in sepsis. J Am Soc Nephrol 2003;14:792–805.

[22] Vijayan A, Miller SB. Acute renal failure: prevention and nondialytic therapy. Semin Nephrol 1998;18(5):523–32.

[23] Nolan CR, Anderson RJ. Hospital-acquired acute renal failure. J Am Soc Nephrol 1998;9(4):710–8.

[24] Shilliday IR, Quinn KJ, Allison MEM. Loop diuretics in the management of acute renal failure: a prospective, double-blind, placebo-controlled, randomized study. Nephrol Dial Transplant 1997;12:2592–6.

[25] Heyman SN, Rosen S, Epstein FH, et al. Loop diuretics reduce hypoxic damage to proximal tubules of the isolated perfused rat kidney. Kidney Int 1994;45:981–5.

[26] Pruchnicki MC, Dasta JF. Acute renal failure in hospitalized patients: part II. Ann Pharmacother 2002;36:1430–42.

[27] Martin SJ, Danziger LH. Continuous infusion of loop diuretics in the critically ill: a review of the literature. Crit Care Med 1994;22(8):1323–9.

[28] Adin DB, Taylor AW, Hill RC, et al. Intermittent bolus injection versus continuous infusion of furosemide in normal adult greyhound dogs. J Vet Intern Med 2003;17(5):632–6.

[29] Adin DB, Hill RC, Scott KC. Short-term compatibility of furosemide with crystalloid solutions. J Vet Intern Med 2003;17(5):724–6.

[30] Bellomo R, Chapman M, Finfer S, et al. Low-dose dopamine in patients with early renal dysfunction: a placebo-controlled randomised trial. Lancet 2000;356:2139–43.

[31] Rudis MI. Low-dose dopamine in the intensive care unit: DNR or DNRx? Crit Care Med 2001;29:1638–9.

[32] Sigrist NE. Use of dopamine in acute renal failure. J Vet Emerg Crit Care 2007;17(2): 117–26.

[33] Halpenny M, Markos F, Snow HM, et al. Effects of prophylactic fenoldopam infusion on renal blood flow and renal tubular function during acute hypovolemia in anesthetized dogs. Crit Care Med 2001;29(4):855–60.

[34] Simmons JP, Wohl JS, Schwartz DD, et al. Diuretic effects of fenoldopam in healthy cats. Journal of Veterinary Emergency and Critical Care 2006;16(2):96–103.

[35] Murray C, Markos F, Snow HM. Effects of fenoldopam on renal blood flow and its function in a canine model of rhabdomyolysis. Eur J Anaesthesiol 2003;20:711–8.

[36] Mathews KA, Monteith G. Evaluation of adding diltiazem therapy to standard treatment of acute renal failure caused by leptospirosis: 18 dogs (1998–2001). J Vet Emerg Crit Care 2007;17(2):149–58.

[37] Smarick SD, Haskins SC, Aldrich J, et al. Incidence of catheter-associated urinary tract infection among dogs in a small animal intensive care unit. J Am Vet Med Assoc 2004;224(12):1936–40.

[38] Wooley JA, Btaiche IF, Good KL. Metabolic and nutritional aspects of acute renal failure in critically ill patients requiring continuous renal replacement therapy. Nutr Clin Pract 2005;20(2):176–91.

[39] Macintire DK. Bacterial translocation: clinical implications and prevention. In: Bonagura JD, editor. Kirk's current veterinary therapy XIII: small animal practice. Philadelphia: W.B. Saunders; 2000. p. 201–3.

[40] Jacob F, Polzin DJ, Osborne CA, et al. Clinical evaluation of dietary modification for treatment of spontaneous chronic renal failure in dogs. J Am Vet Med Assoc 2002;220(8):1163–70.

[41] Ross S, Osborne CA, Polzin DJ, et al. Clinical evaluation of effects of dietary modification in cats with spontaneous chronic renal failure [abstract]. J Vet Intern Med 2005;19(3):433.

[42] Marks SL. The principles and implementation of enteral nutrition. In: Ettinger SJ, Feldman EC, editors. 6th edition, Textbook of veterinary internal medicine, vol 1. St. Louis (MO): Saunders Elsevier; 2005. p. 596–8.

[43] Chan D. Parenteral nutritional support. In: Ettinger SJ, Feldman EC, editors, Textbook of veterinary internal medicine, vol 1. St. Louis (MO): Saunders Elsevier; 2005. p. 586–91.

[44] DiBartola SP. Disorders of sodium and water: hypernatremia and hyponatremia. In: DiBartola SP, editor. Fluid, electrolyte, and acid-base disorders in small animal practice. 3rd edition. St. Louis (MO): Saunders Elsevier; 2006. p. 47–79.

[45] Elliott J, Barber PJ. Feline chronic renal failure: clinical findings in 80 cases diagnosed between 1992 and 1995. J Small Anim Pract 1998;39:78–85.

[46] DiBartola SP, Rutgers HC, Zack PM, et al. Clinicopathologic findings associated with chronic renal disease in cats: 74 cases (1973–1984). J Am Vet Med Assoc 1987;190(9):1196–202.

[47] Lulich JP, Osborne CA, O'Brien TD, et al. Feline renal failure: questions, answers, questions. Compend Contin Educ Pract Vet 1992;14(2):127–53.

[48] Polzin DJ, Osborne CA, Ross S. Chronic kidney disease. In: Ettinger SJ, Feldman EC, editors. 6th edition, Textbook of veterinary internal medicine, vol. 2. St. Louis (MO): Elsevier Saunders; 2005. p. 1756–85.

[49] Rubin SI, LeClerc SM. A practical guide to recognizing and treating hypokalemia. Vet Med 2001;96:462–76.

[50] DiBartola SP. Management of hypokalemia and hyperkalemia. J Feline Med Surg 2001;3: 181–3.

[51] DiBartola SP, de Morais HA. Disorders of potassium: hypokalemia and hyperkalemia. In: DiBartola SP, editor. Fluid, electrolyte, and acid-base disorders in small animal practice. 3rd edition. St. Louis (MO): Saunders Elsevier; 2006. p. 91–121.

[52] Kogika MM, Lustoza MD, Notomi MK, et al. Serum ionized calcium in dogs with chronic renal failure and metabolic acidosis. Vet Clin Pathol 2006;35:441–5.

[53] Schenck PA, Chew DJ. Prediction of serum ionized calcium concentration by use of serum total calcium concentration in dogs. Am J Vet Res 2005;66:1330–6.

[54] Schenck PA, Chew DJ, Nagode LA, et al. Disorders of calcium: hypercalcemia and hypocalcemia. In: DiBartola SP, editor. Fluid, electrolyte, and acid-base disorders in small animal practice. 3rd edition. St. Louis (MO): Saunders Elsevier; 2006. p. 122–94.

[55] Bateman S. Disorders of magnesium: magnesium deficit and excess. In: DiBartola SP, editor. Fluid, electrolyte, and acid-base disorders in small animal practice. 3rd edition. St. Louis (MO): Saunders Elsevier; 2006. p. 210–26.

Fluid and Electrolyte Therapy in Endocrine Disorders: Diabetes Mellitus and Hypoadrenocorticism

Søren R. Boysen, DVM

Department of Clinical Sciences, University of Montreal, CP 5000, Sainte Hyacinthe, Quebec, Canada, J2S 7C6

DIABETES MELLITUS

Diabetic ketoacidosis (DKA) and hyperglycemic hyperosmolar syndrome (HHS) are serious complications of decompensated diabetes mellitus that can result in major fluid and electrolyte imbalances and are associated with substantial morbidity and mortality in dogs and cats [1–3]. The prognosis, however, varies depending on coexisting diseases, which have been identified in 69% to 92% of patients and include infection, neoplasia, heart failure, renal failure, pancreatitis, gastrointestinal tract disease, hyperadrenocorticism, hepatic disease, dermatitis, and uterine disease [1–4]. Drugs that affect carbohydrate metabolism, such as corticosteroids, thiazides, and sympathomimetic agents, also have been reported to precipitate DKA and HHS crises [1,3,5]. The major criteria for the diagnosis of DKA in the veterinary patient is the biochemical triad of hyperglycemia, ketonemia, and acidemia, whereas the diagnosis of HHS requires a glucose concentration greater than 600 mg/dL (33 mmol/L), absence of urine ketones, and a calculated total serum osmolality greater than 350 mOsm/kg [6]. Despite differences in definition, the treatment for both syndromes is similar and overlap exists, with some patients that have DKA being hyperosmolar (>350 mOsm/kg H_2O) and some patients that have HHS having mild ketosis without acidosis [1,2,7].

Pathophysiology

The metabolic derangements of DKA and HHS are complex, and comprehensive reviews are available [5,7]. In summary, the metabolic derangements result from a relative or absolute insulin deficiency combined with increased concentrations of counterregulatory hormones (eg, glucagon, catecholamines, cortisol, growth hormone), which usually are increased in association with a coexisting disease process [1,3,7]. When these hormone imbalances occur, hyperglycemia ensues as a result of increased hepatic glucose production (by means of upregulation of glycogenolysis and gluconeogenesis primarily through the actions

E-mail address: soren.boysen@umontreal.ca

0195-5616/08/$ – see front matter
doi:10.1016/j.cvsm.2008.01.001

of catecholamines and glucagon) and decreased uptake of glucose by peripheral tissues [5].

In DKA, insulin deficiency, combined with increased concentrations of catecholamines, cortisol, and growth hormone, activates hormone-sensitive lipase, which results in lipolysis and the release of free fatty acids. These free fatty acids are taken up by the liver; converted to the ketones acetoacetate, acetone, and β-hydroxybutyrate (the process of which is enhanced by increased glucagon concentration); and released into the circulation [5]. These ketones then are filtered by the kidney and partially excreted in the urine, which causes ketonuria and contributes to osmotic diuresis.

In the case of HHS, a decrease in glomerular filtration rate (GFR) leads to severe hyperglycemia and hyperosmolar syndrome. In people, an inverse relation between increasing glucose concentration and decreasing GFR has been demonstrated [8]. This decrease in GFR may be prerenal or renal in origin. When hyperglycemia of diabetes mellitus occurs and the renal threshold for glucose is exceeded, glucosuria and osmotic diuresis ensue. This may lead to dehydration, hypovolemia, and a decrease in GFR, resulting in decreased glucose clearance by the kidney and exacerbation of hyperglycemia. Coexisting diseases, including shock, renal failure, or heart failure, contribute to decreased GFR, which may explain why these diseases are more commonly identified in patients that develop HHS [2]. Although not well established, it is believed that ketone formation is minimal in HHS because of the presence of low concentrations of insulin, which are sufficient to inhibit lipolysis effectively but insufficient to control blood glucose concentration [5,7].

Associated Complications

Acid-base imbalance

Acidosis is an important complication in dogs and cats that have DKA and HHS and has been shown to correlate with the outcome in dogs that have DKA [1]. The cause of acidosis is likely multifactorial, but a major component is the overproduction of acetoacetic acid and β-hydroxybutyric acid [5]. Acetoacetic acid is the initial ketone produced by the liver, which then may be reduced to β-hydroxybutyric acid or nonenzymatically decarboxylated to acetone [9]. Acetone is chemically neutral, but the other two ketones are organic acids [9]. At physiologic pH, these two ketoacids dissociate completely, resulting in the production of hydrogen ions and ketoanions [5]. Acidosis results when the bicarbonate that buffers accumulated hydrogen ions is overwhelmed. Lactic acidosis also is commonly identified in dogs and cats that have DKA and HHS and can contribute substantially to acidosis [1,2]. In addition, renal failure often is identified in cats that have HHS, which may be associated with renal azotemia and acidosis [2,3]. Finally, hyperchloremic metabolic acidosis also may occur in patients that have DKA and HHS, especially during therapy. This acid-base disturbance occurs as a result of chloride retention when ketoanions are excreted in the urine with sodium and potassium, by intracellular shifting of bicarbonate after therapy, and by administration of chloride-rich fluids (eg, 0.9% saline) during therapy [5,8]. This acidosis usually is self-limiting and of minimal clinical relevance because it tends to correct itself in the 24 to 48 hours after initiation of therapy as a result of enhanced renal acid excretion [5].

Fluid and electrolyte imbalances

Fluid losses in patients that have HHS and DKA are multifactorial in nature, and each patient must be assessed individually and regularly re-evaluated to estimate initial losses and account for ongoing losses. Hyperglycemia and, to a lesser extent, ketosis induce osmotic diuresis and severe fluid loss, which tend to be more severe in patients that have HHS than in patients that have DKA [5]. Gastrointestinal losses through vomiting and diarrhea, which are frequently reported clinical signs in patients that have DKA and HHS, further contribute to fluid losses [1,2]. Coexisting diseases, such as renal failure, vasculitis, liver failure, and hyperadrenocorticism, also may affect fluid losses and must be considered when assessing the patient's fluid therapy plan.

Plasma sodium concentration in dogs and cats with DKA and HHS can be low, normal, or high, but most studies show that uncorrected sodium concentrations are low at the time of presentation [1,2]. Decreased plasma sodium concentration is likely explained by the persistence of hyperglycemia, which pulls fluid into the vascular space, thus diluting the concentration of sodium [7,10]. Because of this osmotic shift of water into the vascular space, it has been suggested that sodium concentration be corrected for the degree of hyperglycemia by adding 1.6 mEq/L (1.6 mmol/L) to the measured sodium level for every 100-mg/dL (5.6-mmol/L) increase in glucose concentration greater than normal. The corrected plasma sodium concentration should more accurately reflect the true hydration status of the patient [5,7,10].

Total body potassium and phosphorus depletion often is profound in patients that have DKA and HHS, despite the fact that some animals are presented with normal to increased plasma concentrations of these electrolytes [1,2]. Extracellular potassium and phosphorus are lost by means of the kidneys as a result of osmotic diuresis and insulin deficiency (insulin is required for normal sodium, chloride, potassium, and phosphorus absorption in renal tubular epithelial cells) [4]. Osmotic diuresis increases delivery of fluid to the distal nephron and dilutes electrolytes within the tubular lumen, resulting in decreased reabsorption of these electrolytes. Further depletion of electrolytes occurs because of anorexia, vomiting, and diarrhea. The loss of ketones in the urine further contributes to osmotic diuresis; because ketoanions are negatively charged (and their dissociated hydrogen ions are buffered by bicarbonate), their excretion in the urine is accompanied by a positive ion other than hydrogen (ie, sodium or potassium), which further contributes to electrolyte depletion. Several events can occur during DKA and HHS to maintain normal to increased plasma potassium and phosphate concentrations, however, despite depletion of total body stores. Hyperglycemia increases plasma osmolality, and consequently draws water into the intravascular space, initially diluting plasma electrolyte concentrations. As water moves out of cells, intracellular potassium and phosphorus concentrations increase (ie, intracellular dehydration) and extracellular concentrations decrease (ie, extracellular dilution), producing a concentration gradient that favors extracellular movement of potassium and phosphorus. This extracellular shift of potassium and phosphorus is enhanced by the presence of acidosis and hypoinsulinemia [1]. As DKA and HHS progress, osmotic diuresis leads to dehydration with decreased renal perfusion and GFR. As GFR decreases, renal excretion of potassium and phosphorus decreases and plasma concentrations can be normal to increased despite substantial total body potassium and phosphorus depletion. Once fluid administration and insulin therapy are started, additional electrolyte depletion can occur as a result of insulin-mediated re-entry of potassium and phosphorus into cells, correction of acidosis (which promotes intracellular shifting of potassium and phosphorus), dilution of electrolytes by extracellular fluid expansion, and continued potassium and phosphorus excretion in urine as a result of ongoing osmotic diuresis [1].

Decreased ionized magnesium concentrations are not common in dogs that have DKA, and serum magnesium concentration does not seem to be correlated with the outcome [5]. Nevertheless, it still should be monitored, because magnesium is lost during osmotic diuresis and patients that have documented hypomagnesemia may develop arrhythmias and refractory hypokalemia or hypocalcemia [11].

Treatment

The primary objectives in the treatment of patients that have DKA and HHS are to restore intravascular volume, correct dehydration, correct electrolyte and acid-base disturbances, and decrease glucose concentrations. It is also important to identify and address any coexisting diseases. Because DKA and HHS are life-threatening emergencies, therapy typically involves hospitalization of the patient.

Fluids

The first priority in patients that have DKA or HHS is to restore intravascular volume by administration of fluids. If the patient is presented in a state of shock, priority is given to achieving cardiovascular stability and reversing shock (see articles elsewhere in this issue related to therapy of shock).

If cardiovascular function is stable, fluid therapy varies according to the degree of dehydration and clinical signs of the patient. An occasional patient that has DKA is presented in a euvolemic state with minimal fluid or electrolyte disturbances [1]. If the patient is alert, eating, and drinking and does not show systemic signs of illness, aggressive therapy is unnecessary, even in the presence of increased ketone concentrations. Control of blood glucose concentration by subcutaneously administered insulin often is sufficient to treat these patients, similar to patients that are presented with uncomplicated diabetes mellitus.

Most patients that have DKA and HHS are presented with moderate to severe fluid and electrolyte imbalances and systemic signs of illness that necessitate aggressive in-hospital therapy, however. Because fluid losses are a major contributing factor to the development of severe hyperglycemia and ketoacidosis, priority is given to expanding the extracellular space (intravascular and interstitial) rapidly and improving renal perfusion before starting insulin therapy [5,7]. The administration of fluids, without concurrent insulin, has been shown to decrease blood glucose concentrations by 30% to 50% in children who have DKA during the first hour of fluid therapy by dilution of blood glucose and increased renal perfusion (increased GFR and renal glucose clearance) [5,7,12]. Fluid therapy also has been shown to decrease concentrations of counterregulatory hormones and serum osmolality, making cells more responsive to insulin [7]. In fact, if insulin therapy is started before restoring intravascular volume and establishing good tissue perfusion, glucose and water may shift from the vascular space into cells, leading to vascular collapse, shock, and death [8,12]. Therefore, insulin therapy should be delayed for 1 to 2 hours after initiation of fluid therapy in critically ill patients that have DKA and HHS, especially when hyperglycemia is severe or hypotension is present. In the absence of shock, heart failure, or oliguric to anuric renal failure, the author prefers to administer fluids at a rate of 15 to 20 mL/kg/h [13], or 20% of the calculated fluid deficit in the first hour of therapy followed by 30% of the calculated deficit over the next 4 to 5 hours. The final 50% of the calculated fluid deficit is corrected over the remaining 18 hours so that the fluid deficit is completely corrected by 24 hours. Maintenance fluid needs ($[BW_{(kg)} \times 30] + 70$), based on body weight (BW), and anticipated ongoing losses (through continued osmotic diuresis, renal insufficiency, vomiting, diarrhea, and fever) also should be added to the fluid therapy protocol.

Although debated in the human literature and not investigated in veterinary medicine, it has been recommended not to decrease the plasma osmolality of patients that have DKA and HHS by more than 3 to 4 mOsm/L/h, because rapid decreases in the serum osmolality may lead to cerebral edema [5,7]. A practical approach to following osmolality clinically is to calculate effective osmolality. Calculation of effective osmolality is determined by the sodium (measured serum sodium concentration $\times$ 2) plus glucose (measured blood glucose concentration in mg/dL $\div$ 18 or glucose in mmol/L) concentrations [7,10]. This change represents a change in total effective osmolality such that a decrease in osmolality of 5 mOsm/L/h caused by a decrease in blood glucose concentration coupled with an increase in osmolality of 4 mOsm/L/h caused by increased serum sodium concentration would decrease effective osmolality only by 1 mOsm/L/h. To follow changes in osmolality, blood glucose concentration should be evaluated hourly and serum electrolyte concentrations checked during the first 2 hours of therapy and every 4 to 6 hours thereafter until normal hydration is restored. If evaluation of serum electrolyte concentrations is not readily available, it is prudent to follow blood glucose concentration hourly to prevent a decrease of more than 100 mg/dL/h (5.5 mmol/L/h) [13]. Dextrose (at a concentration of 2.5%) can be added to the intravenous fluids if the decrease in blood glucose concentration is more than 100 mg/dL/h (5.5 mmol/L/h), or the insulin infusion rate can be adjusted if insulin therapy has already been initiated. Hourly evaluation of blood glucose concentration can be achieved by use of a central venous catheter to allow repeated blood sampling or by use of the marginal ear vein to obtain capillary blood samples [14,15].

Isotonic fluids are recommended in the treatment of patients that have DKA and HHS to prevent a rapid decrease in osmolality, which is more likely to occur if hypotonic fluids are administered. This approach is especially important in cases of HHS, in which a rapid decrease in the glucose or sodium concentration could lead to cerebral edema [2,5]. Fortunately, the risk for clinically relevant cerebral edema seems to be rare, but it still should be considered in patients that fail to respond appropriately to initial therapy. Normal saline currently is the initial isotonic fluid of choice in people and has been recommended in dogs and cats that have DKA and HHS because it provides sodium to correct sodium depletion as glucose is decreased, which may prevent rapid decreases in serum osmolality and subsequent neurologic complications [10]. Administration of 0.9% sodium chloride (NaCl) may contribute to hyperchloremic metabolic acidosis, however, and other isotonic fluids (ie, lactate-, gluconate-, and acetate-containing fluids) have been used effectively in cats and dogs [1,16], although their safety in the initial management of dogs and cats that have DKA and HHS has not been critically investigated. After initial expansion of the extracellular space, the subsequent choice of fluid for replacement depends on the state of hydration, electrolyte concentrations, urine output, ongoing losses and underlying disease conditions.

Potassium

Treatment of patients that have DKA and HHS with fluids and insulin often rapidly decreases serum potassium concentration, especially in the first few hours of therapy. Potassium supplementation therefore is required in most cats and dogs that have DKA or HHS. If serum potassium concentration is increased at the time of presentation, extracellular volume expansion should be initiated with non–potassium-containing fluids until renal perfusion is corrected and underlying oliguric or anuric renal failure is ruled out (ideally by following urine output using an indwelling urinary catheter). Once renal perfusion is restored (based on urine output >2.0 mL/kg/h), fluids should be supplemented with potassium according to serum potassium concentration (Table 1). If potassium concentration is normal or low before starting extracellular volume expansion, potassium should be added to the fluids and insulin administration should be withheld until hydration status is improved (see Table 1). After starting fluid or insulin therapy, serum electrolyte concentrations ideally should be re-evaluated 1 to 2 hours later and then every 4 to 6 hours until normal hydration and adequate glycemic control are achieved. If electrolyte monitoring is unavailable, 20 to 40 mEq/L of potassium can be added to the fluids of patients that have normal renal function. In animals that remain hypokalemic despite aggressive potassium supplementation (up to 0.5 mEq/kg/h), serum magnesium concentration should be evaluated, because correction of serum potassium concentration may not be possible without concurrently correcting

Table 1
Adjustments for potassium supplementation

Serum K$^+$ (mEq/L)	K$^+$ supplement/L
≥3.5	20
3.0–3.5	30
2.5–3.0	40
2.0–2.5	60
≤2.0	80

serum magnesium concentration [17]. If the serum magnesium concentration is low and associated with refractory hypokalemia or arrhythmias, an infusion of magnesium can be started by adding magnesium sulfate to 5% dextrose in water and administering 0.75 to 1.0 mEq/kg/d as a constant rate infusion [18]. The dosage can be reduced by 50% for the next 3 to 5 days [18].

Bicarbonate
Administration of sodium bicarbonate to patients that have DKA has received considerable attention, and although it remains controversial, the current general consensus is that sodium bicarbonate is not of benefit in the therapy of most patients that have DKA [5,7,12]. There are few prospective randomized studies in the human literature and none in the veterinary literature regarding the use of bicarbonate in DKA. Retrospective reviews have not demonstrated any difference in severity of acidosis, mental status improvement, or correction of hyperglycemia whether or not bicarbonate therapy was used [19,20]. Furthermore, detrimental effects associated with administration of sodium bicarbonate include a transient decline in mean arterial pressure and increase in intracranial pressure after rapid intravenous administration, decreased ionized calcium concentration (which may affect left ventricular contractility), decreased potassium concentrations, decreased oxygen delivery caused by decreased unloading of oxygen from hemoglobin at the tissue level (ie, Bohr effect), paradoxical central nervous system acidosis (especially in patients that are hypercarbic because of hypoventilation), and prolongation of ketoanion metabolism [5,21–24]. In addition, overshoot alkalosis may occur when ketoanions and lactate are metabolized (which results in bicarbonate production) after insulin therapy and improved oxygen delivery as a result of resuscitative efforts. Nevertheless, the recommendation in people is to administer bicarbonate if the arterial pH remains lower than 7.0 after 1 hour of fluid therapy. In these cases, sufficient sodium bicarbonate is administered every 2 hours until a pH of 7.0 is achieved. The goal is not to re-establish a normal bicarbonate concentration or arterial pH values. If the arterial pH is higher than 7.0 after 1 hour of fluid therapy, bicarbonate therapy is not recommended [5].

Phosphorus
Phosphorus frequently is supplemented in dogs and cats that have DKA and HHS in the first 12 to 48 hours of therapy [1,3]. Although clinical signs associated with hypophosphatemia are rare and usually limited to hemolytic

anemia in cats, and possibly to stupor and seizures in dogs [3,4], it is recommended to measure serum phosphorus concentration and start phosphate supplementation when the serum phosphorus concentration decreases to lower than 1.5 mg/dL (0.5 mmol/L). Phosphorus supplementation is achieved by administering potassium phosphate at a rate of 0.01 to 0.06 mmol/kg/h in 0.9% saline, although infusions of up to 0.12 mmol/kg/h have been used to increase phosphate concentrations rapidly up to 2.5 mg/dL (0.8 mmol/L) [16]. Caution should be used with higher doses, because overly aggressive phosphorus supplementation may lead to hypocalcaemia, tetany, and soft tissue mineralization [3,5]. Repeated measurements of serum phosphorus and calcium concentrations (every 12–24 hours) are recommended when phosphorus supplementation is instituted.

Insulin

Insulin acts to correct hyperglycemia and decrease ketone production (by reduction in lipolysis and decreased glucagon secretion), and it may augment ketone use [9]. In critically ill patients that have DKA and HHS, regular crystalline insulin should be administered as a low-dose continuous intravenous infusion or by intermittent intramuscular injections. The advantages of low-dose insulin therapy are that it provides a more gradual decrease in blood glucose concentration of 50 to 75 mg/dL/h (2.8–4 mmol/L/h), which minimizes rapid changes in osmolality (that could precipitate cerebral edema) and decreases the risk for hypoglycemia, hypokalemia, and other electrolyte imbalances [5,7]. The intramuscular administration protocol involves an initial regular insulin dose of 0.2 U/kg administered intramuscularly, followed by a dosage of 0.1 U/kg/h administered intramuscularly. Blood glucose concentration is monitored hourly, and once it reaches 250 mg/dL (14 mmol/L), injections are decreased to 0.1 to 0.4 U/kg administered subcutaneously every 4 to 8 hours, and 50% dextrose is added to the fluids to make a 5% solution. Injections are continued subcutaneously at 0.1 to 0.4 U/kg every 4 to 8 hours, with the dosage and dosing interval based on glucose measurements taken every 1 to 2 hours with the goal of maintaining blood glucose concentration between 200 and 300 mg/dL (between 11 and 16.5 mmol/L). The intravenous administration protocol involves adding regular insulin (2.2 U/kg for dogs and 1.1 U/kg for cats) to 250 mL of 0.9% NaCl and adjusting the rate of administration based on hourly evaluation of blood glucose concentration and use of a sliding scale (Table 2). These intramuscular and intravenous protocols are only initial guides, and higher or lower doses of regular insulin may be required based on the response of the animal. If the intramuscular or intravenous protocols described here do not result in a decrease in blood glucose concentration of 50 mg/dL/h (2.8 mmol/L/h) in the first hour, hydration status should be rechecked. If hydration is adequate, the insulin dose should be increased every hour (50%–100%) until a decrease of 50 to 70 mg/dL/h (2.8–3.8 mmol/L/h) in blood glucose concentration is observed. Thereafter, the insulin infusion dose is adjusted to maintain the blood glucose concentrations between 200 and 300 mg/dL (11 and 16.5 mmol/L). Regular

Table 2
Adjustments for intravenously administered regular crystalline insulin and intravenously administered dextrose therapy after initial rehydration

Measured glucose (mg/dL)	Fluid type (250-mL bag)	Fluid rate (mL/h) (dogs: 2.2 U/kg in 250 mL) (cats: 1.1 U/kg in 250 mL)
≥250	0.9% saline	10
200–250	0.9% saline + 2.5% dextrose	7
150–200	0.9% saline + 2.5% dextrose	5
100–150	0.9% saline + 5% dextrose	5
<100	0.9% saline + 5% dextrose	Stop insulin infusion

Adapted from Macintire DK. Emergency therapy of diabetic crisis: insulin overdose, diabetic ketoacidosis, and hyperosmolar coma. Vet Clin North Am Small Anim Pract 1995;25(3):646; with permission.

insulin therapy is continued until the patient is eating and drinking; at that time, the animal can be switched to longer acting insulin administered subcutaneously.

HYPOADRENOCORTICISM

The adrenal gland produces more than 30 hormones, but only 2 are responsible for most glucocorticoid and mineralocorticoid functions of the body: cortisol accounts for more than 95% of glucocorticoid activity, and aldosterone accounts for more than 90% of mineralocorticoid activity [25]. A deficiency in the production or secretion of either of these 2 major hormones, termed *hypoadrenocorticism*, can have profound effects on fluid, electrolyte, and acid-base balance that require prompt recognition and aggressive therapy to prevent death of the patient.

Etiology

Hypoadrenocorticism (Addison's disease) is uncommon in dogs and rare in cats but may result from diseases that directly affect the adrenal glands (primary hypoadrenocorticism) or indirectly affect adrenal gland function (secondary to disease or suppression of the hypothalamic-pituitary axis). Primary hypoadrenocorticism usually results in mineralocorticoid and glucocorticoid deficiency with more pronounced clinical signs. In contrast, secondary hypoadrenocorticism is associated with preserved mineralocorticoid function, and clinical signs often are more subtle, which has given rise to the term *atypical* Addison's disease. Diseases associated with primary and secondary hypoadrenocorticism are listed in Table 3.

Diagnosis

Hypoadrenocorticism is suspected based on history and clinical signs supported by classic electrolyte imbalances and is confirmed with a corticotropin stimulation test. Typical historical findings associated with hypoadrenocorticism include gastrointestinal signs (eg, vomiting, diarrhea possibly with melena),

Table 3
Causes of primary and secondary hypoadrenocorticism in dogs and cats

Primary hypoadrenocorticism	Secondary hypoadrenocorticism
Immune-mediated destruction[a]	Iatrogenic (chronic steroid administration)[a]
Lymphomatous infiltration	Neoplasia of the hypothalamus or pituitary
Metastatic tumors	Trauma
Granulomatous disease	Inflammatory lesions
Amyloidosis	
Trauma	
Infarction	
Iatrogenic causes (surgical removal of the adrenal glands or administration of adrenocorticolytic drugs, such as mitotane or trilostane)	

[a]Reported to be the most common causes.
   Data from Meeking S. Treatment of acute adrenal insufficiency. Clin Tech Small Anim Pract 2007;22:
36–9; and Greco DS. Hypoadrenocorticism in small animals. Clin Tech Small Anim Pract 2007;22:32–5.

lethargy, weakness, and collapse that may wax and wane over time [26]. Biochemical and hematologic abnormalities that should prompt consideration of hypoadrenocorticism include hyponatremia, hypochloremia, hyperkalemia, hypoglycemia, hypercalcemia, eosinophilia, and absolute lymphocytosis (absence of a stress leukogram). When the sodium/potassium ratio is less than 27, hypoadrenocorticism should be considered (although other diseases may cause similar sodium/potassium ratios), and when the ratio is less than 20, hypoadrenocorticism should be strongly suspected [26]. The presence of bradycardia (or an inappropriately normal heart rate) in an animal presented in a state of shock with hypovolemia should prompt consideration of diseases that can cause hyperkalemia, including hypoadrenocorticism. A corticotropin stimulation test (aqueous corticotropin: dogs, 0.5 µg/kg administered intravenously with a maximal dose of 250 µg; cats, 125 µg per cat administered intravenously) with measurement of baseline and 1-hour postinjection plasma cortisol concentrations (an additional 30-minute postinjection plasma cortisol concentration is recommended for cats) should be used to confirm the disease [27]. A postcorticotropin plasma cortisol concentration less than 2 µg/dL (<20 pg/mL) confirms the diagnosis in dogs and cats [26,27].

Mineralocorticoid Deficiency

Aldosterone plays a vital role in maintaining normal sodium, potassium, and water homeostasis by means of sodium, chloride, and water reabsorption and potassium excretion. Its primary site of action is the renal tubule, although it does have some regulatory effects on the gastrointestinal tract, salivary glands, and sweat glands.

Sodium and water homeostasis

Aldosterone acts primarily on the principal cells of the collecting tubule to increase the absorption of sodium [25]. When sodium is reabsorbed through the tubular epithelial cell, negative ions, such as chloride, accompany sodium because of electrical potentials. In addition, because of the concentration difference between the tubular lumen and the renal interstitium created by sodium and chloride absorption, water is passively reabsorbed. It therefore follows that lack of aldosterone secretion results in a tremendous loss of sodium, chloride, and water in the urine. Aldosterone also plays an important role in the absorption of sodium from the gastrointestinal tract, especially in the colon [25]. In the absence of aldosterone, intestinal sodium absorption is diminished, which leads to a parallel decrease in the absorption of chloride and water. The unabsorbed sodium, chloride, and water lead to diarrhea, which often is accompanied by vomiting and further depletion of extracellular fluid volume. As the extracellular fluid volume decreases, intravascular volume falls, cardiac output is decreased, and shock ensues. Death of the patient occurs in 4 days to 2 weeks after complete cessation of mineralocorticoid secretion [25].

Potassium homeostasis
Maintenance of serum potassium concentration primarily depends on renal excretion of potassium by means of the actions of aldosterone and the control of distribution of potassium between the extracellular and intracellular compartments, which also is influenced by aldosterone [25]. Therefore, lack of aldosterone secretion results in marked hyperkalemia. Hyperkalemia is exaggerated by decreased renal perfusion as a result of sodium wasting and hypovolemia, which leads to a decrease in GFR. Finally, shifting of potassium ions out of cells in response to metabolic acidosis, which is common in patients with adrenal crisis, may further contribute to hyperkalemia [28]. Hyperkalemia leads to abnormal cardiac conduction and an increased refractory period, which can result in decreased cardiac output and potentially fatal arrhythmias (eventual ventricular fibrillation or asystole) [26,29].

Acid-base regulation
Aldosterone enhances the secretion of hydrogen ions in exchange for sodium in the intercalated cells of the cortical collecting tubules, and the absence of aldosterone secretion has been associated with mild acidosis [25]. During an adrenal crisis, however, confounding factors, including decreased renal perfusion and hypotension, also can lead to profound acidosis. Decreased renal perfusion occurs as a result of extreme renal sodium and water losses leading to hypovolemia. With decreased renal perfusion, the ability of the kidneys to excrete waste products (including hydrogen ions) is diminished and metabolic acidosis ensues. This acidosis is compounded in patients with hypoperfusion as a result of increased anaerobic metabolism and generation of lactic acidosis.

Glucocorticoid Deficiency
Cortisol has well-known effects on lipid, carbohydrate, and protein metabolism, but its effects on blood pressure, blood volume, and blood glucose concentration contribute to the more serious acute complications of hypoadrenocorticism. Cortisol is a nonspecific stimulant that activates the release of

vasoactive substances, sensitizes blood vessels to the effects of catecholamines, and decreases vascular permeability [25]. A deficiency in cortisol therefore is associated with a decrease in blood pressure, a loss of intravascular volume as a consequence of increased vascular permeability, and hypoglycemia attributable to decreased gluconeogenesis [25].

Although diarrhea, vomiting, and renal sodium losses associated with aldosterone deficiency contribute to total body sodium and water depletion, cortisol deficiency also seems to play an important role in the development of hyponatremia [30]. In fact, hyponatremia may be seen in secondary adrenal insufficiency when mineralocorticoid function is normal [31]. The relation between cortisol and hyponatremia is explained in part by the cortisol's normal inhibitory effects on antidiuretic hormone (ADH) release. In hypoadrenocorticism (in which cortisol secretion is diminished), cortisol's inhibitory effects are lost, resulting in increased ADH secretion. ADH increases free water reabsorption by the kidney, which results in dilution of the plasma sodium concentration [30]. The volume depletion associated with mineralocorticoid deficiency further contributes to ADH release and hyponatremia.

Development of moderate to severe hyponatremia can lead to neurologic signs as a result of osmotic fluid shifts during its development or after initiation of therapy, especially if hyponatremia is chronic and the sodium concentration is corrected too quickly [32]. Proper sodium homeostasis also is required for normal renal medullary function, and hyponatremia with sodium losses can lead to polyuria, polydipsia, and dilute urine in the face of severe dehydration as a result of renal medullary solute washout. It is important not to mistake dilute urine in the face of dehydration, azotemia, and hyperkalemia with acute renal failure, which is a major differential diagnosis in patients presented with an acute adrenal crisis. Most patients that have azotemia as a result of hypoadrenocorticism respond rapidly to aggressive fluid therapy, which should prompt consideration of hypoadrenocorticism, whereas azotemia associated with acute renal failure often takes much longer to correct.

Treatment

The predominant manifestation of acute hypoadrenal crisis is shock, and therapy should be directed toward factors contributing to the development of shock. Treatment should include restoring intravascular volume and establishing normal tissue perfusion, rapidly identifying and treating arrhythmias associated with hyperkalemia, addressing other electrolyte imbalances, correcting hypoglycemia, and providing glucocorticoids. The underlying cause also should be identified and treated.

Fluids

Successful fluid therapy often is the deciding factor in determining if the patient that has acute hypoadrenocorticism lives or dies in the emergency and critical care setting. Rapid intravenous administration of fluids should be initiated at the time of presentation when shock is first identified, and the clinician should not wait for confirmation of a definitive diagnosis. Aggressive fluid therapy restores blood volume and improves renal perfusion, which decreases serum potassium concentration by dilution and promotion of renal potassium excretion. In the absence of underlying heart disease or anuric renal failure, it is recommended to administer one quarter to one third of the calculated "shock dose" of fluids (ie, 20–30 mL/kg using isotonic crystalloids) as a rapid intravenous bolus (over approximately 10 minutes) while continuing to evaluate the animal's perfusion status (eg, heart rate, capillary refill time, blood pressure, blood lactate concentration, urine output, central venous pressure). If the patient remains unstable, 20- to 30-mL/kg boluses should be continued until hemodynamic stability is achieved. Ideally, resuscitation should be achieved within 30 minutes of arrival at the hospital. If gastrointestinal hemorrhage is present (identified in approximately 15% of dogs that have hypoadrenocorticism) [26], a blood transfusion may be required depending on the patient's hematocrit and initial response to fluid therapy.

Normal saline has been recommended as the fluid of choice for volume replacement in patients that have hypoadrenocorticism because it does not contain potassium and is high in sodium compared with other replacement fluids [26,28]. Because osmotic demyelinosis has been reported in hyponatremic dogs after fluid therapy with 0.9% saline [33–35], however, isotonic fluids with lower sodium concentrations may be reasonable alternatives in the initial management of these patients. Because most fluids other than 0.9% saline contain low concentrations of potassium (4–5 mEq/L), the risks and benefits of treating hyponatremia and hyperkalemia must be balanced. Because hyperkalemia is the more immediate life-threatening electrolyte disorder, the author frequently administers 0.9% saline during the first hour of fluid resuscitation and then switches to an alternative isotonic fluid after re-evaluation of the patient's serum electrolyte concentrations.

Hyperkalemia
Treatment of hyperkalemia usually begins with fluid therapy, which decreases serum potassium concentrations by means of dilution and increased GFR. In addition, rapid intravascular volume replacement helps to correct acidosis with resultant transcellular shift of potassium into cells, thereby decreasing serum potassium concentration as pH increases [29]. Isotonic fluids that do not contain potassium (0.9% saline) have been recommended [26,28]. Other isotonic replacement fluids with low concentrations of potassium also decrease serum potassium concentration by the mechanisms described previously, however. In the author's experience, most hyperkalemic patients that have hypoadrenocorticism respond to aggressive fluid therapy alone and do not require additional therapeutic efforts to decrease the serum potassium concentration.

In the few patients that require additional therapy, the decision to treat should be based on the presence of clinically relevant electrocardiographic (ECG) changes consistent with hyperkalemia. As serum potassium concentration increases, classic ECG changes occur as a result of the effect of hyperkalemia on atrial and ventricular depolarization and repolarization. These classic changes include flattened to absent P waves, tented (spiked) T waves, prolongation of the QRS complex, bradycardia, atrial standstill, and sinoventricular complexes [26,29]. The ECG changes typically do not occur until serum potassium concentration exceeds 7 mEq/L; however, there is considerable variation in the severity of hyperkalemia necessary to produce ECG changes [26]. In fact, rarely, serum potassium concentration may reach 9 mEq/L (which normally is associated with life-threatening arrhythmias) with mild or no ECG changes [29]. The variable association between serum potassium concentration and ECG changes is largely attributable to coexisting factors that affect cardiac conduction. Hypocalcemia, hyponatremia, and acidemia can enhance the cardiac toxicity of hyperkalemia, whereas hypercalcemia (observed in 30% of dogs with hypoadrenocorticism) [26] and hypernatremia can counteract the effects of hyperkalemia on cardiac conduction [29]. Other conditions, such as hypoperfusion, pain, and ischemia, also may contribute to the ECG changes in patients that have hypoadrenocorticism and must be considered.

Additional therapy is warranted if the patient is presented with moderate to severe ECG changes as a result of hyperkalemia. Other treatments include glucose administration alone or in combination with insulin and calcium gluconate administration. Although sodium bicarbonate administration (at doses of 1–2 mEq/kg) also has been advocated as a treatment for hyperkalemia, the author has successfully corrected life-threatening hyperkalemia with the treatments mentioned previously and has not found it necessary to administer sodium bicarbonate. In addition, intravenous infusion of sodium bicarbonate can be associated with adverse effects [21–24]. Use of β_2-agonist therapy recently has been investigated as a treatment for hyperkalemia in people [29], but its use in veterinary medicine for this purpose has not been investigated (β_2-adrenergic drugs have been shown to promote intracellular shifting of potassium).

Administration of a bolus of dextrose (0.5–1.0 mL/kg of 50% dextrose diluted to a 25% solution or less with saline) when the intravenous catheter is placed is probably the easiest additional step that can be taken to decrease serum potassium concentration rapidly. In addition, dextrose administration may be required to treat preexisting hypoglycemia, which occurs in approximately 20% of dogs with hypoadrenocorticism [26]. The administration of dextrose alone has been shown to increase endogenous insulin secretion, which results in the movement of potassium from the extracellular space to the intracellular space. This approach has been shown to decrease serum potassium concentration by 0.5 to 1.5 mEq/L within 1 hour, the effects of which may persist for up to 6 hours [26,29]. If insulin is added to the protocol (regular crystalline insulin at a dose of 0.2 U/kg administered intravenously), a more pronounced decrease in serum potassium concentration is noted. If insulin is administered, however, it must be accompanied by a bolus of dextrose, followed by a continuous rate infusion of dextrose (by adding 50% dextrose to the fluids to make a 5% solution) for at least 6 hours to prevent iatrogenic hypoglycemia. Blood glucose concentration should be followed hourly for at least 6 hours if insulin is given.

If hyperkalemia is associated with severe bradycardia and ventricular arrhythmias, 10% calcium gluconate (0.5–1.0 mL/kg administered intravenously to effect over 5 minutes) can be given to antagonize the cardiotoxic effects of hyperkalemia on cardiac conduction. Electrocardiography should be used to monitor cardiac conductivity during intravenous administration of calcium gluconate. The infusion should be given to effect and stopped when the ECG tracing normalizes. The effects of calcium gluconate are almost instantaneous (acting much faster than any other treatment) but short-lived (30–60 minutes) [29]. Its use therefore often is limited to patients with severe arrhythmias caused by hyperkalemia that require immediate cardiac stabilization until fluid therapy and glucose (with or without insulin administration) have a chance to act.

Preliminary evidence suggests that the β_2-adrenergic agonist albuterol (10–20 mg administered by means of a nebulizer in 4 mL of saline over 10 minutes or 0.5 mg administered intravenously) can lower serum potassium concentration by 0.5 to 1.5 mEq/L in people [29]. The peak response is seen within 30 minutes after intravenous administration but does not occur until 90 minutes after inhalation. The potential benefits and adverse effects of administering albuterol to hyperkalemic veterinary patients that have hypoadrenocorticism have not been investigated, and its use cannot be recommended until further studies have been performed.

Acidosis
The acidosis associated with an acute adrenal crisis is more the result of hypoperfusion, with resultant lactic acidosis and decreased renal perfusion, than a consequence of the effects of aldosterone deficiency on hydrogen excretion by the kidney. As such, the acidosis tends to be readily corrected by the initial fluid resuscitation and rarely requires treatment with sodium bicarbonate.

Glucocorticoids
Glucocorticoid deficiency plays a crucial role in the pathogenesis of hypoadrenocorticism, and glucocorticoids should be administered as soon as possible to patients presented in acute adrenal crisis. Although clinical studies investigating the benefits of the different glucocorticoids are lacking, dexamethasone has several theoretic advantages. It is fast acting and can be given intravenously; it can be given before or during corticotropin stimulation testing without altering test results; it provides glucocorticoid activity to help maintain blood pressure, blood glucose concentration, and intravascular volume; and it may have a protective role in the prevention of demyelinosis during correction of hyponatremia [36]. Administration of prednisone, prednisolone, and hydrocortisone may interfere with corticotropin stimulation test results, and therefore should not be administered if the diagnosis is uncertain and a corticotropin stimulation test is required to confirm the diagnosis [26]. The dosage of dexamethasone required for treatment of an adrenal crisis also has not been investigated, and dosages recommended in the veterinary literature vary from 0.1 to 4 mg/kg administered intravenously every 12 to 24 hours [26,28]. The rationale behind lower dosages is that such dosages may prevent some of the

complications associated with higher dosages of dexamethasone, such as gastrointestinal ulceration, the risk for which may be exacerbated in patients with decreased intestinal mucosal perfusion caused by shock. Higher dosages may protect the blood-brain barrier from disruption during rapid correction of hyponatremic states, however [36]. Consequently, the author usually administers dexamethasone intravenously at a dose of 0.25 mg/kg to patients that have mild decreases in serum sodium concentration and at higher doses of up to 2 mg/kg to patients that have moderate to severe hyponatremia (<125 mEq/L). In either case, dexamethasone is given concurrently or within 2 hours of starting aggressive fluid therapy. Electrolyte and acid-base disturbances usually are corrected with these treatments, and the author typically delays mineralocorticoid therapy until the patient is more stable.

Osmotic demyelinosis
The mechanism by which an increase in serum sodium concentration leads to demyelinating lesions has not been fully elucidated but seems to be the result of adaptive changes in the brain in response to the hyponatremic state. Patients that have chronic hyponatremia (≥48 hours in people [30]) are at greater risk because their brain cells have adapted to the hyponatremic state by incorporating transporters to extrude osmolytes (including cations, such as potassium, and organic osmolytes, such as myoinositol, phosphocreatine, and glutathione) from the cell [35]. When the serum sodium concentration rapidly increases, these adaptations may result in rapid fluid loss from brain cells [31,33]. In this setting, the rapid increase in serum sodium concentration draws fluid out of adapted brain cells, leading to osmotic shrinkage of axons, severing their connections within the surrounding myelin sheaths [31]. The diagnosis of osmotic demyelination generally is suspected from the clinical findings of depression, weakness, ataxia, quadriparesis, and decreased sensory perception. Because adrenal insufficiency without demyelination can result in similar signs, this condition may be underreported in the veterinary literature. MRI confirms the diagnosis, although characteristic lesions may not be detectable for up to 4 weeks [30]. Therefore, negative MRI results do not rule out the possibility of osmotic demyelination in the early stages of the disease.

Because of the paucity of studies investigating therapy for hyponatremia in hypoadrenal patients, recommendations regarding its management in veterinary patients cannot be made with certainty. Experimental studies in dogs and clinical experience in human beings suggest that the degree of change in the sodium concentration over 24 hours is more important than the change that occurs over a given hour or period of hours [30,37]. Consequently, serum sodium concentration in asymptomatic patients should not be increased more than 10 to12 mEq/L on the first day and not more than 18 mEq/L over the first 2 days [30,32,37]. Unfortunately, an occasional patient still may develop demyelinosis with this protocol [30]. If, however, a patient is experiencing clinical signs of hyponatremia, such as seizures or other severe neurologic signs, a more rapid correction of serum sodium concentration is recommended, because the risk for untreated hyponatremia and cerebral edema is thought to outweigh the potential risk for harm from overly rapid correction. Experimental studies in rats have demonstrated that high doses of dexamethasone, when administered within 3 hours of initiating correction (using 3% hypertonic saline) of a chronic hyponatremic state, can significantly decrease the incidence and severity of osmotic demyelinosis. Dexamethasone may prevent disruption of the blood-brain barrier that otherwise occurs during overly rapid correction of serum sodium concentration in chronic hyponatremic states [36]. Given that dexamethasone already is necessary for treatment of the adrenal crisis, it seems reasonable to administer it within 3 hours of starting fluid therapy. In contrast, early use of mineralocorticoids in the treatment of hypoadrenocorticism may predispose to faster correction of hyponatremia and development of demyelinosis [28]. Therefore, it may be prudent to withhold mineralocorticoid supplementation until initial stabilization and correction of electrolyte imbalances have been achieved by means of fluid therapy.

Maintenance therapy

Long-term mineralocorticoid supplementation in dogs is provided by oral administration of fludrocortisone (0.02 mg/kg given every 24 hours, with a daily increase of 0.05–0.1 mg until serum electrolyte concentrations are stabilized) or deoxycorticosterone pivalate (DOCP; 2 mg/kg given every 25 days) [27]. If DOCP is used, prednisone (0.22 mg/kg) usually is given concurrently, because DOCP does not possess glucocorticoid activity. Fludrocortisone possesses some glucocorticoid activity, but some dogs still may require additional prednisone supplementation [26]. Cats generally are treated with DOCP (12.5 mg per cat every 3–4 weeks) and prednisone (0.22 mg/kg). Some investigators advocate injectable corticosteroids, such as methylprednisolone acetate (Depo-Medrol; 10 mg per cat every 3–4 weeks) in place of daily oral administration of glucocorticoids for cats [26]. The dosing interval for DOCP in dogs and cats usually is based on serum electrolyte measurements taken every 2 to 4 weeks during the initial induction phase. Doses are increased by 5% to 10% if serum potassium concentration remains high and serum sodium concentration is low and are decreased when serum potassium concentration is low and serum sodium concentration is high. In the event of a stressful situation (eg, illness, surgery, plane travel, boarding), dogs and cats should receive additional prednisone therapy at up to 5 to 10 times the physiologic maintenance dosage.

References

[1] Hume DZ, Drobatz KJ, Hess RS. Outcome of dogs with diabetic ketoacidosis: 127 dogs (1993–2003). J Vet Intern Med 2006;20(3):547–55.

[2] Koenig A, Drobatz KJ, Beale B, et al. Hyperglycemic, hyperosmolar syndrome in feline diabetics: 17 cases (1995–2001). J Vet Emerg Crit Care 2004;14(1):30–40.

[3] Bruskiewicz KA, Nelson RW, Feldman EC, et al. Diabetic ketosis and ketoacidosis in cats: 42 cases (1980–1995). J Am Vet Med Assoc 1997;211(2):188–92.

[4] Panciera DL. Fluid therapy in endocrine and metabolic disorders. In: DiBartola SP, editor. Fluid therapy in small animal practice. 3rd edition. Philadelphia: WB Saunders; 2006. p. 478–89.

[5] Chiasson JL, Aris-Jilwan N, Bélanger R, et al. Diagnosis and treatment of diabetic ketoacidosis and the hyperglycemic hyperosmolar state. Can Med Assoc J 2003;168(7): 859–66.

[6] Feldman EC, Nelson RW. Diabetic ketoacidosis. In: Feldman EC, Nelson RW, editors. Canine and feline endocrinology and reproduction. 2nd edition. Philadelphia: WB Saunders; 1996. p. 392–421.

[7] Kitabchi AE, Umpierrez GE, Murphy MB, et al. Management of hyperglycemic crisis in patients with diabetes mellitus. Diabetes Care 2001;24:131–53.

[8] Kandel G, Aberman A. Selected developments in the understanding of diabetic ketoacidosis. Can Med Assoc J 1983;128:392–7.

[9] Rose DB, Post T. Hyperosmolal states-hyperglycemia. In: Rose DB, Post T, editors. Clinical physiology of acid-base and electrolyte disorders. 5th edition. New York: McGraw Hill; 2001. p. 794–821.

[10] Schermerhorn T, Barr SC. Relationships between glucose, sodium and effective osmolality in diabetic dogs and cats. J Vet Emerg Crit Care 2006;16(1):19–24.

[11] Bateman S. Disorders of magnesium: magnesium deficit and excess. In: DiBartola SP, editor. Fluid therapy in small animal practice. 3rd edition. Philadelphia: WB Saunders; 2006. p. 210–26.

[12] Vanelli M, Chiarelli F. Treatment of diabetic ketoacidosis in children and adolescents. Acta BioMed 2003;74:59–68.

[13] Felner E, White PC. Improving management of diabetic ketoacidosis in children. Pediatrics 2001;108(3):735–40.

[14] Macintire DK. Emergency therapy of diabetic crisis: insulin overdose, diabetic ketoacidosis, and hyperosmolar coma. Vet Clin North Am Small Anim Pract 1995;25(3):639–50.

[15] Thompson MD, Taylor SM, Adams VJ, et al. Comparison of glucose concentrations in blood samples obtained with a marginal ear vein nick technique versus from a peripheral vein in healthy cats and cats with diabetes mellitus. J Am Vet Med Assoc 2002;221(3):389–92.

[16] Nichols R, Crenshaw KL. Complications and concurrent diseases associated with diabetic ketoacidosis and other severe forms of diabetes mellitus. Vet Clin North Am Small Anim Pract 1995;25(3):617–24.

[17] Whang R, Whang DD, Ryan MP. Refractory potassium repletion. A consequence of magnesium deficiency. Arch Intern Med 1992;152(1):40–5.

[18] Kerl ME. Diabetic ketoacidosis: treatment recommendations. Compend Contin Educ Pact Vet 2001;23(4):330–9.

[19] Morris LR, Murphy MB, Kitabchi AE. Bicarbonate therapy in severe diabetic ketoacidosis. Ann Intern Med 1986;105:836–40.

[20] Biallon A, Zerri F, LaFond P, et al. Does bicarbonate therapy improve the management of severe diabetic ketoacidosis? Crit Care Med 1999;27(12):2690–3.

[21] Forsythe SM, Schmidt G. Sodium bicarbonate for the treatment of lactic acidosis. Chest 2000;118:882–4.

[22] Cooper DJ, Walley KR, Wiggs BR, et al. Bicarbonate does not improve hemodynamics in critically ill patients who have lactic acidosis: a prospective, controlled clinical study. Ann Intern Med 1990;112:492–8.

[23] Heseby JS, Gumprecht DG. Hemodynamic effects of rapid bolus hypertonic sodium bicarbonate. Chest 1981;79:552–4.

[24] Lang RM, Fellner SK, Neumann A, et al. Left ventricular contractility varies directly with blood ionized calcium. Ann Intern Med 1988;108:524–9.

[25] Guyton AC, Hall JE. Adrenocortical hormones. In: Guyton AC, Hall JE, editors. Textbook of medical physiology. 11th edition. Philadelphia: Elsevier Saunders; 2006. p. 944–60.

[26] Greco DS. Hypoadrenocorticism in small animals. Clin Tech Small Anim Pract 2007;22(1): 32–5.

[27] Lathan P, Tyler J. Canine hypoadrenocorticism: diagnosis and treatment. Compend Contin Educ Pract Vet 2005;27(2):121–32.

[28] Meeking S. Treatment of acute adrenal insufficiency. Clin Tech Small Anim Pract 2007;22(1):36–9.

[29] Rose BD, Post T. Hyperkalemia. In: Rose DB, Post T, editors. Clinical physiology of acid-base and electrolyte disorders. 5th edition. New York: McGraw Hill; 2001. p. 888–930.

[30] Rose BD, Post T. Hypoosmolal states—hyponatremia. In: Rose DB, Post T, editors. Clinical physiology of acid-base and electrolyte disorders. 5th edition. New York: McGraw Hill; 2001. p. 696–745.

[31] Shulman DI, Palmert MR, Kemp SF, et al. Adrenal insufficiency: still a cause of morbidity and death in childhood. Pediatrics 2007;119(2):e484–94.

[32] Lauriat SM, Berl T. The hyponatremic patient: practical focus on therapy. J Am Soc Nephrol 1997;8(10):1599–607.

[33] Brady CA, Vite CH, Drobatz KJ. Severe neurologic sequelae in a dog after treatment of hypoadrenal crisis. J Am Vet Med Assoc 1999;215:222–5.

[34] Churcher RK, Watson ADJ, Eaton A. Suspected myelinolysis following rapid correction of hyponatremia in a dog. J Am Anim Hosp Assoc 1999;35:493–7.

[35] O'Brien DP, Kroll RA, Johnson GC, et al. Myelinolysis after correction of hyponatremia in two dogs. J Vet Intern Med 1994;8(1):40–8.

[36] Murase T, Sugimura Y, Takefuji S, et al. Mechanisms and therapy of osmotic demyelination. Am J Med 2006;119(7):S69–73.

[37] Laureno R, Karp BI. Myelinolysis after correction of hyponatremia. Ann Intern Med 1997;126(1):57–62.

Fluid Therapy in Patients with Pulmonary Disease

Sophie Adamantos, BVSc, CertVA, MRCVS[a],*,
Dez Hughes, BVSc, MRCVS[b]

[a]Department of Veterinary Clinical Sciences, Royal Veterinary College,
Hawkshead Lane, North Mymms, Hatfield AL9 7TA, UK
[b]55 Hume Street, Greensborough, Victoria 3088, Australia

Fluid therapy in patients with pulmonary disease is challenging. By the time pulmonary edema is present, the mechanisms that protect the lung against fluid accumulation already have been overwhelmed, and fluid therapy is likely to result in further increases in pulmonary capillary hydrostatic pressure, fluid extravasation, and worsening of pulmonary dysfunction [1]. Patients at risk for developing pulmonary dysfunction include those that have suffered blunt thoracic trauma and those at risk for developing acute respiratory distress syndrome (ARDS). These include patients with sepsis or systemic inflammatory response syndrome and patients at risk for or suffering from pneumonia. Many of these patients also have hypoperfusion and require ongoing fluid therapy to maintain tissue oxygen delivery. The difficulty lies in providing necessary fluid therapy while limiting ongoing pulmonary leakage and worsening of pulmonary edema.

For many years the debate on fluid therapy has focused on the type of fluid to give rather than the volume [2], and the accepted practice in human medicine has been based on aggressive fluid therapy protocols to maximize cardiovascular function [3]. Use of these liberal fluid therapy protocols, however, has been associated with widespread body system dysfunction, including pulmonary dysfunction [4–7]. Respiratory compromise is especially important in veterinary compared with human patients because of the availability, difficulty, and expense of artificial ventilation. More recent recommendations in human medicine suggest fluid therapy directed toward euvolemia, particularly in the presence of ARDS or traumatic brain injury [2,8–11].

OVERVIEW OF FLUID DYNAMICS IN THE LUNG

The healthy pulmonary parenchyma is well protected against the effects of intravascular volume overload. As in other tissues, fluid fluxes in the lung are

*Corresponding author. E-mail address: sadamantos@rvc.ac.uk (S. Adamantos).

0195-5616/08/$ – see front matter
doi:10.1016/j.cvsm.2008.01.005

subject to Starling forces [12]. Formation of extravascular lung water (EVLW) can be described by the following equation [13]:

$$EVLW = kA\,[(Pc{-}Pi) - \sigma(\pi c{-}\pi i)] - lymph\ flow$$

where k represents capillary permeability to water, A represents capillary surface area, *(Pc-Pi)* represents the hydrostatic pressure gradient between the capillary and interstitium, σ represents vascular permeability to macromolecules, and $\pi c{-}\pi i$ represents the colloid osmotic pressure gradient between the capillary and interstitium.

The forces responsible for return of fluid to the vascular space are $(\pi c{-}\pi i)$ and lymph flow.

The primary factor promoting fluid filtration in the lung is hydrostatic pressure, which in turn is determined by capillary flow, arterial resistance, venous resistance, and venous pressure [14]. Various protective strategies limit increases in hydrostatic pressure that otherwise would result in the formation of pulmonary edema, some of which are described in the following sections.

Capillary hydrostatic pressure can increase substantially without causing pulmonary edema [15]. Additional increases cause fluid to move into the alveolar interstitium, which is unable to expand in response to increased filtration from the pulmonary capillaries, resulting in higher interstitial pressure. Increased alveolar interstitial pressure encourages movement of fluid toward the more distensible peribronchiovascular interstitium near the hilus and around larger vessels and encourages higher rates of lymph flow, thus protecting the alveoli from flooding [16]. Lymphatic drainage is effective in the presence of increased hydrostatic pressure and can increase up to 15 times to remove excess capillary filtrate [15,17,18]. The pulmonary capillary endothelium also is relatively permeable to plasma proteins, which results in a low colloid osmotic pressure gradient between the pulmonary interstitium and intravascular space [16]. This low colloid osmotic pressure gradient protects against pulmonary edema caused by hypoproteinemia and hemodilution during massive fluid resuscitation and is re-established rapidly during acute hypoproteinemia, rapidly restoring lymph flow in these circumstances [19]. These mechanisms limit the effects of increased capillary hydrostatic pressure in healthy animals. They may be easily overcome in the presence of a pre-existing reduction in colloid osmotic pressure or increased permeability of the microvascular barrier, however [1,20]. Once the capacity for interstitial fluid retention is overcome, water begins to spill into the alveoli. Once this process has begun, it is difficult to halt [21,22].

Diseases such as pneumonia and ARDS are associated with damage to the capillary endothelium that results in increased capillary leakage of proteins and water (so-called increased permeability edema). Evidence suggests that fluid filtration occurs at lower capillary hydrostatic pressures in the presence of increased permeability. Resolution of pulmonary edema depends on the type of fluid, with pure water being more rapidly reabsorbed than fluids that contain macromolecules and cells.

FLUID THERAPY IN PULMONARY DISEASE

The choice of fluid in a particular clinical situation remains a contentious issue. Little evidence suggests that one type of fluid is more beneficial than another in most situations. In fact, when considering patients with pulmonary disease, it seems more sensible not to question what fluid to use but rather how much. In veterinary medicine, the choice of fluid to use is based on experimental evidence, studies in human patients, and personal clinical experience, because little clinical evidence is available in the veterinary literature. Given the evidence available, a limited fluid therapy strategy that ensures euvolemia may be advisable in patients with pulmonary dysfunction. Fluid restriction at the expense of tissue perfusion, however, may increase the risk of ARDS and multi-organ failure.

Pulmonary dysfunction is an important cause of patient morbidity and mortality in critically ill human patients, and a wealth of clinical and experimental information is available on this subject. Many of these studies show little difference when comparing types of fluid for resuscitation of patients with hypoperfusion. Evidence suggests that fatal pulmonary edema is associated with large volume intraoperative fluid administration [7]. It also has been observed that patients with ARDS had a smaller positive fluid balance than patients without ARDS in the same intensive care unit [8]. Some evidence suggests that resuscitation with hydroxyethyl starch or albumin is accompanied by less EVLW accumulation than resuscitation using isotonic fluids, but deterioration of pulmonary function is similar for resuscitation with all types of fluids [23,24].

The use of a pulmonary arterial (Swan-Ganz) catheter allows measurement of a full array of cardiovascular function parameters. Titrating fluid administration to the best filling pressure-stroke volume relationship may be the best way to avoid deterioration in pulmonary function [25,26], but this approach is not practical in most veterinary situations. In human medicine, use of pulmonary arterial catheters is falling out of favor in intensive care units because there is little difference in patient outcome regardless of their use, and they are associated with increased cost and patient morbidity [27,28].

FLUID THERAPY IN PATIENTS WITH PULMONARY CONTUSIONS

Patients with severe injury often require fluid therapy to replace hemorrhagic losses and avoid prolonged hypoperfusion. Experimental studies on dogs subjected to pulmonary contusions and hemorrhagic shock have shown no difference in EVLW between volume resuscitation with plasma or moderate rates of crystalloid fluid administration. Faster rates (> 30 mL/kg/h) of isotonic crystalloid fluid infusion were associated with increases in EVLW and histologic evidence of worsening of pulmonary contusions [29]. The available evidence and clinical experience suggest that patients with pulmonary contusions after trauma should be resuscitated conservatively by maintaining mean arterial blood pressure of more than 70 mm Hg to ensure adequate tissue perfusion [30]. The choice of fluid seems to make little difference, although less volume is required when using colloids compared with crystalloids to achieve the same cardiovascular endpoints [30]. Careful reassessment should be performed regularly after cessation of fluid therapy to monitor for deterioration in pulmonary function. Delayed resuscitation from hemorrhagic shock is associated with increased pulmonary capillary permeability [31], which makes prompt management of hypoperfusion with carefully titrated fluid therapy important [32].

FLUID THERAPY IN ACUTE LUNG INJURY AND ACUTE RESPIRATORY DISTRESS SYNDROME

Acute lung injury and ARDS are challenging diagnoses to make antemortem in veterinary patients. Criteria for clinical diagnosis in human patients may be difficult to apply to veterinary patients. Both of these conditions have been increasingly recognized in critically ill dogs and cats, however. Patients who have acute lung injury and ARDS have increased permeability of the alveolar-capillary barrier as a result of inflammation [33]. Increased permeability results in loss of the colloid osmotic pressure differential between the capillary and interstitium. In these situations, small increases in capillary hydrostatic pressure result in fluid exudation into the interstitium at a lower pressure than in the absence of increased permeability [13].

In these patients, whether to pursue a liberal or conservative fluid therapy plan continues to be debated in human medicine [11]. A recent prospective study that compared liberal and conservative approaches to fluid therapy in patients with acute lung injury failed to show a difference in 60-day mortality, although there was a trend toward easier ventilatory management [11]. This study was limited by the fact that patients were not subjected to different fluid management strategies unless they had stable cardiovascular function, adequate urine output, and normal central venous and pulmonary artery occlusion pressures.

Maintaining intravascular volume at the lowest level consistent with adequate systemic perfusion remains a reasonable objective in these patients [33]. If systemic perfusion cannot be maintained after restoration of intravascular volume, treatment with vasopressors or positive inotropes should be initiated sooner rather than later [33]. Accurate measures of systemic perfusion are not readily available for clinical use in veterinary patients. In the absence of renal disease, urine output provides an estimate of renal (and therefore systemic) perfusion and may be used as a readily available indicator of adequate perfusion in critically ill patients.

No evidence suggests that any type of fluid modulates pulmonary capillary permeability. Experimental evidence suggests that colloids such as albumin and dextran-40 can extravasate into the interstitium with water and contribute to increased EVLW [34,35], but this has not been observed clinically [36]. In patients with early ARDS, colloid infusion improves hemodynamic and oxygen transport variables more effectively and is not associated with deleterious pulmonary effects [36]. In the terminal stages of ARDS, any fluid administered worsens pulmonary function and the patient's condition [36]. Although there is a trend toward lower EVLW after resuscitation with colloid as compared with resuscitation with crystalloid, there is little difference in respiratory function [23,24,37,38]. Reluctance to provide mechanical ventilation in veterinary patients limits our ability to apply findings from studies in human patients to veterinary species. If mechanical ventilation is not available, a conservative approach to fluid therapy seems prudent when systemic perfusion remains compromised despite administration of vasopressors or positive inotropes to correct intravascular volume.

Little clinical evidence is available to guide fluid therapy in cases of pneumonia without ARDS. Given the presence of inflammatory changes, suggestions for fluid therapy in patients with ARDS likely would be applicable to patients with pneumonia.

SUMMARY

When managing these challenging cases, clinicians should remember that pulmonary function may deteriorate with any type of fluid administration. One also must consider the fact that once alveolar flooding occurs, it is difficult to reverse. It is vital to avoid overperfusion in patients with pulmonary dysfunction; if hypoperfusion persists, it should be treated with vasopressors and positive inotropes to enhance tissue oxygen delivery. Although a single set of rules cannot be applied to every patient, the following guidelines can be used when managing these cases. Euvolemic patients with adequate tissue perfusion (as determined by blood pressure, urine output, and serum lactate concentration) should be given sufficient isotonic fluid volume to balance insensible losses. If severe pulmonary compromise is present, cessation of all fluid therapy should be considered if the patient is able to match its insensible losses with voluntary intake of water. In hypovolemic or hypotensive patients, small boluses of isotonic crystalloids or colloids should be given to restore perfusion, avoiding rates of more than 30 mL/kg for isotonic crystalloids. If perfusion is not restored by adequate volume resuscitation, vasopressors or positive inotropes should be administered sooner rather than later to prevent fluid overload.

It is unlikely that the dilemma about fluid therapy in patients with pulmonary disease will be resolved soon, considering the divergent recommendations for liberal or restricted fluid administration. Currently, considerable evidence suggests that unrestricted fluid therapy is detrimental to patients with compromised pulmonary function.

References
[1] Guyton AC, Lindsey AW. Effect of elevated left atrial pressure and decreased plasma protein concentration on the development of pulmonary edema. Circ Res 1959;7(4): 649–57.
[2] Cotton BA, Guy JS, Morris JA Jr, et al. The cellular, metabolic, and systemic consequences of aggressive fluid resuscitation strategies. Shock 2006;26(2):115–21.
[3] Shoemaker WC, Appel P, Bland R. Use of physiologic monitoring to predict outcome and to assist in clinical decisions in critically ill postoperative patients. Am J Surg 1983;146(1): 43–50.

[4] Shah KJ, Chiu WC, Scalea TM, et al. Detrimental effects of rapid fluid resuscitation on hepatocellular function and survival after hemorrhagic shock. Shock 2002;18(3):242–7.

[5] Vassar MJ, Moore J, Perry CA, et al. Early fluid requirements in trauma patients: a predictor of pulmonary failure and mortality. Arch Surg 1988;123(9):1149–57.

[6] Lowell JA, Schifferdecker C, Driscoll DF, et al. Postoperative fluid overload: not a benign problem. Crit Care Med 1990;18(7):728–33.

[7] Arieff AI. Fatal postoperative pulmonary edema: pathogenesis and literature review. Chest 1999;115(5):1371–7.

[8] Bishop MH, Jorgens J, Shoemaker WC, et al. The relationship between ARDS, pulmonary infiltration, fluid balance, and hemodynamics in critically ill surgical patients. Am Surg 1991;57(12):785–92.

[9] The Acute Respiratory Distress Syndrome Network. Ventilation with lower tidal volumes as compared with traditional tidal volumes for acute lung injury and the acute respiratory distress syndrome. N Engl J Med 2000;342(18):1301–8.

[10] Dutton RP, McCunn M. Traumatic brain injury. Curr Opin Crit Care 2003;9(6):503–9.

[11] Wiedemann HP, Wheeler AP, Bernard GR, et al. Comparison of two fluid-management strategies in acute lung injury. N Engl J Med 2006;354(24):2564–75.

[12] Starling E. On the absorption of fluid from connectvie tissue spaces. J Physiol 1896;19: 312–26.

[13] Rosenberg AL. Fluid management in patients with acute respiratory distress syndrome. Respir Care Clin N Am 2003;9(4):481–93.

[14] Demling R. Effect of plasma and interstitial protein content on tissue edema formation. Curr Stud Hematol Blood Transfus 1986;53:36–52.

[15] Taylor AE. The lymphatic edema safety factor: the role of edema dependent lymphatic factors (EDLF). Lymphology 1990;23(3):111–23.

[16] Demling RH, LaLonde C, Ikegami K. Pulmonary edema: pathophysiology, methods of measurement, and clinical importance in acute respiratory failure. New Horiz 1993;1(3): 371–80.

[17] Erdmann AJ 3rd, Vaughan TR Jr, Brigham KL, et al. Effect of increased vascular pressure on lung fluid balance in unanesthetized sheep. Circ Res 1975;37(3):271–84.

[18] Zarins CK, Rice CL, Smith DE, et al. Role of lymphatics in preventing hypooncotic pulmonary edema. Surg Forum 1976;27(62):257–9.

[19] Harms BA, Kramer GC, Bodai BI, et al. Effect of hypoproteinemia on pulmonary and soft tissue edema formation. Crit Care Med 1981;9(7):503–8.

[20] Gaar KA Jr, Taylor AE, Owens LJ, et al. Effect of capillary pressure and plasma protein on development of pulmonary edema. Am J Physiol 1967;213(1):79–82.

[21] Zumsteg TA, Havill AM, Gee MH. Relationships among lung extravascular fluid compartments with alveolar flooding. J Appl Physiol 1982;53(1):267–71.

[22] Bachofen H, Schurch S, Michel RP, et al. Experimental hydrostatic pulmonary edema in rabbit lungs. Morphology. Am Rev Respir Dis 1993;147(4):989–96.

[23] Finch JS, Reid C, Bandy K, et al. Compared effects of selected colloids on extravascular lung water in dogs after oleic acid-induced lung injury and severe hemorrhage. Crit Care Med 1983;11(4):267–70.

[24] Cryer HM, Self SB, Carillo E, et al. Effects of electrolyte or colloid infusion on the injured lung. Am Surg 1983;49(12):645–50.

[25] Matejovic M, Krouzecky A, Rokyta R Jr, et al. Fluid challenge in patients at risk for fluid loading-induced pulmonary edema. Acta Anaesthesiol Scand 2004;48(1):69–73.

[26] Rutili G, Parker JC, Taylor AE. Fluid balance in ANTU-injured lungs during crystalloid and colloid infusions. J Appl Physiol 1984;56(4):993–8.

[27] Harvey S, Young D, Brampton W, et al. Pulmonary artery catheters for adult patients in intensive care. Cochrane Database Syst Rev 2006;3:CD003408.

[28] Shah MR, Hasselblad V, Stevenson LW, et al. Impact of the pulmonary artery catheter in critically ill patients: meta-analysis of randomized clinical trials. JAMA 2005;294(13): 1664–70.
[29] Richardson JD, Franz JL, Grover FL, et al. Pulmonary contusion and hemorrhage: crystalloid versus colloid replacement. J Surg Res 1974;16(4):330–6.
[30] Kelly ME, Miller PR, Greenhaw JJ, et al. Novel resuscitation strategy for pulmonary contusion after severe chest trauma. J Trauma 2003;55(1):94–105.
[31] Herndon DN, Traber DL, Traber LD. The effect of resuscitation on inhalation injury. Surgery 1986;100(2):248–51.
[32] Wisner DH, Sturm JA. Controversies in the fluid management of post-traumatic lung disease. Injury 1986;17(5):295–300.
[33] Ware LB, Matthay MA. The acute respiratory distress syndrome. N Engl J Med 2000;342(18):1334–49.
[34] Holcroft JW, Trunkey DD. Pulmonary extravasation of albumin during and after hemorrhagic shock in baboons. J Surg Res 1975;18(2):91–7.
[35] Holcroft JW, Trunkey DD, Lim RC. Further analysis of lung water in baboons resuscitated from hemorrhagic shock. J Surg Res 1976;20(4):291–7.
[36] Appel PL, Shoemaker WC. Evaluation of fluid therapy in adult respiratory failure. Crit Care Med 1981;9(12):862–9.
[37] Haupt MT, Teerapong P, Green D, et al. Increased pulmonary edema with crystalloid compared to colloid resuscitation of shock associated with increased vascular permeability. Circ Shock 1984;12(3):213–24.
[38] Meredith JW, Martin MB, Poole GV Jr, et al. Measurement of extravascular lung water in sheep during colloid and crystalloid resuscitation from smoke inhalation. Am Surg 1983;49(12):637–41.

Maintaining Fluid and Electrolyte Balance in Heart Failure

Teresa C. DeFrancesco, DVM

Department of Clinical Sciences, North Carolina State University College
of Veterinary Medicine, 4700 Hillsborough Street, Raleigh, NC 27606, USA

Heart failure is defined as the inability of the heart to generate sufficient cardiac output to meet the metabolic needs of the body at rest and exercise [1]. The term is sufficiently broad to include functional and structural heart diseases of varying severities and causes. Most veterinarians often associate heart failure exclusively with the later stages of heart failure when clinical signs of water and sodium retention are evident. Classically, these clinical signs of congestive heart failure in the dog and cat include pulmonary edema, ascites, and pleural effusion. Heart failure can also be asymptomatic (modified New York Heart Association functional classes I and II and International Small Animal Cardiac Health Council class I) or associated with relatively mild symptoms, however. Many veterinarians often recognize these animals as having heart disease but not necessarily heart failure. This distinction between different severities of heart failure is important. Maintenance and management of fluid and electrolyte balance are contingent on understanding the animal's heart failure severity and on detecting comorbid conditions and identifying heart failure therapeutic agents previously administered. To illustrate this point, the management of fluid and electrolyte abnormalities in a hypotensive dog with severe pancreatitis and concurrent well-compensated mild mitral valve regurgitation involves different fluid management strategies than in a dog with advanced mitral valve disease on chronic furosemide and enalapril therapy. The dog with mild mitral valve regurgitation benefits mostly from cautiously aggressive intravenous replacement fluid administration, whereas the dog with severe congestive heart failure secondary to chronic mitral valve regurgitation needs a more conservative fluid therapy strategy, combined with a transient decrease or discontinuation of diuretics and possibly the vasodilator. Optimizing cardiac output with other strategies, such as positive inotropes, may also be important in the dog with advance heart disease. Independent of comorbid conditions, however, advanced heart failure and its treatment are often associated with a variety of hemodynamic, fluid, and electrolyte derangements. This article gives the practitioner an overview of pathophysiology of common

E-mail address: teresa_defrancesco@ncsu.edu

0195-5616/08/$ – see front matter
doi:10.1016/j.cvsm.2008.02.005

fluid and electrolyte changes present in animals with heart failure, highlighting specific clinical correlates. Additionally, specific therapeutic interventions to manage these abnormalities are discussed. A list of drugs used to re-establish fluid and electrolyte homeostasis is provided at the end of the article (Appendix).

UNDERSTANDING AND MANAGEMENT OF FLUID ACCUMULATION IN HEART FAILURE

Understanding the pathophysiology of fluid accumulation in heart failure is vital to proper management. Cardiogenic pulmonary and systemic edema occurs when increased venous or capillary hydrostatic pressures cause increased transudation of fluid across the capillaries, resulting in a net accumulation of fluid in the lungs, body cavities, or peripheral tissues. Increased lymphatic drainage in the lungs provides a safety margin, especially in chronic heart failure, allowing higher hydrostatic pressures to be tolerated [1]. Despite the geared-up pulmonary lymphatic system, however, edema accumulates in the interstitial space, progressing to the alveolus and, eventually, the bronchi as pressure increases. The increased hydrostatic and venous pressure results typically from the combined effects of high ventricular filling pressures and renal retention of sodium and water. Ventricular systolic or diastolic failure increases venous pressure behind the failing heart. This can be the predominant mechanism for fluid accumulation in a dog with acute chordae tendineae rupture and fulminant pulmonary edema. In this acute decompensated heart failure case scenario, the compensatory neurohumoral response has not yet developed [1]. When heart failure develops more slowly, however, sodium and water retention is the predominant contributor to edema formation. Increased total body water and sodium result from a complex combination of initially appropriate, although long-term maladaptive, compensatory mechanisms.

Important maladaptive compensatory mechanisms resulting in fluid accumulation in heart failure are as follows:

1. Increased sympathetic nervous system activation
2. Activation of the renin-angiotensin-aldosterone system (RAAS)
3. Release of other vasoactive peptides (eg, endothelin-1, natriuretic peptides) and arginine vasopressin (eg, antidiuretic hormone [ADH])
4. Myocardial remodeling resulting in hypertrophy, fibrosis, and altered β-receptor function
5. Renal adaptations resulting in redistribution of renal blood flow and sodium and water resorption

Simply stated, the renal response to the failing heart, largely influenced by increased activation of the RAAS and vasopressin (ADH), leads to increased tubular sodium and water resorption, decreasing urinary sodium and water excretion. This increased sodium and water resorption increases plasma volume, which, over the long term, leads to the pulmonary edema and cavitary effusion.

Management

The relative contribution of sodium retention causing increased plasma volume and subsequent edema formation depends on the time course of spontaneous heart failure. A dog with fulminant pulmonary edema attributable to acute chordae tendineae rupture (acute heart failure) may not necessarily have an increased plasma volume, and thus may be more predisposed to acute ischemic renal injury with the typically aggressive diuretic therapy. Rapidly decreasing or minimizing the furosemide dose as dyspnea improves, optimizing vasodilator and inotropic therapy, and even administering cautious intravenous fluids (if the animal is not drinking on its own) may be prudent to minimize hypovolemia and renal injury in this case. That said, the use of diuretics, particularly furosemide, is a mainstay for managing symptomatic pulmonary edema and body cavity effusions. Furosemide, a potent loop diuretic, blocks sodium, potassium, chloride, and, subsequently, water resorption. By shrinking plasma volume, it decreases the hydrostatic pressure and edema formation. The clinical challenge with furosemide is accurate dosing during initial and chronic management. The best dose of furosemide is the minimum dose that controls the symptoms of heart failure without side effects. Long term, this dose is determined during periodic evaluations of the patient at the clinic and with telephone rechecks. Owners can assist in titrating the dose of diuretics by counting the respiratory rate and determining cough frequency at home. Once trained in how to become a critical observer of their animal's respirations, most owners are helpful in the management of their animal's heart failure. This article is not intended to be a detailed narrative of how to treat heart failure; nonetheless, it is important to emphasize that the ideal management of heart failure should include an angiotensin-converting enzyme inhibitor (ACE-I) in addition to furosemide. An ACE-I (eg, enalapril, benazepril) has been shown to improve morbidity and decrease mortality in dogs with congestive heart failure attributable to dilated cardiomyopathy and mitral valve disease [2–6]. The use of an ACE-I, which is a balanced vasodilator, typically allows a reduction in the furosemide dose by decreasing systemic vascular resistance and improving cardiac output. In addition to the ACE-I and furosemide, pimobendan, a new oral inodilator drug, should be added in the management of canine heart failure of all causes. Recent studies have shown that pimobendan also improves survival and quality-of-life scores in dogs with heart failure attributable to dilated cardiomyopathy and mitral valve disease [7–9]. Pimobendan has a dual mechanism of action: it is a calcium-sensitizing drug and a phosphodiesterase III inhibitor, resulting in vasodilation and positive inotropic effects. By its vasodilating and inotropic properties, it consistently improves cardiac output and the clinical signs of heart failure.

Advanced heart failure

Heart failure is a progressive condition. Increasing drug doses and adding medications are common procedures over the long course of managing an animal with congestive heart failure. As the heart disease worsens and medical management intensifies, the risk for fluid and electrolyte abnormalities also increases. Familiarity with the drug's actions and anticipated complications is essential to managing advanced and, often, refractory edema and effusions. In canine heart failure, pimobendan, ACE-I, and furosemide should be the foundation of medical management. Additional vasodilators and diuretics and other drugs that optimize cardiac output (eg, antiarrhythmic drugs) may be helpful in the management of refractory heart failure. Deciding which drug to add or which drug dose to increase is challenging even for an experienced cardiologist. In general, however, improving cardiac output and attempting to minimize the increase in diuretic doses are good goals for therapy. Eventually, increasing the dose and adding diuretics are necessary to manage chronic refractory heart failure successfully. In fact, additional diuretics, rather than maximizing the furosemide dose, may improve diuresis by sequential nephron blockage [10]. Spironolactone and hydrochlorothiazide are oral diuretics that can be useful as "to-go-home medications" in nonazotemic, refractory, or recurrent heart failure cases, in which animals are already on high-dose furosemide. By adding a diuretic with a different and more distal site of action (eg, hydrochlorothiazide in the distal tubule, spironolactone in the collecting ducts), the diuretics can have a synergistic diuretic effect. Spironolactone, an aldosterone antagonist and potassium-sparing diuretic, improves survival and quality of life in human patients with heart failure [11]. The reasons for the survival benefit are not clearly understood, but minimizing hypokalemia, which may translate to a decreased rate of arrhythmic sudden death in addition to its neurohumoral antialdosterone benefits, has been theorized. Although the survival benefit of spironolactone has not been demonstrated in dogs that have heart failure, adding spironolactone to an ACE-I and furosemide seems to be well tolerated and has been shown to decrease hypokalemia [12,13].

UNDERSTANDING AND MANAGEMENT OF COMMON METABOLIC DERANGEMENTS

Azotemia

The finding of increased blood urea nitrogen (BUN) and serum creatinine levels is always concerning in the setting of heart failure because it reflects a reduction in glomerular filtration rate as a result of organ dysfunction (heart or kidney) or as a complication of heart failure therapy. Renal impairment in human patients who have heart failure is common and is increasingly recognized as an independent risk factor for morbidity and mortality [14,15]. The Acute Decompensated Heart Failure National Registry (ADHERE), a large database of more than 100,000 human patients who have heart failure, reported that approximately 30% of the patients had concurrent chronic renal disease at admission [16]. Furthermore, approximately one quarter of human patients hospitalized for treatment of heart failure experience significant worsening of their renal function. In a recent canine study, the prevalence of renal dysfunction in chronic valvular disease was also surprisingly high—50% overall. Additionally, as the functional class of heart failure increased, so did the percentage of azotemic dogs, which may suggest that azotemia may be a poor prognostic indicator [17]. In another canine study of spontaneous heart failure, an increase in BUN was associated with worsening severity of heart failure and diuretic use [12]. Common causes of azotemia associated with heart failure can be divided into prerenal and renal etiologies (Table 1). It is important to emphasize that the renal impairment may result from a combination of causes and that concomitant renal disease and advanced heart disease are not uncommon. Additionally, severe hypoperfusion of the kidneys (prerenal azotemia), regardless of the cause, can lead to acute and potentially irreversible renal failure as a result of ischemic injury if the insult is severe and sustained.

Renal function, electrolytes, and blood pressure should be assessed before and after initiation of therapy for heart failure. The time interval between assessments depends on the severity of heart failure and the intensity of management. For the typical case of outpatient heart failure, reassessment in 5 to 7 days is sufficient, whereas the management of an intense inpatient heart failure case requiring high-dose diuretics may require daily or every other day reevaluation of BUN, creatinine, and electrolytes until the patient is stabilized.

Management of azotemia in heart failure depends somewhat on understanding its etiology. In general, however, improving cardiac output and, if possible, decreasing diuretic dose are vital to improving renal function. If the renal impairment is primarily attributable to poor cardiac output, immediate maneuvers directed at improving cardiac output are necessary. For example, urgent removal of pericardial effusion causing cardiac tamponade and intravenous fluid therapy should improve the azotemia. Similarly, azotemia associated with severe and symptomatic complete heart block should improve with urgent pacing to increase heart rate and initiating intravenous fluids. The rate of fluid administration depends on the acuteness of the illness (ie, how long the animal has not been eating or drinking properly) and if any previous diuretic or vasodilating therapy had been overzealously administered. Aside from these previous examples of primarily low-output heart failure, most heart failure associated with azotemia has a combination of congestion (eg, edema, effusion) and low cardiac output. In these cases, it is important to decrease diuretic dose to a minimum and to optimize cardiac output. In the author's experience, for in-hospital management of severe congestive heart failure with azotemia, the furosemide dose can be minimized by constantly reassessing the patient's respiratory rate and titrating the dose accordingly. After an initial intravenous bolus, continuous rate infusion (CRI) of furosemide is an effective way to control and titrate the dose to the patient. The CRI can be stopped as soon as the animal's respiratory rate is approaching normal and is superior to giving several large scheduled bolus doses. In some cases of erroneously diagnosed pulmonary edema, the diuretics can be stopped entirely. Occasionally, a dog with respiratory disease, pulmonary hypertension, and cor pulmonale is misdiagnosed with left-sided congestive heart failure. These dogs are especially at risk for developing azotemia if aggressive diuretic therapy is used. They are usually older dogs, often with some underlying renal

Table 1
Etiology of azotemia commonly associated with heart failure

Category of azotemia	Etiology	Comments
Prerenal	Severe low-output heart failure	• Advanced end-stage heart disease, cardiac tamponade attributable to pericardial effusion, and symptomatic complete heart block are examples of heart diseases that can cause low-output heart failure and azotemia • Many times, the combination of low cardiac output attributable to advanced heart disease and preexisting renal disease can lead to azotemia
	Hypovolemia and volume contraction associated with diuretic administration	• Diuretics, particularly furosemide, can lead to potent diuresis and volume contraction and subsequent azotemia • Consider preexisting occult renal disease when azotemia develops with appropriate diuretic therapy • Reduction in diuretic dose, if possible, usually improves azotemia
	Decreased renal perfusion pressure associated with excessive vasodilation	• Hypotension associated with vasodilators can lead to azotemia • As with diuretics, reduction in dose can improve azotemia
	Vomiting, diarrhea, and anorexia causing dehydration and hypovolemia associated with heart failure drugs or noncardiac condition	• Some cardiac drugs, especially digoxin, can lead to anorexia and vomiting, resulting in dehydration and hypovolemia • Comorbid conditions, such as gastroenteritis or pancreatitis, can complicate heart failure management
Renal	Preexisting chronic renal disease	• May be more common than previously recognized, particularly in older animals with heart disease • Many times, becomes apparent with heart failure drug therapy
	Acute renal failure attributable to ischemic renal ischemic renal injury	• If the prerenal azotemia of any cause is severe and sustained, it can lead to ischemic renal injury
	Renal thrombosis associated with feline arterial thromboembolism	• Many cats with arterial thromboembolism have evidence of previous renal infarcts leading to renal impairment
	GN associated with advanced HWD	• Many dogs with severe HWD have proteinuria associated with GN • Severe GN can lead to renal tubular loss and azotemia

Abbreviations: GN, glomerulonephropathy; HWD, heartworm disease.

insufficiency. Additionally, many of these dogs also have pulmonary hypertension severe enough to compromise left heart preload and cardiac output. These dogs with pulmonary hypertension also may benefit from pulmonary arterial vasodilation to improve cardiac output. Vasodilators, such as sildenafil, pimobendan, and amlodipine, all ameliorate clinical signs associated with pulmonary hypertension [18–20].

Therapeutic removal of pleural effusion or ascites also helps to lower the diuretic dose during initial and chronic management of heart failure in animals prone to azotemia. Nevertheless, in the long term, ascites and pleural effusion should ideally be managed medically. Animals with concurrent renal disease may not tolerate high-dose diuretics, and periodic removal of body cavity effusions provides relief of symptoms and extension of quality life. Other strategies to improve cardiac output and azotemia include the cautious use of vasodilators (ACE-I) and positive inotropic drugs. The author's experience suggests that pimobendan is helpful in managing azotemia in patients that have heart failure. The addition of pimobendan should be considered in all cases of symptomatic canine heart failure, especially in the face of azotemia. Pimobendan allows reductions in the diuretic dose and even the ACE-I, if needed. Although not approved for use in cats, pimobendan has been used by the author in cats that have severe refractory heart failure, generally with good results. Dobutamine, an intravenous catecholamine, is another positive inotrope that can lead to short-term improvement of cardiac output and azotemia, especially if the patient is unable to take oral medications. Appropriate use of vasodilators, particularly ACE-I, also improves cardiac output and renal blood flow. Adjusting the dose of vasodilators in the presence of azotemia and heart failure can be challenging. It is important to emphasize that vasodilators, in general, improve cardiac output by decreasing systemic vascular resistance. One should be a bit hesitant to discontinue using the vasodilator, especially ACE-I, unless severe azotemia (creatinine >3 mg/dL) or hypotension (systolic blood pressure <100 mm Hg) develops. The author is more likely to reduce the dose of the vasodilators than to discontinue them in mild to moderate azotemia. Additionally, the diuretic dose is carefully examined and, if possible, decreased. Remember, diuretics never improve cardiac output. Vasodilator therapy is particularly important in managing the dog that has acutely decompensated heart failure with chordae tendineae rupture. As previously stated, these dogs are generally not markedly hypervolemic and may be more predisposed to azotemia secondary to aggressive diuretic therapy. Their fulminant and severe pulmonary edema is primarily attributable to increased pulmonary venous pressure from sudden worsening of mitral valve regurgitation. In the author's experience, intravenous nitroprusside, a balanced vasodilator, is helpful in these cases to improve the dyspnea, reduce the diuretic dose, and improve cardiac output.

In addition to manipulating preload, afterload, and cardiac output with cardiac medications, the management of azotemia in a patient that has heart failure may include the use of parenteral fluids. In general, one is hesitant to administer subcutaneous fluids or intravenous fluids in an animal that has heart failure but is eating or drinking on its own. There are several instances when parenteral fluids may be needed, however. In general, intravenous fluids serve two purposes. One is to replace or maintain intravascular fluid volume, and the other is to maintain or replace free water, electrolytes, blood components, or protein. Ultimately, the purpose of fluid administration is to maintain cardiac preload and cardiac output, oxygen delivery, and tissue perfusion to ensure adequate cellular homeostasis. Most animals that have heart failure are hypervolemic when showing clinical signs. Thus, initial management, with some exceptions, should not include intravenous fluids. In addition to selecting the rate and amount of fluids to administer carefully, consideration should be given to the sodium concentration of the fluids. For example, intravenous fluids given to a patient that has heart failure primarily to maintain hydration or to replenish potassium should have a lower sodium concentration (eg, 0.45% sodium chloride [NaCl] + 2.5% dextrose).

A solution containing 5% dextrose in water is often used to deliver intravenous drugs, such as nitroprusside or dobutamine. In this setting, fluids should ideally be given at a low rate (eg, 1–10 mL/h) delivered with a fluid or syringe pump. This situation is contrasted to a patient that has heart failure with severe gastrointestinal fluid loss attributable to digoxin toxicity, which should initially be given a fluid with a higher sodium content (eg, lactated Ringer's solution) to replace fluid losses caused by vomiting and diarrhea. The fluids can be switched to a lower sodium-containing fluid as soon as the vomiting and diarrhea cease and the patient is well hydrated. The rate and amount of parenteral fluids to administer are considered on a case-by-case basis. Although there are no studies to support this claim, many experienced cardiology clinicians consider subcutaneous or even oral fluids less likely to worsen clinical signs of congestion. Some patients are sick enough with concurrent disease or overzealous off-loading medications (eg, diuretics, vasodilators), however, such that administering intravenous fluids is needed. Vascular volume and cardiac output should be monitored to minimize the risk for volume overload. This can also help to determine the rate and amount of fluids to administer. The "gold standard" for evaluation of pulmonary venous pressure and cardiac output is pulmonary artery catheterization with thermodilution cardiac output monitoring. This technique has been associated with some morbidity [21] and is not readily available at most veterinary practices and referral centers. Other more practical and frequently used monitoring techniques include respiratory rate and effort, body weight, urine output, central venous pressure (CVP), systemic blood pressure, echocardiography, and thoracic radiography. Closely monitoring respiratory rate and breath sounds by an experienced veterinary nurse or clinician may facilitate early detection of pulmonary edema or pleural effusion in a patient that has heart failure and is receiving fluids. Two or three times the daily body weight measurement on an accurate scale may be useful in intravenous fluid management, because acute changes in body weight are most likely attributable to acute changes in body water. Knowledge of CVP can be helpful in administering fluids to a patient that has heart failure, but it also has some significant drawbacks. It is important to recognize that CVP measures the preload of the right heart and that there can be significant disconnection between CVP and left-sided filling pressures in a patient that has heart disease [1]. In other words, a patient that has heart failure can develop severe pulmonary edema without a detectable increase in CVP. Overreliance on CVP monitoring can lead to overzealous fluid administration and accumulation of pulmonary edema in a patient that has heart disease. A normal CVP measurement is 0 to 5 mm Hg, but it can be greater than 5 mm Hg in a patient that has heart failure. In the author's experience, the goal for fluid administration in a patient that has heart failure is not to increase the baseline CVP unless the initial CVP is markedly decreased. In addition to monitoring systemic and venous pressures, periodic imaging of the heart and lungs with an echocardiogram or radiograph may provide valuable information regarding heart size, edema or effusion formation, and venous tone. Both techniques are noninvasive; however, the echocardiogram has the advantage of being a potentially "cage-side" technique. For most noncardiologist echocardiographers, the most important images are those that assess left atrial and ventricular size. Many charts of normal chamber dimensions relative to body size exist. If the size of the left atrium is normal in an azotemic dog with chronic mitral valvular heart disease, this suggests that cautious intravenous fluids may be well tolerated. Alternatively, if the echocardiogram shows a marked enlarged left atrial size with dilation of the pulmonary veins, intravenous fluids may worsen pulmonary edema and this dog's azotemia may be better served with manipulation of cardiac output with drugs like positive inotropes and vasodilators. The echocardiogram is also helpful in assessing accumulation of cavitary effusions. Similarly, the thoracic radiograph helps to evaluate heart size and pleural effusion reaccumulation. Additionally, the thoracic radiograph assesses pulmonary parenchyma and pulmonary venous size and may identify impending pulmonary edema before overt clinical signs. This information can be useful in monitoring the patient that has heart failure and is receiving intravenous fluids.

Sodium Derangements

The most common sodium disorder in heart failure is hyponatremia. Hyponatremia has been associated with increased severity of heart failure and higher mortality in human beings and dogs [12,22,23]. Most animals with well-compensated heart failure are not hyponatremic, however. The primary mechanism for hyponatremia in heart failure is a nonosmotic release of ADH, causing an increase in free water absorption in the renal collecting ducts, which results in an increase in extracellular and plasma water and "dilutes" the concentration of plasma sodium [24]. Although counterintuitive, total sodium content is actually increased in patients that have heart failure and hyponatremia. The finding of hyponatremia usually indicates severe heart failure in which the kidneys perceive "effective hypovolemia" from poor cardiac output, resulting in ADH release. Many of the patients that have heart failure and hyponatremia are also azotemic. Independently or concurrently with advanced heart failure, another possible mechanism for hyponatremia is the use of diuretics in high doses or in combination with other diuretics. The mechanism for hyponatremia with combination diuretic therapy is attributable, at least in part, to marked natriuresis. Typically, the hyponatremia associated with excessive diuretic use is associated with hypokalemia and hypochloremia. As with the previously discussed patients that have azotemic heart failure, improving cardiac output and minimizing diuretic doses are central to successful management.

Potassium Derangements

Hypokalemia and hyperkalemia are not uncommon in patients that have advanced heart failure. Hypokalemia can result in muscular weakness and can have serious effects on the cardiac action potential, increasing the risk for ventricular arrhythmias [25]. Arrhythmogenesis secondary to hypokalemia results primarily from QT interval prolongation and facilitation of early after-depolarizations. Hypokalemia may also interfere with antiarrhythmic therapy (particularly sodium channel blockers, such as lidocaine) because it hyperpolarizes the cell membrane. Hypokalemia may also potentiate the effects of digoxin toxicity and exacerbate digitalis-related arrhythmias. In addition to its cardiac effects, recent studies have linked hypokalemia to systemic hypertension in human patients [26]. Experimental animal studies and one clinical study in cats that had renal failure have also identified a link between hypokalemia and hypertension [26,27]. Several canine surveys have associated hypokalemia in dogs that have heart failure with diuretic use, particularly loop diuretics [12,28]. The mechanism for hypokalemia with loop diuretics is a somewhat anticipated effect, considering its direct action to inhibit sodium, potassium, and chloride resorption at the ascending loop of Henle. Interestingly, a canine study showed amelioration of hypokalemia with the addition of spironolactone [12]. Additionally, hypokalemia can result from prolonged anorexia or severe vomiting and diarrhea. Severe gastrointestinal loss, together with diuretics, may quickly result in hypovolemia and depletion of electrolytes, such as sodium, potassium, and chloride. Hypokalemia is actually perpetuated when it is associated with renal sodium avidity, chloride depletion, and metabolic alkalosis. Thus, correction of chloride and sodium deficits is needed to correct the potassium deficit in these cases. The route and dose of potassium supplementation depend on the severity of the deficit and associated conditions. Intravenous potassium supplementation is recommended if the animal is potentially symptomatic from hypokalemia (eg, arrhythmias, weakness) or has severe hypokalemia (<3.0 mg/dL). The rate of intravenous potassium supplementation (typically with potassium chloride) ranges from 0.05 to 0.5 mEq/kg/h. The lower end of this range (0.05–0.1 mEq/kg/h) is considered the hourly maintenance supplementation, wherein 0.5 mEq/kg/h is the maximum rate of supplementation that might be required in severe and symptomatic hypokalemia. If higher rates of potassium supplementation are used, frequent re-evaluation (every 6–12 hours as needed) of serum potassium is recommended to ensure appropriate dosing. Oral supplementation with potassium gluconate is more commonly performed in chronic management of mild and asymptomatic hypokalemia in heart failure. The dosing, in the author's opinion, is somewhat empiric, usually starting low and titrating upward based on periodic laboratory and clinical evaluations.

Hyperkalemia in the setting of heart failure is sometimes present in cats that have aortic thromboembolism. Life-threatening hyperkalemia is likely associated with reperfusion of ischemic muscle tissue and release of intracellular potassium into the extracellular space. Decreased renal blood flow from poor cardiac function and possible renal thrombosis may also contribute to severe hyperkalemia. Hyperkalemia is often the terminal factor in cats that have aortic thromboembolism. Emergency treatments with insulin-dextrose, sodium bicarbonate, or calcium infusions are required to manage the severe and life-threatening hyperkalemia (see the article by Schaer elsewhere in this issue). In the author's experience, continuous electrocardiographic monitoring is helpful to recognize and evaluate the response to therapy for hyperkalemia in this patient population. The classic electrocardiographic changes associated with hyperkalemia include tall tented T waves, loss of P waves, and broadening of the QRS complex. Mild hyperkalemia is sometimes identified in animals treated concurrently with potassium-sparing diuretics (spironolactone) and ACE-I. In the Randomized Aldactone Evaluation Study Investigators (RALES) trial in human patients, severe hyperkalemia was experienced in approximately 3% of the spironolactone-treated group [11]. The risk for hyperkalemia associated with spironolactone may increase with increased dose [29]. ACE-I alone also can rarely cause mild hyperkalemia secondary to its antialdosterone effects [30]. Mild hyperkalemia may be associated with advanced heart failure as a result of poor renal blood flow and subsequent decreased delivery to the distal renal tubules and decreased excretion of potassium. The management of mild hyperkalemia usually involves a dose reduction of the potassium-sparing diuretic and, sometimes, the ACE-I. In a patient that has heart failure and moderate to severe hyperkalemia associated with severe azotemia, acute ischemic renal failure and a poor outcome are likely.

Magnesium Derangements

Magnesium, comparable to potassium, has an important role in the maintenance of resting membrane potential and in the regulation of ion shifts within the cardiac muscle cell. Low magnesium also increased the frequency and severity of arrhythmias in human patients [31]. Hypomagnesemia, similar to hypokalemia, has been associated with systemic hypertension in human and animal models [32]. Hypomagnesemia has been encountered in human and canine patients that have cardiovascular disease and in dogs receiving diuretics [28], whereas mild hypermagnesemia was identified in another study of dogs receiving spironolactone and ACE-I [13]. Mild asymptomatic magnesium deficits probably exist in more patients that have heart failure than we recognize, because serum magnesium does not accurately reflect total body magnesium content. That said, magnesium supplementation in patients that have heart failure at our institution is almost exclusively performed in the management of severe refractory ventricular arrhythmias or severe concurrent hypokalemia [33]. For refractory symptomatic ventricular arrhythmias, a slow intravenous infusion of magnesium chloride or magnesium sulfate is given after dilution into approximately 3–10 mL of 5% dextrose in water or sterile water. After the urgent loading, a slower rate infusion is implemented over the next 12 to 24 hours.

Acid-Base Derangements

Patients that have heart failure can present with a variety of simple and mixed acid-base disturbances. Although no clinical studies have documented the frequency or severity of these disorders in veterinary medicine, the author's clinical experience suggests that advanced and symptomatic heart failure is not uncommonly associated with acid-base disorders. Additionally, blood gas analysis can be helpful in assessing other electrolyte disorders and the severity of ventilatory compromise. Keeping that in mind, acid-base disorders are usually not severe and do not require specific therapy aside from standard heart failure management. Moreover, performing blood gas analysis is usually not crucial to the diagnosis or management of the patient that has symptomatic heart failure. In fact, some would argue that in a dyspneic patient with a high probability of having heart failure, arterial blood gas analysis may be too stressful for the diagnostic and management benefit. For the purposes of a patient with a high probability of having heart failure, venous blood gas measurement is much less stressful and can provide the added information needed to assess electrolytes and ventilatory status (Pco_2).

The presence of metabolic acidosis, which is recognized by acidemia associated with a lower than normal bicarbonate concentration in a patient that has heart failure, may represent advanced disease and poor cardiac output; metabolic acidosis is caused by lactic acidosis and tissue ischemia. Another supporting finding for low cardiac output on a venous blood gas report is low central venous Po_2 (<30 mm Hg). The low venous Po_2 suggests that the capillary bed is extracting a larger than usual quantity of oxygen because of heart pump failure, resulting in lower than normal venous oxygen content. Respiratory acidosis, which is recognized by acidemia associated with higher than normal Pco_2, in a patient that has symptomatic heart failure is usually a red flag for ventilatory failure generally attributable to respiratory muscle fatigue. Severe pleural effusion, which decreases tidal volume, may also be associated with respiratory acidosis. Although not performed commonly, mechanical ventilation may be indicated in a first-time patient that has heart failure, is not responding to heart failure medications, and is showing signs of fatigue, as evidenced by the physical examination and hypercarbia. Respiratory alkalosis, recognized by alkalemia associated with lower than normal Pco_2, is not uncommon in the patient that has symptomatic left-sided heart failure. Pulmonary edema causes stretch and nociceptive receptors in the lungs to increase respiratory rate. Additionally, stretch receptors in the left atrium induce tachypnea and lead to respiratory alkalosis [1]. Alkalemia, which is associated with a higher than normal bicarbonate concentration, suggests metabolic alkalosis. Metabolic alkalosis is often associated with volume contraction that is coupled with chloride depletion. This scenario is not uncommon in patients that have heart failure and received aggressive diuretic (usually furosemide) therapy, possibly overzealously. Vomiting and diarrhea are also commonly associated with metabolic alkalosis. Thus, metabolic alkalosis should alert the clinician to volume contraction associated with sodium avidity and to chloride and potassium depletion. Management of metabolic alkalosis typically involves transient discontinuation of diuretics and administration of high-sodium– and high-chloride–containing fluids (eg, lactated Ringer's solution) with potassium chloride supplementation.

Glucose Derangements

Hyperglycemia has been recognized in human and canine patients that have heart failure, in addition to other causes of severe systemic disease, as a marker of poor outcome [23,34]. In one canine clinical study, survivors of acutely decompensated heart failure had lower blood glucose (median of 101 mg/dL) as compared with the nonsurvivors (median of 120 mg/dL) [23] The reason for the hyperglycemia is likely multifactorial and not clearly understood. Proposed mechanisms include insulin receptor antagonism, impaired insulin-mediated glucose uptake, and signal transduction. Activation of the sympathetic nervous system may also play a role in the insulin resistance and hyperglycemia. The insulin resistance recognized in heart failure may have several detrimental effects, including increasing extracellular water and impaired myocardial energy use that may eventually be damaging to the heart cells.

Related to hyperglycemia and heart failure is a recently described condition called corticosteroid-associated congestive heart failure. Corticosteroids have been associated as a risk factor for development of heart failure in human beings [35]. A few feline but not canine studies have also identified an association of previous corticosteroid administration potentially precipitating heart failure [36,37]. The mechanism by which corticosteroids may induce heart failure is not clearly understood and is likely multifactorial. Increased sodium and water retention, plasma volume expansion from hyperglycemia, increased systemic vascular resistance (afterload), and direct myocardial remodeling effects have all been considered. In one small prospective study of cats with skin disease receiving high-dose methylprednisolone, serum glucose, sodium, and chloride concentrations decreased significantly a few days after steroid administration [38]. Estimated plasma volume in that study increased by 13% (>40% in 3 cats). This study suggested that plasma volume expansion is a result of intracellular-to-extracellular fluid shift secondary to corticosteroid-mediated hyperglycemia.

Plasma Protein and Red Blood Cell Derangements

Mild hypoalbuminemia is not an uncommon serum biochemical finding in animals that have advanced heart disease. The mechanisms of hypoalbuminemia in heart failure are most likely related to a dilutional effect from plasma volume expansion and increased loss of albumin attributable to an edematous gastrointestinal system in animals that have right-sided heart failure. Chronic repeated body cavity centesis removing high-protein fluid from pleural effusion or

ascites may also lead to or worsen hypoalbuminemia. Usually, no specific therapy is required to manage hypoalbuminemia aside from attempts to decrease
the frequency of repeated centesis.

Relevant to the discussion of fluid balance in heart failure is a brief explanation of hyperviscosity syndrome. Increased blood viscosity, caused by an excessive increase in red blood cells, plasma proteins, or other blood components,
can cause sludging and decreased perfusion through the microvascular capillary beds. Hypergammaglobulinemia, typically caused by a myeloproliferative
disorder, is the most common cause of hyperviscosity syndrome in human
beings [39]. Case reports and a case series have documented hyperviscosity
syndromes in dogs and cats with multiple myeloma and myeloma-like conditions [40,41]. Although ocular, neurologic, and bleeding manifestations are
more common, cardiac hypertrophy and congestive heart failure associated
with hyperviscosity syndrome have also been described. Cardiac hypertrophy
was observed in 30% of cats in which thoracic imaging was performed in one
case series of myeloma-like disorders [40]. Moreover, the author has personal
experience with two cats in congestive heart failure and severe monoclonal
hyperglobulinemia. Heart failure may develop secondary to expanded plasma
volume and the increased systemic vascular resistance attributable to increased
blood viscosity. The management of congestive heart failure in an animal that
has hyperviscosity syndrome is directed at urgent reduction of the blood
viscosity, usually with plasmapheresis to remove excessive protein from the
plasma rapidly. Medical management of the myeloproliferative disorder is
needed for long-term control of the hyperviscosity syndrome, but medical management of the heart disease may also be needed.

Anemia has recently emerged as a relatively common and independent risk
factor for worse outcome in human patients who have heart disease [42]. Even
small reductions in hemoglobin concentration are associated with a less favor-
able prognosis [43]. The causes of anemia in advanced heart failure are not
entirely clear. Renal dysfunction and neurohormonal and proinflammatory
cytokine activation seem to contribute to the anemia of chronic disease. In normal conditions, tissue hypoxemia attributable to poor cardiac output would
stimulate the bone marrow to increase red blood cell production; however,
erythropoiesis seems to be defective in heart failure. Chronic anemia, regardless of the etiology, induces a vasodilation-mediated high cardiac output state
associated with plasma volume expansion and neurohormonal activation.
The high cardiac output state initially helps to increase oxygen transport.
The hemodynamic and neurohumoral alterations have long-term deleterious
effects, however, and may lead to congestive heart failure. Our understanding
of the prevalence and clinical significance of anemia in animals that have heart
disease is poor. There is one case report of a kitten that had severe flea infes-
tation and anemia-associated congestive heart failure [44]. Dogs that have moderate to severe congestive heart failure have been shown to have decreased
hematocrits when compared with normal healthy controls [45]. Additionally,
one recent canine study failed to demonstrate a link between anemia and

worsening of heart failure severity [12]. Nevertheless, familiarity with the cardiovascular effects of chronic normovolemic anemia is important in the management of a patient that has heart failure and concurrent anemia. Patients that have heart failure and normovolemic anemia are at high risk for developing pulmonary edema with blood transfusions. A couple of classic examples are the middle-aged cocker spaniel that has immune-mediated hemolytic anemia with concurrent compensated mitral valve disease and the older cat that has chronic anemia as a result of long-standing renal disease with concurrent hypertrophic cardiomyopathy. Despite the decline in hematocrit and oxygen-carrying capacity in these patients, they should be euvolemic if no concurrently bleeding or fluid losses are present. Thus, if these patients require a blood transfusion, slow administration of packed red blood cells with close monitoring of respiratory rate is recommended. Packed red blood cells deliver the component of the blood that is most needed and minimize the risk for volume overload, whereas whole blood does not.

APPENDIX

Drugs useful in the management of fluid and electrolyte disorders in heart failure			
Drug	Species	Route	Dosage
Diuretics			
Furosemide	Dog	IV, SQ	1–4 mg/kg q 6–12 hours PRN (maximum: 12 mg/kg/d)
Furosemide	Dog	PO	1–4 mg/kg q 8–24 hours PRN (maximum: 12 mg/kg/d)
Furosemide	Dog	CRI	0.25–0.5 mg/kg/h × 4–8 hours after bolus
Furosemide	Cat	IV, SQ	1–4 mg/kg q 8–24 hours
Furosemide	Cat	PO	1–4 mg/kg q 12–48 hours
Spironolactone	Both	PO	0.3–1 mg/kg q 24 hours for ALD blockade
Spironolactone	Both	PO	1–2 mg/kg q 12–24 hours for diuresis
Hydrochlorothiazide plus spironolactone	Dog	PO	0.5 mg/kg dosed based on spironolactone q 12–48 hours
ACE-I			
Enalapril	Dog	PO	0.5 mg/kg q 12–24 hours (start at even lower dosage if azotemic)
Enalapril	Cat	PO	0.5 mg/kg q 24–72 hours
Benazepril	Both	PO	0.5 mg/kg q 24 hours (start low if azotemic)
Vasodilators			
Nitroglycerin 2% ointment	Both	Skin	0.25 inch per 5–10 kg q 8 hours (for first 24 hours typically)

(continued on next page)

Appendix
(continued)

Drug	Species	Route	Dosage
Nitroprusside	Dog	IV	0.25–5 µg/kg/min CRI (direct BP monitoring ideal)
Amlodipine	Cat	PO	0.625 mg q 24 hours; titrate up PRN with BP monitor
Amlodipine	Dog	PO	0.1 mg/kg q 12–24 hours initially; titrate upward PRN to maximum of 0.25 mg/kg q 12 hours and monitor BP
Hydralazine	Dog	PO, IV	0.5 mg/kg q 12–24 hours initially; titrate PRN 1–3 mg/kg q 12 hours and monitor BP
Sildenafil	Dog	PO	0.5–1 mg/kg q 12–24 hours, perhaps q 8 hours; extremely expensive
Electrolytes			
Potassium chloride	Both	IV	0.05–0.5 mEq/kg/h
Potassium gluconate	Both	PO	2 mEq q 12–24 hours; titrate upward PRN in bigger dog
Magnesium sulfate	Dog	IV	30 mg/kg slow (15–20 minutes) and then 30 mg/kg over 12–24 hours
Magnesium chloride	Dog	IV	0.15 mEq/kg slow (15–20 minutes) and then 0.3 mEq/kg over 24 hours
Regular insulin/dextrose	Both	IV	0.5–1 U/kg of insulin with dextrose at a rate of 2 g/U of insulin
Sodium bicarbonate	Both	IV	1–2 mEq/kg
Calcium gluconate 10%	Both	IV	1 mL per 5 kg (10 lb) slowly monitoring ECG
Inotropes			
Digoxin (Cardoxin)	Dog	PO	0.003 mg/kg q 12 hours (target levels: 0.5–1.2 ng/mL)
Digoxin	Dog	IV	0.0025 mg/kg q 1 hour × 4 hours (total of 0.01 mg/kg)
Digoxin	Cat	PO	0.01 mg/kg q 48 hours (one quarter of a 0.125 mg- tablet q 48 hours)
Pimobendan	Dog	PO	0.25 mg/kg q 12 hours (can increase to TID in refractory HF)
Dobutamine	Dog	IV	1–10 µg/kg/min CRI (need ECG monitoring, VPCs)
Dobutamine	Cat	IV	1–3 µg/kg/min CRI (VPCs and seizures are adverse effects)

Abbreviations: ALD, aldosterone; BP, blood pressure; ECG, electrocardiogram; HF, heart failure; IV, intravenous; PO, per os; PRN, as needed; q, every; SQ, subcutaneous; TID, three times daily; VPCs, ventricular premature complexes.

References

[1] Guyton AC, Hall JE. Textbook of medical physiology. Philadelphia: W.B. Saunders; 1996. p. 265–74, 496–7.

[2] Acute and short-term hemodynamic, echocardiographic, and clinical effects of enalapril maleate in dogs with naturally acquired heart failure: results of the Invasive Multicenter PROspective Veterinary Evaluation of Enalapril study. The IMPROVE Study Group. J Vet Intern Med 1995;9:234–42.

[3] Controlled clinical evaluation of enalapril in dogs with heart failure: results of the Cooperative Veterinary Enalapril Study Group. The COVE Study Group. J Vet Intern Med 1995;9:243–52.

[4] Hamlin RL, Benitz AM, Ericsson GF, et al. Effects of enalapril on exercise tolerance and longevity in dogs with heart failure produced by iatrogenic mitral regurgitation. J Vet Intern Med 1996;10:85–7.

[5] Ettinger SJ, Benitz AM, Ericsson GF, et al. Effects of enalapril maleate on survival of dogs with naturally acquired heart failure. The Long-Term Investigation of Veterinary Enalapril (LIVE) Study Group. J Am Vet Med Assoc 1998;213:1573–7.

[6] Pouchelon JL. The effect of benazepril on survival times and clinical signs of dogs with congestive heart failure: results of a multicenter, prospective, randomized, double-blinded, placebo-controlled, long-term clinical trial. J Vet Cardiol 1999;1:7–18.

[7] Fuentes VL, Corcoran B, French A, et al. A double-blinded, randomized, placebo-controlled study of pimobendan in dogs with dilated cardiomyopathy. J Vet Intern Med 2002;16: 255–61.

[8] Smith PJ, French AT, Van Israel N, et al. Efficacy and safety of pimobendan in canine heart failure caused by myxomatous mitral valve disease. J Small Anim Pract 2005;46:121–30.

[9] Lombard CW, Jons O, Bussadori CM. Clinical efficacy of pimobendan versus benazepril for the treatment of acquired atrioventricular valvular disease in dogs. J Am Anim Hosp Assoc 2006;42:249–61.

[10] Rose BD, Post TW. Clinical use of diuretics. In: Rose BD, editor. Clinical physiology of acid-base and electrolyte disorders. New York: McGraw-Hill; 2001. p. 447–77.

[11] Pitt B, Zannad F, Remme WJ, et al. The effect of spironolactone on morbidity and mortality in patients with severe heart failure. Randomized Aldactone Evaluation Study Investigators. N Engl J Med 1999;341:709–17.

[12] Boswood A, Murphy A. The effect of heart disease, heart failure, and diuresis on selected laboratory an electrocardiographic parameters in dogs. J Vet Cardiol 2006;8:1–9.

[13] Thomason JD, Rockwell JE, Fallaw TK, et al. Influence of combined angiotensin-converting enzyme inhibitors and spironolactone on serum K^+, Mg^{2+}, and Na^+ concentrations in small dogs with degenerative mitral valve disease. J Vet Cardiol 2007;9:103–8.

[14] Hillege HL, Nitsch D, Pfeffer MA, et al. Renal function as a predictor of outcome in a broad spectrum of patients with heart failure. Circulation 2006;113:671–8.

[15] Smith GL, Lichtman JH, Bracken MB, et al. Renal impairment and outcomes in heart failure: systematic review and meta-analysis. J Am Coll Cardiol 2006;47:1987–96.

[16] Adams KF Jr, Fonarow GC, Emerman CL, et al. Characteristics and outcomes of patients hospitalized for heart failure in the United States: rationale, design, and preliminary observations from the first 100,00 cases in the Acute Decompensated Heart Failure National Registry (ADHERE). Am Heart J 2005;149:209–16.

[17] Nicolle AP, Chetboul V, Allerheiligen T, et al. Azotemia and glomerular filtration rate in dogs with chronic valvular disease. J Vet Intern Med 2007;21:943–9.

[18] Humbert M, Sitbon O, Simonneau G. Treatment of pulmonary hypertension. N Engl J Med 2004;351:1425–36.

[19] Sahara M, Takahashi T, Imai Y, et al. New insights in the treatment strategy for pulmonary hypertension. Cardiovasc Drugs Ther 2006;20:377–86.

[20] Kellum HB, Stepien RL. Sildenafil citrate therapy in 22 dogs with pulmonary hypertension. J Vet Intern Med 2007;21:1258–64.

[21] Binanay C, Califf RM, Hasselblad V, et al. Evaluation study of congestive heart failure and pulmonary artery catheterization effectiveness: the ESCAPE trial. J Am Med Assoc 2005;294:1625–33.

[22] Gheorghiade M, Rossi JS, Cotts W, et al. Characterization and prognostic value of persistent hyponatremia in patients with severe heart failure in the ESCAPE trial. Arch Intern Med 2007;167:1998–2005.

[23] Brady CA, Hughes D, Drobatz KJ. Association of hyponatremia and hyperglycemia with outcome in dogs with congestive heart failure. Journal of Veterinary Emergency and Critical Care 2004;14:177–82.

[24] Rose BD, Post TW. Regulation of the effective circulating volume. In: Rose BD, editor. Clinical physiology of acid-base and electrolyte disorders. New York: McGraw-Hill; 2001. p. 258–84.

[25] Podrid PJ. Potassium and ventricular arrhythmias. Am J Cardiol 1990;65:33E–44E.

[26] Adrogue HJ, Madias NE. Sodium and potassium in the pathogenesis of hypertension. N Engl J Med 2007;356:1966–78.

[27] Syme HM, Barber PJ, Markwell PJ, et al. Prevalence of systolic hypertension in cats with chronic renal failure at initial evaluation. J Am Vet Med Assoc 2002;220:1799–804.

[28] Cobb MA, Mitchell AR. Plasma electrolyte concentrations in dogs receiving diuretic therapy for cardiac failure. J Small Anim Pract 1992;33:526–9.

[29] Effectiveness of spironolactone added to an angiotensin-converting enzyme inhibitor and a loop diuretic for severe chronic congestive heart failure (the Randomized Aldactone Evaluation Study (RALES)). Am J Cardiol 1996;78:902–7.

[30] de Denus S, Tardif JC, White M, et al. Quantification of the risk and predictors of hyperkalemia in patients with left ventricular dysfunction: a retrospective analysis of the Studies of Left Ventricular Dysfunction (SOLVD) trials. Am Heart J 2006;152:705–12.

[31] Hollifield JW. Magnesium depletion, diuretics and arrhythmias. Am J Med 1987;82:30–7.

[32] Laurant WF, Touyz RM. Physiological and pathophysiological role of magnesium in the cardiovascular system: implications in hypertension. J Hypertens 2000;18:1177–91.

[33] Zipes DP, Camm AJ, Borggrefe M, et al. ACC/AHA/ESC 2006 guidelines for the management of patients with ventricular arrhythmias and the prevention of sudden death—executive summary. Eur Heart J 2006;27:2099–140.

[34] Capes SE, Hunt D, Malmberg K, et al. Stress hyperglycaemia and increased risk of death after myocardial infarction in patients with and without diabetes: a systemic overview. Lancet 2000;355:773–8.

[35] Souverein PC, Berard A, Van Staa TP, et al. Use of oral glucocorticoids and risk of cardiovascular and cerebrovascular disease in a population based case-control study. Heart 2004;90:859–65.

[36] Smith SA, Tobias AH, Fine DM, et al. Corticosteroid-associated congestive heart failure in 12 cats. International Journal of Applied Research in Veterinary Medicine 2004;2(3):159–70.

[37] Rush JE, Freeman LM, Fenollosa NK, et al. Population and survival characteristics of cats with hypertrophic cardiomyopathy: 260 cases (1990–1999). J Am Vet Med Assoc 2002;220(2):202–7.

[38] Ployngam T, Tobias AH, Smith SA, et al. Hemodynamic effects of methylprednisolone acetate administration in cats. Am J Vet Res 2006;67(4):583–7.

[39] Mehta J, Singhal S. Hyperviscosity syndrome in plasma cell dyscrasias. Semin Thromb Hemost 2003;29:467–71.

[40] Mellor PJ, Haugland S, Murphy S, et al. Myeloma-related disorders in cats commonly present as extramedullary neoplasms in contrast to myeloma in human patients: 24 cases with clinical follow-up. J Vet Intern Med 2006;20:1376–83.

[41] Matus RE, Leifer CE, Gordon BR, et al. Plasmapheresis and chemotherapy of hyperviscosity syndrome associated with monoclonal gammopathy in the dog. J Am Vet Med Assoc 1983;183:215–8.

[42] Horwich TB, Fonarow GC, Hamilton MA, et al. Anemia is associated with worse symptoms, greater impairment in functional capacity and a significant increase in mortality in patients with advanced heart failure. J Am Coll Cardiol 2002;39:1780–6.

[43] Anand I, McMurray JJ, Whitmore J, et al. Anemia and its relationship to clinical outcome in heart failure. Circulation 2004;110:149–54.

[44] Yaphe W, Giovengo S, Moise NS. Severe cardiomegaly secondary to anemia in a kitten. J Am Vet Med Assoc 1993;202:961–4.

[45] Farabaugh AE, Freeman LM, Rush JE, et al. Lymphocyte subpopulations and hematologic variables in dogs with congestive heart failure. J Vet Intern Med 2004;18:505–9.

INDEX

A

Acid(s), weak, acid-base disorders and, 560

Acid-base abnormalities
  fluid therapy in vomiting and diarrhea
    for, 663
  vomiting and diarrhea and, 658

Acid-base analysis, blood gas results and,
  543–544

Acid-base derangements, management of,
  738–739

Acid-base disorders
  hypoalbuminemic alkalosis and,
    562
  hypochloremic alkalosis and, 562
  metabolic, in CCU, **559–574**
  metabolic acidosis and, 562–571. See
    also *Metabolic acidosis, causes of.*
  metabolic alkalosis and, 561–562
  strong ions and, 560
  weak acids and, 560

Acid-base imbalance
  diabetes mellitus and, 700–701
  fluid therapy complications related to,
    610

Acidemia, blood gas results and, 546

Acidosis
  hyperchloremic, metabolic acidosis due
    to, 565
  hyperphosphatemic, metabolic acidosis
    due to, 564–565
  hypoalbuminemic, acid-base disorders
    and, 562
  in glucocorticoid deficiency
    management, 713
  lactic, metabolic acidosis due to,
    568–571
  metabolic. See *Metabolic acidosis.*
  respiratory. See *Respiratory acidosis.*
  toxin-induced, metabolic acidosis due
    to, 566–567
  uremic, metabolic acidosis due to,
    565–566

Acute lung injury, fluid therapy in patients
  with, 722–723

Acute respiratory distress syndrome (ARDS),
  fluid therapy in patients with, 722–723

Adolescent(s), fluid therapy in, 626–627

Albumin
  described, 595–598
  fluid therapy complications related to,
    613–614
  in critically ill dogs and cats, **595–605**
    costs of, 598
    indications for, 599
  25% human serum, in critically ill dogs
    and cats, 600–602
    administration of, 601
    adverse effects of, 601–602
    delayed immune-mediated
      reactions due to, treatment
      for, 602–603

Alkalemia, blood gas results and, 546

Alkalosis
  hypochloremic, acid-base disorders and,
    562
  metabolic. See *Metabolic alkalosis.*
  respiratory. See *Respiratory alkalosis.*

Alveolar gas equation, 423

Alveolar-arterial oxygen difference, 424

Anion gap
  analysis of, 444–446
  changes in, causes of, 445, 447
  described, 443
  quick reference for, **443–447**

ARDS. See *Acute respiratory distress syndrome
  (ARDS).*

Azotemia, management of, 730–735

B

Bicarbonate, for DKA or HHS in diabetes
  mellitus, 705

Blood gas analysis
  clinical examples of, 553–556
  results of
    acid-base vs. respiratory function
      and, 543–544
    acidemia and, 546

Note: Page numbers of article titles are in **boldface** type.

0195-5616/08/$ – see front matter
doi:10.1016/S0195-5616(08)00095-8